D1154573

The World of Soy

THE FOOD SERIES

A list of books in the series appears at the back of this book.

The World of Soy

Edited by
CHRISTINE M. DU BOIS
CHEE-BENG TAN AND
SIDNEY W. MINTZ

UNIVERSITY OF ILLINOIS PRESS
Urbana and Chicago

Manufactured in the United States of America
C 5 4 3 2 1

∞ This book is printed on acid-free paper.

Library of Congress Cataloging-in-Publication Data
The world of soy / edited by Christine M. Du Bois,
Chee-Beng Tan and Sidney W. Mintz.
p. cm.
Includes bibliographical references and index.
ISBN 978-0-252-03341-4 (cloth : alk. paper)
1. Soyfoods.
2. Cookery (Soybeans)
3. Food habits.
I. Du Bois, Christine M., 1962– II. Tan, Chee Beng. III. Mintz, Sidney Wilfred,
1922–
TX558.S7W67 2008
641.3'5655—dc22 2007046950

Contents

Acknowledgments vii

Introduction: The Significance of Soy 1
Sidney W. Mintz, Chee-Beng Tan, and Christine M. Du Bois

Section One: Acceptance of Soy in Global and Historical Context

1. Legumes in the History of Human Nutrition 27
   Lawrence Kaplan
2. Early Uses of Soybean in Chinese History 45
   H. T. Huang
3. Fermented Beans and Western Taste 56
   Sidney W. Mintz
4. Genetically Engineered Soy 74
   Christine M. Du Bois and Ivan Sergio Freire de Sousa

Section Two: Ethnographic Studies of Soy's Acceptance

5. Tofu and Related Products in Chinese Foodways 99
   Chee-Beng Tan
6. Tofu Feasts in Sichuan Cuisine 121
   Jianhua Mao

7. Fermented Soybean Products and Japanese Standard Taste 144
Erino Ozeki

8. Fermented Soyfoods in South Korea:
The Industrialization of Tradition 161
Katarzyna J. Cwiertka and Akiko Moriya

9. Tofu in Vietnamese Life 182
Can Van Nguyen

10. Soyfoods in Indonesia 195
Myra Sidharta

11. Social Context and Diet: Changing Soy Production and Consumption in the United States 208
Christine M. Du Bois

12. Soybeans and Soyfoods in Brazil, with Notes on Argentina: Sketch of an Expanding World Commodity 234
Ivan Sergio Freire de Sousa and Rita de Cássia Milagres Teixeira Vieira

13. Soy in Bangladesh: History and Prospects 257
Christine M. Du Bois

14. Soybeans and Soybean Products in West Africa: Adoption by Farmers and Adaptation to Foodways 276
Donald Z. Osborn

Conclusion: Soy's Dominance and Destiny 299
Christine M. Du Bois and Sidney W. Mintz

Appendix A. Scientific Names for Plants and Edible Fungi 315
Appendix B. More on Tofu in Chengdu 320

Contributors 325

Index 329

Acknowledgments

A book of this scope owes its existence to a multitude of individuals and institutions. Many have been thanked in the first endnote at the end of each chapter. But some had an impact on the book as whole, and to them we express our special appreciation here.

All three editors wish first to thank the Chiang Ching-kuo Foundation for International Scholarly Exchange (located in Taipei, Taiwan, and McLean, Virginia) for generously funding the 2003 conference that marked the beginnings of this book. We also wish to thank the Foundation of Chinese Dietary Culture (located in Taipei) for making the soybean conference part of its 8th Symposium, which took place in Chengdu, China. We are grateful to the foundation for providing us with accommodations and extraordinary food. In particular we thank Board Chairman George C. S. Wong and May Chang for their help and encouragement.

Sidney Mintz and Christine Du Bois thank in addition the Center for a Livable Future, Bloomberg School of Public Health, Johns Hopkins University, and the Salus Mundi Foundation for their generous support of our ongoing research. Their encouragement and confidence in us greatly helped to make this book possible.

We wish as well to thank Dr. Felicity Northcott, Holly Martin, Sara Brownschidle, and Jessi Koch, whose research on the retailing of soyfood products was financed by the Salus Mundi Foundation and undertaken in connection with our own work.

Sidney Mintz and Christine Du Bois have benefited from the time and hospitality of numerous people who shared their viewpoints and expertise with us. At the University of Illinois, we wish to thank Dr. Barbara Klein and Dr. Keith Cadwallader of the Illinois Center for Soy Foods, Dr. Karl Weingartner of INTSOY, and Dr. Pradeep Khanna of the National Soybean Research Center for explaining their work to us in depth. At the Solae Company, we thank Charlotte Korte, Geri Burdak, Sandra Herring, Dr. Charlie Kolar, Dr. Matthew McMindes, Dr. Kathryn Greaves, and Dr. Leon Kelly. At the Monsanto Company, we thank Karen Marshall, Kathy Sehnert, Dr. Timothy Conner, Dr. Robert Horsch, Walter Mayhew, Dr. Bob Beuhler, Kim Magin, and Dr. Harvey Glick for their time and hospitality. We also thank Professor Glenn Stone at Washington University, St. Louis, for his help and advice.

Christine Du Bois wishes to thank Jim Hershey at the World Initiative for Soy in Human Health for his patience with her many questions. She also heartily thanks Missouri farmer Dave Bonderer for similar patience with her queries. From Greenpeace, she thanks Charles Margulis for information. For providing her with endless news clippings about soy, she thanks Bob March and George March. She also thanks Steve Demos at White Wave, Peter Golbitz at Soyatech, and Yat Sun Wen and Richard Chung with Nature Soy in Philadelphia.

Sidney Mintz thanks his research assistant, Brian Buta; William Shurtleff of the Soyfoods Center in Lafayette, California; and the staff of the Milton Eisenhower Library at the Johns Hopkins University.

Multiple portions of the manuscript benefited from readings by Jackie Mintz and Dr. Larry Buxbaum. Professor Andrew Smith and Dr. Ted Hymowitz read the entire text as peer reviewers and provided very valuable feedback. Dr. Willis Regier, director of the University of Illinois Press, and Rebecca Crist, the managing editor, have nursed this book through to completion, and we thank them.

We wish that we could extend our thanks personally to the many others who helped us in countless ways: librarians, activists, industry representatives, soybean associations, federal employees, friends, and our ever helpful families. To those we have not had the space to name, we extend our sincerest appreciation.

Note: Asian contributors' names are listed in English, with the family name last. Within the articles, however, writers use the traditions for writing names that pertain to the cultures they are analyzing.

The World of Soy

INTRODUCTION

The Significance of Soy

SIDNEY W. MINTZ, CHEE-BENG TAN,
AND CHRISTINE M. DU BOIS

Soy and History

This collection of essays on the soybean and the various foods made from it extends across Earth's surface and over many centuries.[1] The domestication of the soybean itself took place more than three thousand years ago in Asia. But the essays in this book also tell a story of modernity, because in today's world it would be fair to say that hardly any other food plant is as modern as the soybean. The spread of its cultivation, the uses to which it is put, and its global economic, medical, and even political significance set it apart from all of the other major food plants of humankind. The contributors of the essays that follow aim to capture both the antiquity and the modernity that have marked the soybean's spread and the multiplication of its uses.

Of course, the history of the soybean is preceded by other equally remarkable stories about food. Soy's modern diffusion has been extraordinary, yet to put its global expansion in perspective we must pause to consider the first great diffusions of the modern era, what Crosby (1972) dubbed the "Columbian Exchange." Anthropologists and historians of the Americas have long boasted about the agricultural achievements of the indigenous Americas, and those achievements were astonishing indeed. The plants domesticated and the foods produced by the native pre-Columbian peoples of the Western Hemisphere would eventually play a central role in feeding the globe. Such edibles included potatoes, peppers, and tomatoes in Europe; maize and manioc in Africa; and sweet potatoes, peanuts, christophine (*chayote*), and yam beans (*jícama*) in Asia. Pineapples, papaya, allspice, arrowroot starch, and endless other unusual and delicious contributions to diet and nutrition spread from the Americas across the whole world.

Both from and to the hemisphere and over the centuries, these diffusions transformed the diets of countless millions, so much so that it is difficult now to imagine French cuisine without potatoes or string beans; Italian cuisine without tomatoes, peppers, or polenta; rural life in China without sweet potatoes; or the daily fare of West Africans without maize or manioc. Chocolate and vanilla, Jerusalem artichokes, a remarkably rich assemblage of bean species and varieties, and much else were to cross the Atlantic from west to east.

Yet equally important for world agricultural history were the parallel successes of Old World cultivars in the New World. As Old World conquerors and settlers spread through the Americas, the peoples of the New World learned about not only cattle, swine, sheep, horses, and goats but also wheat, olives, rice, and grapes, not to mention bananas, mangoes, citrus fruits, and much else. The creation of what are today considered classic regional cuisines involved many foods from elsewhere, as much with pork or beef or goat cheese or wheat bread in the Americas as with potatoes in France, tomatoes in Italy, or peppers in Spain and Hungary. All of these changes involved the transfer of new crops to old regions of settlement, the gradual incorporation of new substances, and the transmutation of what were initially exotic tastes into familiar and beloved flavors and foods. Once a new substance is integrated into a coherent food system, it loses its exoticism and becomes native, as have, for instance, raw tuna, pasta, pizza, bagels, quesadillas, and goat cheese in the diet that millions of North Americans now quite routinely eat.[2]

Such monumental transfers of plants, animals, and tastes have always marked the history of human spread and conquest. But in the perspective of agricultural history, an equally important part of the Columbian expansion was the implantation of Old World cultivars in the Americas, where they had been brought to launch the mass production of food commodities for export rather than for local consumption. It was one thing for European colonists in this hemisphere to learn to eat corn on the cob or tortillas, drink chocolate, and plant pineapples and papayas and quite another to develop in the hemisphere the overseas production of sugarcane, for example, from which to manufacture sugar, rum, and molasses for export. Sugar became a pioneering Old World crop in the Americas, blazing an economic trail for other crops, including eventually the soybean.

The amazing success of sugar production in the New World relied on the abundance and fertility of land, wood, and water, wrested from native peoples, and on a vast reservoir of enslaved labor, dragged out of Africa to the Americas over the course of more than 350 years. This was an early—and hideously brutal—triumph of European overseas farming, based on a plant first domesticated in New Guinea and then eventually processed into three highly desirable products for Western consumption.[3] Although New World peoples as well would become enthusiastic consumers of all three of those products, the plantations were created not for them but rather for masses of consumers living elsewhere, particularly in Europe (Mintz 1985a).

The successes of plantations in sugar, tobacco, indigo, coffee, and cotton in the Americas were early stages in the development of a global agricultural system of production to serve an emerging world market, the very market that would eventually trade in soybeans on a vast scale. Those plantation crops would be followed some centuries later by the rise of the enormous wheat and meat factories of the Argentine pampas and Canadian and North American prairies (Friedmann and McMichael 1989), enterprises that McMichael (1995, xiii) describes as the "relocation of capitalist agriculture in the New World . . . the new site of temperate food production for industrializing Europe." In these cases, decisive factors included appropriate climate; abundant water supply; the intermittent but massive migration of more Old World peoples, both forced and voluntary, to the New World; the gradual displacement and destruction of indigenous populations; and what seemed like the Americas' infinite supply of fertile lands and timber.

Such developments inevitably take on a curious character. They are fundamentally rural, yet they manage somehow to seem detached from rural life. That detachment is not obvious because of the continuous need to service living things and the presence of the personnel who do the work. People purchased or hired to care for growing plants will not be primarily concerned with the destiny of the harvest. Whether they are indentured servants, slaves, migrant laborers, or local landless casual labor, their tasks are to hoe, water, cultivate, pick, and ship, to do the harsh stoop labor that large-scale agricultural production requires. They have no share in what happens to the fruits of their labors and, to that extent, no interest either.

But for those who own and run such farms, although they must concern themselves in a general way with the success of cultivation and processing, their prevailing interest has much more to do with the market than with growing things or with what becomes of those who do the work. From the sugar plantations of the seventeenth century to the wheat farms of the twentieth century, capitalistic New World farms have of course always been oriented to the sale of their products, and since the beginning most of it has been aimed overseas. Such estates or plantations were large; they usually grew a single commercial crop, such as sugarcane or cotton; their labor force, either free or coerced, was massed, seasonal, and mostly unskilled; and their success depended heavily on the vagaries of the weather and the world market. Rural life in and around such farms was no less genuine for these reasons. But it was a far different rural life from that of any family farm. When the plant that was being produced was itself a foreign transplant, it was likely to remain detached and foreign in some ways, at least until its use as a food or otherwise became part of local life, culture, and tastes.

In the twentieth century yet another stage in the agricultural history of the Americas was to take shape, and it would be based on the foreign plant of concern here, the soybean. There would be similarities with previous agricultural transformations in the Americas—the introduction of an Old World plant on highly capitalized farms, the importance of exports, and a long process of incorporating the crop into local diets—but there would also be fundamental differences. From its early years in America, soy would be intimately associated with the young field of modern chemistry.

Although soybeans had actually been planted for the first time in North America in 1765 (Hymowitz and Shurtleff 2005, 473), for the most part North American farmers and scientists ignored them until the end of the nineteenth century and the early years of the twentieth century. To be sure, some prescient agricultural scientists had been aware of their potential. It was known that they had been a staff of life for countless millions of Asians for millennia and that their richness in protein and oil was unmatched. Henry Ford and others touted their promise for industry. But although Ford in his enthusiasm threw a many-course soybean feast for his friends, no one really knew soybeans as a food. And even without soybeans, oil and protein were both available in the North American diet. In the scheme of things, then, soybeans were perceived not primarily as human food but rather as an industrial crop that could best be exploited by breaking it down into its components, more like an inedible oilseed, such as cotton, than like a food containing oil, such as maize or peanuts.

The story of the soybean's successful incorporation into the North American economy is hence different from that of many other introductions. A noteworthy aspect of the plant's usefulness, one that attracted attention early, resides in a characteristic shared with other legumes. Bacterial species of the *Rhizobiacae* family inhabit its roots. These bacteria get their food via the plant, but they reciprocate by breaking down nitrogen in the soil to a form that plants can assimilate. It is for this reason that soybean plants were first used in the United States as a forage crop to enrich the soil. Frequently the plants were plowed under—as green manure—without any of the beans being harvested.

But since soybeans are also rich in oil, many of their subsequent uses in the United States became tied to their oil content. Soy oil is used to this day in the manufacture of paints and plastics and for other industrial purposes; the lecithin in soybeans is also extracted as a highly useful ingredient for food processing and industry. The major use of the oil today—as a human food—only emerged over time in relation to wartime shortages of other more familiar oils. A persistent scientific and engineering effort improved the oil's taste and usage qualities, further contributing to soy's rise in the American economy. The wartime necessity of consuming soy oil thus became an agreeable and economical convenience during peacetime. In addition, a titanic legal and political struggle to win acceptance of margarine—which by then had come to be composed primarily of soy oil—was finally won. Soy oil is now the most important edible fat in the United States. And yet this major cooking oil in American kitchens is hardly ever marketed with the word "soybean" on the front label. This is minor evidence, although we think persuasive evidence, of the widespread, if unspoken, American perception of soybeans as a nonfood item, more suitable for industry and animal feed than for humans.

Nonetheless, the production history of soybeans in North America is unmatched, and their importance in the world economy is extraordinary. In the decade following the worldwide depression of 1929, U.S. soybean production more than quintupled (Soyatech 2001, 355). World War II was a powerful lever for further increases. In one year (1941–42), production doubled in order to fill a rocketing demand for oil and soy by-products. All the beans were harvested rather than plowed under, and the United States became the world's leading soybean producer. It has held that position ever since except for a single year: 1947. By 1956, "the center of world production shifted to the western hemisphere as the United States passed Asia in total production" (Shurtleff and Aoyagi 2007, 1).

From that year until 2006, the United States was the world's leading exporter of whole soybeans. (Since 2006 it has been locked, with modest fluctuations, in a statistical tie with Brazil.) By 1973, soybeans had surpassed both wheat and maize to become the country's most important cash crop (Shurtleff and Aoyagi 2007, 2). But success led to international rivalry, and

Brazil and Argentina became big producers. Together with the United States, these countries now produce about 80 percent of the world's soybeans. It is perhaps worth remembering that the vast and fertile lands of all of the New World, and not only of the United States, have counted heavily in the buildup of hemispheric production, but that buildup would not have occurred were it not for the specific uses to which soybeans could be put.[4]

So far, utilization of soybeans as food has been referred to mostly in passing. The contributions to this volume, however, are primarily concerned with foods, not with the other uses of soybeans. Those food uses of the beans and their products are quite complex. On the one hand, they harken back to ancient practices, as in the manufacture of bean curd (tofu), soy sauce, and bean pastes. On the other hand, they involve highly modernized, industrial processes for the extraction of the oil, the manufacture of animal feed (a use that ultimately leads to human food in the form of meat), the fabrication of extruded soy protein for use in new food analogues such as veggie burgers, the preparation of infant formula and health-promoting nutraceuticals, and so on. In this enumeration as well, the contrast of ancient and modern is pronounced.

The essays in this volume focus on foods in which soy protein is a primary ingredient (soyfoods). But it must not be forgotten that in industrialized countries soy also appears in myriad foods as an additive, albeit often in tiny quantities. Just a little soy protein or lecithin can inexpensively change the texture, consistency, moisture retention, or shelf life of a food. For this reason, soy is constantly used in the manufacture of America's processed groceries. Sometimes it is also used as an economical extender of more expensive ingredients (e.g., meat) or as one of several sources of protein within a processed food. Soy appears in these ways in hospital meals, vegetarian foods, sports drinks and snacks, pizza toppings, seafood, diet products, frozen desserts, dietary supplements, and myriad other ordinary grocery items.

Thus, on a random day in the kitchen of one of the authors the following foods contained soy oil, soy lecithin, or soy protein: grain products (hot dog rolls, whole wheat bread, breakfast cereals, crackers, animal cookies, brownie mix, and fig bars); canned goods, including soups, tuna, and cat food; peanut butter; powdered drinks (breakfast drinks, hot cocoa mix, and nondairy creamer); turkey sausage; tofu; chocolate products (candy and chocolate ice cream); sauces and condiments, including whipped dessert topping, margarine, salad dressing, mayonnaise, barbecue sauce, teriyaki sauce, cilantro sauce, Worcestershire Sauce, and beef bouillon cubes;

and frozen foods, including waffles, chicken nuggets, ravioli, pierogies, and eggplant parmigiana. Clearly, soy has become a nearly ubiquitous although often unnoticed presence in many diets, notably the American diet. In the United States, soy has moved far beyond being an exotic Oriental ingredient and has penetrated many ethnic cuisines, at least in their American versions. Moreover, soy's popularity as a nutraceutical means that it very likely will appear in ever more products in years to come.

The often hidden, nearly invisible presence of soy is significant in part because it is embroiled in struggles over the future of genetic engineering. But this is not the place to deal at great length with either soybean uses or genetic engineering, which are addressed elsewhere in the book. We need instead to reflect now on how people deal with new foods. Many of the cases considered in this book concern changes in food patterns: how they come about and what factors can facilitate or hinder such processes of change. These matters deserve a look here.

Soy and Dietary Change

A variety of perspectives must be considered when examining changes in food-related behavior. If you start with the human organism's life-or-death need for nourishment, then it is reasonable to hypothesize that consciously or not, over time human groups would select certain foods because of their positive biological consequences. This by no means negates the role of culture in shaping cuisines. The wide diversity of human foods, the patterning of foods that typifies specific human groups, and the socialization process by which many food preferences become deeply rooted in particular societies are all evidence of the bulking role of culture in the arena of food choice. But to recognize a biological level is to accord analytical respect to the functioning of the human body without reducing human food choice simply to biology.

Biology can affect food choices through, for example, urgent physical needs, the affective power of taste, or individual differences. To note one case of physical need, British sailors were encouraged to eat limes and other types of citrus because of the role of vitamin C in preventing scurvy, a disease that can be excruciatingly painful and even fatal. In a wholly different case involving taste, we know that when humans consume chili peppers (*Capsicum spp.*), their bodies can create endorphin feedback loops capable of transforming over time what might begin as a painful experience into a pleasurable one (Rozin 1990). Yet again, individual genetic differences will determine which persons are able to taste certain bitter compounds (Rozin 2000). This means that there is a biological basis for the presumption that such persons are more likely to avoid the bitter compounds than are individuals who simply cannot taste them.

Biology has to do with change in the realm of food as in every other arena that evolution touches. Like Kaplan (1973), Mintz (1985b, 1998, 2001) takes the view that agrarian societies learned over time to combine a core cereal such as rice with a legume (such as soy), thereby enhancing chances for survival, unlike those societies that acquired no experiential evidence of the protein value of legumes. Indeed, natural selection may well have favored the development of cuisines that routinely offered a complete array of essential amino acids, whether through combinations of plants or through animal foods. Of course, biological evolution left a great deal of room for human creativity and the gradual emergence and stabilization of cultural differences in food systems.

Food choices also turn on the ecological and agricultural constraints that can make particular foods available or ecologically desirable (Harris 1985). Prior to the Columbian Exchange—and our present era of massive and near-constant globalization—local environmental constraints played major roles in the development of geographically specific cuisines (Mintz 1996). Yet neither environments nor cuisines ever stand still.[5] Soil conditions, weather patterns, the availability of hunted animals, the diseases of plants, and the technological changes that mark human history together with migration, trade, and cultural variation have affected the emergence of cuisines, which occurs at variable rates. Chapters in this volume illustrate some of the ecological constraints and incentives that have affected soybean cultivation as well as soy's rich and complex history within many cuisines.

More striking today than in early times[6] and in spite of the world's growing affluence, dietary choices are significantly affected by food prices, particularly for those who must feed their families on restricted budgets. For example, in the Ecuadorian Andes in the 1980s as purchased foods were gradually supplanting indigenous foods, we are told that children constantly pleaded with their parents for more of a coveted treat: bread. These were people for whom bread was not a traditional food; it had entered into local life as an indulgence. As one ethnographer explains, parents were "forced into conflict with their children on this issue: they simply [could not] afford to provide bread at every morning meal" (Weismantel 1988, 110, 156). The economic component of shifting dietary patterns—often in synch with changes toward wage labor, declining local farming, and urbanization—is poignantly clear in such situations.

But the wheels of food history are driven by far more than biology and economics: food patterns are shaped in both obvious and covert ways by cultural norms. People in some societies knowingly and customarily eat some foods—such as mushrooms or blowfish (*fugu*) or even shellfish from polluted waters—that can be toxic and sometimes kill. Indigenous Amazonian horticulture was actually built largely around one food (cassava: *Manihot esculenta* Crantz) that, without proper processing, can be deadly poisonous when eaten. Unless we wish to attribute all such behavior to a suicidal drive or psychosis, we have to concede that cultural forces have great power over food choices.

Religious beliefs and practices encourage the consumption of certain foods in certain ways, such as fish on Fridays among generations of Roman Catholics. Such beliefs and practices also help create or reinforce culinary taboos, including those against pork among Muslims and Jews, beef among Hindus, and meat of any kind among many Buddhist monks. Food choices are also patterned by age, gender, ethnicity, kin or totem group, class or caste, and numerous other criteria of social assortment. Culture significantly shapes those foods that are considered prestigious, healthful, positively medicinal, ethical, or patriotic to eat and those foods that are perceived as the opposites of these. Humans constantly use food as a vehicle for culturally patterned, symbolic expression, a language of a kind for dealing with the social, physical, and supernatural worlds. The "grammar" of this language so affects food choice that "if one wanted to guess as much as one could about a person's food attitudes and preferences, the best question to ask would be: What is your native culture or ethnic group? Not only would this response be very informative but there is also no other question one could ask that would be remotely as informative" (Rozin 2000, 1479). Even this statement might be refined. Seventh-day Adventists in Jamaica and Rastafarians in Baltimore, for example, make socially defined food choices that clearly surmount their ethnic status or native group. Thus, membership in subcultural groups must be strongly taken into account as well.

In the realm of food, as in so many other realms, cultural background can deeply affect even individual psychology (see chapter 7 in this volume). All the same, individual variation in preference does exist within groups that share cultural norms (e.g., some French people just do not like wine; some Americans hate soft drinks). Such variation matters to food psychologists, who study the ways people experience particular foods (the effects of boredom, aversion following nausea, preference following satiety, pathologies of food choice, and so on) and how varying associations affect food choices (Rozin 2000).

It should be noted in this connection that individual psychology can sometimes have larger impacts, as when the consumption preferences or beliefs of a revered leader become fashionable in society at large.[7] On the domestic level, research has shown that living with a highly skilled cook can lead to greater appreciation of soyfoods (Wansink 2005, 50–52). The household cook, in other words, can function as a gatekeeper of food preferences (Wansink 2003, 2005), passing on not only cultural norms but also sometimes her or his personal tastes.

All of these approaches to food habits must take stock of history, which makes clear that although foods are often chosen, sometimes they are instead foisted on a population, as in the case of slaves and soldiers who must take what they can get, or are withheld or prohibited, as in some cases with women and girls in developing countries (for material on South Asia, see Miller 1997; for case studies in Africa, see Aunger 1994 and O'Laughlin 1974). The idea of choice, although useful at times, is not always the most relevant key for uncovering what people may usually or commonly eat.

Historical approaches to diet must take into account both chosen and imposed food patterns, as these are affected by strictly local conditions as well as by large-scale events such as wars, trade, government policies and their outcomes, technological changes in food processing, immigration, and the effects of exposure to mass media. The importance of history for all analytical approaches to dietary patterns is evident in the essays in this volume. In a very real sense, historical perspectives highlight the value of these other perspectives. Each of the approaches discussed above has something to contribute to a history of human eating that avoids attributing change to any single type of cause. Historical analysis, in fact, often shows the intertwining of different factors shaping diet (see, for instance, Orlove 1997 on how class differences, the price of meat, and meat's symbolic associations influenced the politics of a Chilean food riot).

But these many approaches are not merely "good to think" (Lévi-Strauss 1963, 89). An applied anthropology that addresses food inequality and hunger worldwide must be based on a serious understanding of food patterns and how they can change. Such an understanding is vital to an evaluation of the future of soyfoods. We know that soy has played a positive role in relieving malnutrition—for example, as a common food in famine relief supplies—and that it has the potential to contribute far more if it can become a viable local crop and an accepted low-cost and accessible food among protein-deficient populations. The need for foods of this kind is serious and real. The United Nations Food and Agriculture Organization estimates that worldwide during the period 2000–2002, some 852 million people suffered from malnutrition (FAO 2005). Most of them were undernourished in protein as well as other nutrients, and the potentiality of soyfoods for attacking this problem is enormous. But to be effective, solutions to malnutrition will work better if they take into account what people are now eating and how they can change.

We see the soyfood potential in terms of a twofold approach to world hunger. On the one hand, addressing the root causes of hunger is essential. This requires the promotion of more equitable and just treatment of all people so that societies no longer tolerate hunger within or even outside their borders or use or condone food deprivation as a weapon or side effect of war. Addressing the causes of hunger also usually requires the reduction of population pressures as well as specific technological adaptations. Among those adaptations, soy can often play a role in long-term agriculture.

On the other hand, while we engage in the lengthy struggle against inequalities so severe that children regularly perish, are permanently stunted, or are cognitively damaged by hunger-related factors, in crisis situations we have to focus too on short-term survival. Here soy can continue to play a rapid, practical role in keeping bodies alive and healthy. In distressed regions, however, care must be taken to avoid having foreign donations of soy protein undermine the prices of locally grown protein sources. Ideally, locally grown soy could be promoted through long-term agricultural strategies and then supported with donor purchases and distribution in the event of a food crisis. The distribution would take into account local preferences for how to prepare soy.

The chapters in this volume are meant to report on the place of soyfoods in world diet but also to provoke thought and discussion about dietary change. There are no simple answers. In introducing soyfoods to particular human groups, it will be practical to work as much as possible within the contours of local cuisines (within what Ozeki labels in her essay "standard taste"; see also Rozin 1983). But while this recommendation is widely acknowledged by experts in food change, the possibilities themselves remain open-ended. We believe that the questions our chapters may provoke have to be answered differently for each population of eaters.

Diversity and Unity

The essays that compose this book were not commissioned. Each represents the specific interests of its author(s), although most were written for a 2003 conference in Chengdu, Sichuan (China), sponsored by the Foundation of Chinese Dietary Culture and the Chiang Ching-Kuo Foundation. The editors' aim has been to assemble in one work the thinking of many specialists so that interested readers could get an overarching but diverse view of the history and nature of the single food source that concerns us. The materials are diverse both because the contributors worked on different geographical areas and with people of differing cultures and because they share no single perspective in regard to their data.

Yet we realized in the course of our work that despite the diversity of the essays' topics, every author had to deal, in one way or another, with change. What had happened to the world food system and with soybeans and soyfoods—and was still happening as we watched—became our volume's subject.

Although the essays are arranged in two sections and the substantive content of every essay stands on it own, we have endeavored to put together an integrated and coherent assemblage. Such integration inheres in certain thematic unities, which unfold within the essays themselves when they are read as one. It may be useful to deal here with five of those unities. Readers may wish to pursue the ideas that they carry as they read on.

In the opening essay, Lawrence Kaplan provides a broad and useful general background to understanding legumes, which remain globally important human foods although unfortunately they may now be losing ground to other foods. The soybean is, of course, a legume, one of a large number domesticated by humans. But at our request Kaplan only touches lightly on soy in his essay because soy is in many ways a unique case. By contrast, all of the remaining essays are devoted to the soybean and its by-products alone. Hence we begin exploring the book's themes with the unity implicit in our focus on a single legume that is anciently domesticated; extraordinarily rich in calories, fat, and protein; highly nourishing; and ecologically advantageous.

During a lengthy period after its domestication, the mature seed of the soybean plant was not readily digestible by humans. Even so, and despite the difficulties that the soybean posed for the human gut, it was to become a vital food, one of the essential five plant foods (and of them, the only legume) in the Chinese food system. As H. T. Huang points out in his essay on soy's early history, this was because of advantages that it provided both cultivator and consumer, such as its hardiness, its benefits to the soil, and its rich protein. These advantages motivated the Chinese to find creative ways to prepare soy. Huang details techniques of cooking, fermenting, sprouting, and grinding.

Then, long after soy's domestication, the Chinese devised a quite simple process that made possible the creation from the soybean of many new foods. That process involves soaking the beans; grinding them into a slurry; cooking and filtering the milk; adding gypsum, salt, an acid, or some other coagulant; and filtering and skimming off the coagulated product. That product, called bean curd in English, subsequently gave rise to a wide variety of other products, differing in their textures, flavors, preservability, and uses. The liquid (or milk), the curd separated from the whey, and the lees or waste remaining all have food uses.

Once institutionalized in Chinese cultivation and cuisine, this process for creating different foods made more likely and worthwhile the subsequent diffusion of the soy plant itself and of the various products made from the beans. That original process also underlay novel elaborations in soyfoods production both in China and elsewhere within Asia. In other words, as with the rest of culture, when good objects and ideas travel, they are likely to result in new products in the hands of others who bring to them differently formed ideas and needs of their own and in this way appropriate them culturally and psychologically. In his essay, Chee-Beng Tan notes that while this processing of soybeans is now highly modernized in some places, it remains simple in nature, can still be carried out in nearly any home kitchen, and is practiced in many Asian households even today. It resembles closely the technique used during the Ming dynasty many centuries ago as described by the Chinese physician Li Shizhen (see Huang 2000, 303).

Tan points out that the process used in modern bean curd factories is strikingly similar, differing mostly in the use of machines and the scale and speed of production. This relatively basic procedure means that small-scale family-level production can survive, as it does in China and in Chinese communities overseas. Added elaborations, including fermentation of tofu, are similarly available to ordinary cooks, and not surprisingly, this simplicity has led in turn to a large number of subsidiary food practices and products.

Note, however, that the technological innovations described here took place over the course of two millennia. Huang's essay points out that the soybean had apparently been domesticated by around 1000 BC (see also Hymowitz 1970) and that the process of bean curd manufacture was not invented until around AD 900, nearly two thousand years later. Yet through their enormous importance in daily life in Asia, soybeans affected the lifeways of millions (today, hundreds of millions if not billions) of people. These developments took place primarily (but not exclusively) in what Tan refers to in his essay as "the core tofu culture area" (China, Japan, Korea and Vietnam), and the essays concerned with these four nations deal in good measure with the development of differentiated soyfood usages that arose after the diffusion of soybean cultivation to their territories.

By contrast, the essay by Christine M. Du Bois and Ivan Sergio Freire de Sousa thrusts the examination of soy's transformations squarely into the twenty-first century. In the past decade, farmers in the United States, Brazil, and Argentina have undertaken the cultivation of genetically engineered (GE) soy at an astonishing rate. The commercial success of GE soy and other crops has given rise to social tensions and intense debates over the effects of GE crops on human health, natural environments, farmer livelihoods, and the plight of the poor in developing countries. The essay discusses recent developments in politics, law, and science that pertain to genetic engineering, presenting a balanced perspective on this sensitive and complex topic. Unlike most discussions of GE crops, the essay focuses specifically on soy.

Beyond the importance of this plant and its transformations, some of the essays also confront the issue of taste, which plays a vital role in the story. As Erino Ozeki points out in her essay on Japan, most food scholars have neglected to study taste, focusing instead on other details about foodstuffs. Taste merits reflection not only from the point of view of human biology but also from that of particular cultures, within each of which taste is significantly shaped by social learning. In an original contribution that resonates with the flavor principle of Rozin's (1983[1973]) pioneering cookbook, Ozeki ties her conception of Japanese food choices to what she defines as standard taste in Japanese culture. In her view, Japanese taste standards center on the use of dashi (stock made from kelp or dried fish) and fermented soybean products (soy sauce or miso paste). In Japan these foods have traditional importance, going back in the case of miso to the Muromachi era (ca. AD 1333–1573). Shoyu (soy sauce) only became popular later, probably in the late sixteenth century, for it was more costly for ordinary folks to produce in small quantities. In her overview of these products in Japan, Ozeki sees these early achievements as directly relevant to the taste predispositions of the modern Japanese.

The essays on Korea and Vietnam also deal in varying degree with the issue of taste, as does Jianhua Mao's pathbreaking essay on the soyfoods of Chengdu (Sichuan). In his essay, Mao describes the joys of eating tofu prepared in myriad ways. While Sichuan food is superficially known to be spicy and hot, Mao reveals the nuanced complexity of flavors in its cuisine.

His recital of tofu cuisines in the city of Chengdu, past and present, is quite remarkable. The challenge to translators was that most of the recipe names evoke verses from ancient and modern Chinese literature, fictional and historical. Mao's essay here may very well be the first comprehensive English-language study that records by name multiple tofu recipes from a single Chinese city. In that city, an intense rivalry among restaurants is expressed not only in their foods, decor, and architecture but also in the cultural styles of eating, which are loosely imputed to China's past (such as the ritual of washing customers' hands before they eat), and in a vibrant and surprising restaurant subculture, one that instantly recalls Hobsbawm and Ranger's (1983) "invention of tradition." The cultural packaging of tofu dishes so as to evoke historical images exemplifies this. For example, Mao mentions the dish "Overlord Saying Farewell to His Concubine," from the famous opera story of the rebel leader Xiangyu (232–202 BC). In this dish, the cosmetic makeup of Xiangyu the Overlord is so delicately "painted" in the food that diners hesitate to begin using their chopsticks to eat it.

Probably because Vietnam was contiguous with China, the Vietnamese learned tofu-making technology early but perhaps not as early as might be assumed. Although Can Van Nguyen tells us that in Vietnam "it would be hard to find someone who eats rice but never eats tofu," Vietnamese texts suggest that tofu did not become popular in Vietnam until around the eighteenth century. The popularization of soybeans and tofu there may exist in part because of the migrations of Chinese Buddhists southward. Certainly Buddhism and the emphasis on vegetarianism contributed to both the popularity and diffusion of tofu and soybean products throughout soy-using Asia (see also Huang 2000 and the essays in this volume by Tan and Ozeki).

Nguyen describes the tofu making of monks and farming families. But instead of using gypsum for coagulation, the Vietnamese prefer sour water, concocted from lemon and star fruit, from sour leaves, or from locally made vinegar. We find that each subregion has its own distinctive flavors. In Vietnam there is lemon grass–flavored fried tofu, a deep-fried tofu that has been marinated for an hour before frying in minced lemon grass, chili, and saffron. Those who know tofu only in its Western guise can imagine how different this must taste.

Within the confines of taste, fermentation has a part to play as it did in the case of Japan, and as a processing technique it constitutes here a third unifying theme. While people in the West probably see soyfoods mainly as processed yet fresh, an important sector of the world soyfood repertory actually consists of dried, smoked, and especially fermented products, many of which have long been integrated within local Asian cuisines and few of which are well known outside Asia. As Sidney W. Mintz indicates in his essay, the soybean is "the legume most improved as human food by fermentation." Fermentation transforms a food's nature, changes its taste, and can much enhance its preservability. Quite striking in the case of Asia, fermented soyfoods emerged over time as important in sauces and dressings, as breakfast foods, and in other ways that remain quite alien to historic Western food categories. Indeed, Mintz notes that with one conspicuous exception (soy sauce), fermented legumes have been almost wholly absent from Western food history.

Not only in Japan but also in Korea fermented soyfoods (*chang*) play an essential part in defining the standard taste. Katarzyna Cwiertka and Akiko Moriya describe the Korean "soybean trinity": *kanjang* (soy sauce), *yoenjang* (soybean paste), and *koch'ujang* (hot red pepper paste). These three together "play an equally important role in providing Korean cuisine with its distinctive taste."

Koreans have a long history of soyfood consumption.[8] Korean cuisine includes roasted soybeans and roasted soybean flour, several kinds of tofu, and soymilk. Cwiertka and Moriya deem fermented soyfoods most important for Koreans, however: "the taste of food is the taste of *chang*." As Korean cuisine has become a potent national symbol, South Koreans are ever prouder of their homemade *chang*.

The essay by Cwiertka and Moriya exemplifies the ways that forces for change inflect and complicate food systems. While domestic manufacture of fermented foods was once criticized in Korea as old-fashioned, today such products enjoy reenhanced respect. On the one hand, factory-produced soy sauce has lost favor; on the other hand, it is still marketed in large quantities. In the Korean case, issues of identity compete with convenience, shaping whether people choose the mass-produced soy or not and in what circumstances. Food traditions have also been given special support and attention, as various government entities in Korea have awakened to the need to preserve old-time food processing and local culinary distinctions. These examples show that change does not simply proceed along some undifferentiated continuum from past to future. Instead, culinary issues today are segregating people into groups with diverse opinions and attitudes in relation to food. New forms of differentiation among people within single societies may indeed be one of the broader consequences of contemporary changes in food systems.

In two different regards, Indonesia stands apart from the picture we have provided so far. First, when compared with Vietnam, Japan, or Korea, Indonesia lies outside the core group of traditional tofu users to which Tan refers. Second, it has developed foods based on the soybean that in spite of possible links to the Chinese past merit consideration as indigenous local creations.[9]

Indonesia's most distinctive soyfoods are *oncom* and *tempe,* the first made from the dregs of tofu processing and the second by fermenting dehulled and soaked soybeans. Note that *tempe* is associated exclusively with Indonesia, where it was invented. One of the country's main sources of both protein and calories, *tempe* is still consumed on almost a daily basis by the poor and with startling frequency by the rich as well. Soy sauce and soybeans are widely used but, as elsewhere, with distinctive local flavors. For example, Myra Sidharta tells us in her essay that in Central Java, fermented black soybean sauce gains a special flavor with the addition of brown palm sugar. In ethnic Chinese areas star anise and cinnamon flower are used, and on the west coast fish oil is sometimes an ingredient in soy sauces. In this fourth most populous nation on earth and second most populous among those nations that regularly eat soy protein, soyfood creativity abounds.

A fourth unifying theme involves the links (or lack thereof) between production and consumption, a central and ancient relationship in Asia. (The integration of production and consumption has barely begun to take shape outside Asia; we will describe it presently.) In the United States, increases in soyfood consumption have been led by the successes of energy bars and, notably, of soymilk (in an odd simulacrum to the triumph of soy oil margarine over butter, once again creating anguish for the dairy industry). As Du Bois shows in her essay, various other soyfoods have made quite steady progress, particularly in the quasi-medical sphere of infant formulas and nutraceuticals. But the direct consumption of soy, other than its oil, is minor in the West when compared to the scale of production. Nonetheless, the health food movement and growing awareness of soy protein as a nutritious, nonfattening food in the United States have noticeably popularized the consumption of what were once ethnic Asian soyfoods such as tofu and soymilk.

We note that in the United States there is a curious equivalence or conceptual rivalry between protein-rich legumes and animal protein, a situation to which this book points though without any confident explanation. For many in the West, for example, soyfoods are perceived as substitutes for meat. Yet in much of Asia, such a simple equivalence does not always figure in how people think about their foods.[10] What meat can mean in a society that regularly eats meat is not the same as what it means in societies where meat is eaten only very selectively or not at all. Accordingly, the perception of foods that can serve nutritively in place of meat also varies. In many contemporary Asian societies, soy is not now seen as a meat substitute; indeed, it is not a substitute for anything at all. It stands on its own as a taken-for-granted foodstuff.

Soybean agriculture in Brazil and Argentina, as described by Ivan Sergio Freire de Sousa and Rita de Cássia Teixeira Vieira, joins U.S. soy production in moving readers from the level of familial production and consumption to that of the world market, broadly conceived. Although families of Asian origin in Latin America may sometimes eat and even process tofu at home and although Asian restaurants there may advertise it occasionally on their menus, the gap between production and consumption in these two nations is more readily compared to the situation in the United States than to that of Asia. Changes in American trade policy in the 1970s, during Richard Nixon's presidency, afforded Brazil and then Argentina the opportunity to compete with the United States in soy production. They did so with zest, were rewarded handsomely, and together now produce nearly half of the world's soybeans.

The success of the soy crop in Brazil and Argentina owes much to modern technology and standardization, including genetic modification. This path of development is not free of controversy, when savannahs are turned into areas of soy cultivation and large profits go to multinational conglomerates. Local consumption cleaves mostly to the use of cooking oil and animal feed. Sousa and Vieira report that "in contemporary Brazil, about 90% of consumed oil comes from soybeans," and chickens fed on soybeans are called "soybeans with wings." While tofu and soyfoods in general are popular in Brazil among persons of Japanese and Chinese descent, they cannot be said to be part of Brazilian cuisine.

Finally, there is the thematic unity suggested by the essays by Christine Du Bois and Donald Z. Osborn. They confront another more problematic aspect of change. By examining the introduction of soyfoods in Bangladesh and Africa, these essays afford us insights into how soyfoods are perceived and the efforts made to introduce and localize them. Although they deal with instances of local production, they also suggest how new habits of consumption can be acquired.

In countries where there is neither a common practice of meat consumption nor a tradition of soyfoods, stimulating popular acceptance of soy can present a special set of challenges. Du Bois's second essay compares the U.S. case with that of Bangladesh, tracing the work of the Mennonite Central Committee, a North American Christian development organization that for decades was Bangladesh's most active promoter of soybean cultivation and consumption. The local climate and soil pose serious problems for soy production, but at least as difficult was persuading local people to experiment seriously with preparing soyfoods. Currently, the only soy protein foods that are widely accepted are roasted soybeans, eaten as a snack, and soy-fortified biscuits served in schools. These two soy protein foods are complemented by consumption of imported soybean oil. Yet in spite of the limited Bangladeshi acceptance of soyfoods, the nitrogen-fixing qualities of soy cultivation and soy's nutritional value make it a commendable crop for this protein-poor country.

Osborn's essay on soy in West Africa looks at the acceptance of soy and soyfoods as a creative adaptation within local cuisines. The first pressures for soy production in West Africa came from the colonial powers, which were simply focused on European demand for edible oils. Only due to the efforts during the 1970s of the International Institute of Tropical Agriculture (ITTA), established in Nigeria in 1967, were there signs of rising acceptance by farmers of soy as a crop. As for consumption, the first successful adaptation to local foodways is highly instructive about changes in food behavior. The African locust bean (*Parkia biglobosa*) is traditionally used to make a fermented condiment, *daddawa*. (Once again we confront a fermented legume, this time outside both Asia and the West.) It turned out that cooking down soybeans to make *daddawa* takes about half the time as when the legume used is locust beans. As locust beans became scarce and more costly, soybeans began rapidly to replace them in *daddawa* processing.

Yet another such success provides a similar lesson. Osamu Nakayama, a soyfoods expert from the Japanese International Cooperation Agency (JICA) who worked with the IITA during 1989–91 succeeded in adapting a traditional African technique for making an unripened dairy cheese (*wagashi*) to the making of bean curd. Bean curd made from this process resembles the local dairy cheese and is less expensive than the cheese.

These details provide interesting insights. In introducing a new food, it is useful to capitalize on its resemblance to a food already being eaten; to insert a new ingredient in food making, let it be not only similar (in taste, odor, texture, and/or appearance) but also quicker to use and/or cheaper.

Recent marketing of locally made bean curd has been observed in Nigeria and Niger, taking place along traditional Hausa trade networks. There are processing differences in the Niger case from what we learn from China and Vietnam (see Tan's and Nguyen's essays in this volume). In Niger at the family-production level, the beans are not soaked first but instead are ground into flour. The bean flour is then soaked in water before filtering and heating. Unlike China where gypsum is used as a curdling agent, in Niger pearl millet washing water, water with tamarind, or a potassium salt is used as curdling agent. In this respect the African case brings to mind the Vietnamese preference for a sour water made from fruits, leaves, or vinegar. Comparisons of this sort through time (as in China) or across cultures suggest how the simple bean curd–making process can be inflected by local innovation, leading to somewhat different final products.

We have not referred here to the issue of gender raised by some of the essays, particularly in relation to family production of soyfoods. In the essays on China and Korea, we have noted only briefly the gender perspective, discussing the role of women in the traditional production of soyfoods at home. In Africa, as described by Osborn, women's role is very significant in contemporary production and marketing of a local form of bean curd. Women learn from other women about how to make it. In fact, Osborn tells us that "the techniques for *daddawa* and bean curd have been passed on mainly among women," and so he concludes that "their ability to find ways to use the crop would seem to have been critical to its spread." Du Bois's essay suggests that women could also eventually play a pivotal role in promoting soyfood consumption in Bangladesh. The articles thus point to the need for anyone studying dietary change to look carefully at women's attitudes and behaviors in promoting or inhibiting such change.

The Relevance of Soy

We hope that these essays help to document the immense potentialities of a remarkably versatile and rich human food source that remains for half the world undeservedly strange, exotic, or suitable mostly as animal feed. But while soyfoods can be delicious and satisfying, our collective aim is surely not that of converting our readers into soyfood eaters. Our purpose instead is to consider how important soyfoods are and how important they might become in the world arena, a focus that will be taken up again in the book's conclusion. Throughout, we confront the whole issue of change.

So far, the anthropology of food lacks any confident understanding of how and why food systems change. Yet social scientists recognize that such understanding is much needed if we mean to play a part in improving world eating from an environmental or human health perspective. In today's world where malnourishment on the one hand and unhealthy overeating on the other are simultaneously threatening large segments of the world's population and where food adequacy has to be sustained and enlarged in the light of population growth, even as local environments become progressively degraded, soyfoods in all of their variety are acquiring a growing relevance to the world's food future.

Although it is not an exhaustive survey of the contemporary place of soyfoods in modern food systems, we believe that this volume provides a useful and suggestive sampling, both contemporary and historical, of soy's role in human diet. Because these case studies also afford us a closer view of how food uses become stabilized and how they can change, they can help us draw a bead on soyfoods' possible future in human diets as well.

Notes

1. The soybean is *Glycine max* (L.) Merr. See Appendix A for the Latin names of plants and fungi mentioned throughout this volume. The authors are grateful to Eric Ross, Ted Hymowitz, and George B. Du Bois Jr. for thoughtful readings of an earlier draft. We also thank Bill George of the U.S. Department of Agriculture for help with statistics. The contents are, of course, solely our responsibility.

2. In her book on Mexican Indians, Friedlander (1975, 98) shows how eleven of the sixteen ingredients in a traditional mole are in fact not Indian but foreign, mute evidence of the way foods change even when they are not expected to.

3. From time to time in this volume, such words and phrases as "the West," "Western," "the non-Western world," etc., will appear. We are aware of the conceptual problems with this usage, but to make our point sometimes requires this risky generalization.

4. Barkin, Batt, and Dewalt (1990) convincingly demonstrate the usually appalling results of shifting farmland from the production of local subsistence to the production of animal feed for export. This kind of substitution has become more and more global, with dismal consequences in many cases for local agricultural self-sufficiency.

5. In a fine essay on the history of swine in Scotland, Ross (1983) shows how background ecological conditions such as deforestation can impact the food choices people make and how those choices can change over time.

6. We refer here to early times when most people grew their own food rather than bought it.

7. For example, dual Nobel Prize winner Linus Pauling greatly influenced Americans to consume vitamin C supplements.

8. Some Korean scholars suppose that fermented soyfoods originated in Korea. Comprehensive historical research on soy in Korea is needed, comparable to what Huang (2000) has done for China, to investigate fully the origins of soy products outside present-day China itself.

9. As Sidharta's essay in this volume explains, the oral tradition in Kediri, East Java, attributes the introduction of tofu to Indonesia to the soldiers of Kublai Khan in the thirteenth century. Kediri is so identified with tofu that it celebrated its 1,123rd anniversary with a tofu that weighed three hundred kilograms.

10. This is often true even though soyfoods long ago arose in Asia partly to replace meat that had been given up for religious reasons or where meat was scarce or costly.

References

Aunger, R. 1994. "Are Food Avoidances Maladaptive in the Ituri Forest of Zaire?" *Journal of Anthropological Research* 50: 277–310.

Barkin, David, Rosemary Batt, and Billie DeWalt. 1990. *Food Crops vs. Feed Crops.* Boulder, CO: Lynne Rienner.

Crosby, Alfred W., Jr. 1972. *The Columbian Exchange.* Westport, CT: Greenwood.

FAO (Food and Agriculture Organization of the United Nations). 2005. "Committee on World Food Security." 31st session, Rome, May 23–26. http://www.fao.org/docrep/meeting/009/J4968e/j4968e00.htm.

Friedlander, Judith. 1975. *Being Indian in Hueyapan.* New York: St. Martin's.

Friedmann, Harriet, and Philip McMichael. 1989. "Agriculture and the State System: The Rise and Decline of National Agricultures, 1870 to the Present." *Sociologia Ruralis* 29(2): 93–117.

Harris, Marvin. 1985. *Good to Eat: Riddles of Food and Culture.* New York: Simon and Schuster.

Hobsbawm, E., and T. Ranger, eds. 1983. *The Invention of Tradition.* Cambridge: Cambridge University Press.

Huang, Hsing Tsung. 2000. *Fermentations and Food Science,* Vol. 6, *Science and Civilisation in China,* Pt. 5. Cambridge: Cambridge University Press.

Hymowitz, Theodore. 1970. "On the Domestication of the Soybean." *Economic Botany* 24: 408–21.

Hymowitz, T., and W. Shurtleff. 2005. "Debunking Soybean Myths and Legends in the Historical and Popular Literature." *Crop Science* 45: 473–76.

Kaplan, Lawrence. 1973. "Ethnobotanical and Nutritional Factors in the Domestication of American Beans." In C. Earle Smith Jr., ed., *Man and His Foods,* 75–85. Tuscaloosa: University of Alabama Press.

Lévi-Strauss, Claude. 1963. *Totemism.* Boston: Beacon Press.

McMichael, Philip, ed. 1995. *Food and Agrarian Orders in the World Economy.* Westport, CT: Praeger.

Miller, B. D. 1997. "Social Class, Gender, and Intrahousehold Food Allocations to Children in South Asia." *Social Science & Medicine* 44(11): 1685–95.

Mintz, Sidney W. 1985a. *Sweetness and Power: The Place of Sugar in Modern History.* New York: Penguin.

———. 1985b. "The Anthropology of Food: Core and Fringe in Diet." *India International Centre Quarterly* 12(2): 193–204.

———. 1996. *Tasting Food, Tasting Freedom: Excursions into Eating, Culture, and the Past.* Boston: Beacon.

———. 1998. "Core, Fringe and Legume: Agrarian Societies and the Concept of the Meal." In *The Fifth Symposium on Chinese Dietary Culture,* 377–85. Taipei, Taiwan: Foundation of Chinese Dietary Culture.

———. 2001. "Food Patterns in Agrarian Societies: The Core-Fringe-Legume Hypothesis." Paper for the Johns Hopkins University's Center for a Livable Future Conference, Dietary Protein: Options for the Future.

O'Laughlin, Bridget. 1974. "Mediation and Contradiction: Why Mbum Women Do Not Eat Chicken." In M. Rosaldo and L. Lamphere, eds., *Women, Culture and Society,* 301–18. Stanford: Stanford University Press.

Orlove, Benjamin S. 1997. "Meat and Strength: The Moral Economy of a Chilean Food Riot." *Cultural Anthropology* 12(2): 234–68.

Ross, Eric. 1983. "The Riddle of the Scottish Pig." *Bioscience* 33(2): 99–106.

Rozin, Elizabeth. 1983[1973]. *Ethnic Cuisine: The Flavor-Principle Cookbook,* rev. ed. Brattleboro, VT: Stephen Greene.

Rozin, Paul. 1990. "Getting to Like the Burn of Chili Pepper: Biological, Psychological, and Cultural Perspectives." In B. G. Green, J. R. Mason, and M. L. Kare, eds., *Irritation.* New York: Marcel Dekker.

———. 2000. "The Psychology of Food and Food Choice." In Kenneth F. Kiple and Kriemhild Coneè Ornelas, eds., *The Cambridge World History of Food,* Vol. 2, 1476–86. Cambridge: Cambridge University Press.

Shurtleff, William, and Akiko Aoyagi. 2007. "History of World Soybean Production and Trade," Pts. 1 and 2. http://www.soyinfocenter.com/HSS/production_and_trade1.php.

Soyatech. 2001. *Soya & Oilseed Bluebook 2001.* Bar Harbor, ME: Soyatech, Inc.

Wansink, Brian. 2003. "Profiling Nutritional Gatekeepers: Three Methods for Differentiating Influential Cooks." *Food Quality and Preference* 14(4): 289–97.

———. 2005. *Marketing Nutrition: Soy, Functional Foods, Biotechnology, and Obesity.* Urbana and Chicago: University of Illinois Press.

Weismantel, Mary J. 1988. *Food, Gender, and Poverty in the Ecuadorian Andes.* Philadelphia: University of Pennsylvania Press.

SECTION ONE

Acceptance of Soy in Global and Historical Context

1

Legumes in the History of Human Nutrition

LAWRENCE KAPLAN

The two plant families of greatest importance to world agriculture and human nutrition are the grass family (*Poaceae*), which includes the cereal grains, and the legume family (*Fabaceae*). The legume family includes about 650 genera and 18,000 species. In terms of production volume, the cereals are the most important because they furnish the carbohydrates and much of the protein that constitute the major portion of human and domestic animal diets worldwide. On the other hand, in terms of sheer numbers of genera and species used by humans, the legumes are by far the most utilized plant family (Isely 1982). Among these uses are animal feed, human food, chemicals, ornamentals, timber, cooking fuel, pasture crops, and soil enrichment. The herbaceous agricultural legumes used for human food are pulses or food grain legumes. Their principal nutritional significance for humans has been as a protein source—especially as a source of amino acids such as lysine, and a few others—complementary to those of cereal grains. It should be said, however, that in cereal grain- and legume-based diets, most of the protein is supplied by the cereal grain.

The peanut (*Arachis hypogea*), a native of South America, is certainly an important food in parts of Africa and elsewhere, but as yet there is only scant evidence for its early history. It is often considered along with oilseed crops rather than pulses and is not included in this essay. The soybean, because of its distinctive processing for preparations such as an extracted food (e.g., tofu and soy milk) and a fermented flavoring (e.g., soy sauce) and soup base (miso) rather than as a whole-seed food, is in a class by itself and is the subject of later chapters in this volume. Through examining other legumes, this essay provides the historical, comparative context for understanding the adoption of soybeans discussed in the rest of this book.

Legumes in Early Prehistoric Nutrition

Although universally recognized throughout recorded history for their value as food grains, legumes must have presented our early ancestors of the genus *Homo* with some serious problems. Suppose that you were a hardworking gatherer and hunter busy collecting edibles for yourself and perhaps for sharing with other members of your community. Your hominid origins would probably have you seeking roots and tubers for digestible starches and young leaves, insects, and bits of other animal food for protein. Seeds, of course, are good sources of these nutrients.

But the cereal grains and legume seeds may present a technology-poor hominid with some serious problems. Trypsin (or protease) inhibitors are present in both families and are concentrated in the seeds. These substances, unless deactivated by heat, inhibit the ability of digestive enzymes to break down complex protein molecules into smaller structures that can be absorbed and utilized by humans and many other animals. Some other compounds present in legume seeds are the cyanogenic glucosides of some West Indies lima bean varieties, which release toxic hydrocyanic acid in contact with acidic conditions in the stomach, and lathyrogens found in insufficiently cooked chickling peas (*Lathyrus sativus*). Both of these toxins and similar compounds are inactivated or removed by cooking. During times of famine the chickling pea, probably undercooked because of fuel shortage, has been consumed in amounts sufficient to cause paralysis of the limb joints (Aykroyd and Doughty 1964, 119). Some legume seed components are more acutely toxic; the saponin toxin abrin, found in a single seed of *Abrus precatorius* (the rosary pea), is sufficient when masticated to cause the death of an adult human (Isely 1982).

Substances that interfere with digestion and some other substances that may be classed as toxins are not necessarily damaging to humans in small quantities. Indeed, Stahl (1984) points out that immature leaves, although they contain some toxins, also have relatively high amounts of high-quality protein and tolerable amounts of fibrous complex polysaccharides. Thus, a kind of trade-off may exist in which a nutritionally significant amount of protein may be obtained from immature leaves that are ingested at a level below what might be dangerous insofar as the accompanying toxins are concerned. Perhaps the same was true of cereal grains and legume seeds for our remote ancestors. However, whatever creative tension might exist between avoidance of deleterious substances such as toxins, trypsin inhibitors, and the like and securing dietary protein, it is unlikely that sufficient daily protein could be obtained from wild gathered cereal grains, legume seeds, or immature leaves by hominids without protein from animal sources or controlled fire and some rudimentary cooking technology. These issues are provocatively discussed by Stahl (1984) and her commentators.

Heat at cooking temperatures is effective in denaturing the antimetabolites, especially when the seed tissues are thoroughly wet. Estimates of how recently or how remotely in time hominids might have used fire range as far back as 460,000 years ago in the Zhoukoudian Caves near Beijing. The hominids in this instance would have been our close relative *Homo erectus*. Charcoal, burned bone fragments, and ash provide evidence for the use of fire (Fagan 1995, 87), which appears to have been used in food preparation. Plant foods such as roots and tubers may have been roasted in these early hearths, and seeds may have been parched in the hot earth surrounding the fire.

Not until long after the use of fire in food preparation had spread throughout the world with migrating humans do we begin to find verifiable archaeological remains in habitations such as campsites, rock shelters, and caves. After this great dispersal, in different places and at different times, *Homo sapiens* societies developed ceramic containers that could be placed in the fire or in the hot coals to cook gathered or hunted food in water. Bits of organic material sifted or floated out of the dust and soil of the ancient habitations, and the residues in cooking pots can sometimes tell us something about dietary components. The separated-out organic remains may be seeds or fragments of other plant parts, sometimes only microscopic in size, or human fecal remains. Some types of plant remains are clearly wild gathered resources, but others show evidence of human selection in the process of changing wild plants into what we call domesticates.

Legume history begins in this long period of subsistence by means of food gathering and hunting. There is wide agreement among prehistorians that patterns of food gathering and human insight into the natural history of food plants eventually led to selective domestication of certain plants among the many that were exploited in the food-getting process. In Africa south of the Sahara, the Mediterranean Basin, the Near East and Southwest Asia, the Indian subcontinent, China, and North, Central, and South America, cereal grains and legumes were domesticated. With some important exceptions, indigenous cultures in each of these areas have domesticated and made as the basis of their nutrition the combination of cereal grains and legumes.

Both cereal grains and pulses have genetic and structural systems that under human selection have enabled the suppression of the normal (wild) type of seed dispersal. In the cereal grains this has been accomplished by the strengthening of tissues (the rachis) that hold the grain in the fruiting structure or ear. In the food grain legumes, the suppression of seed dispersal has been accomplished by the reduction of pod tissues that cause opening and twisting of the pod valves, an event that scatters the seed. These two mechanisms retain the seeds and facilitate harvesting. Because of harvest practices in the Near East (the ripe pods are threshed outside of the dwelling), legume pods are seldom encountered in archaeological sites. Legume pods in most Western Hemisphere sites are infrequently encountered, but in some sites they make up the majority of the legume remains.

Among the many wild species of legumes that have been gathered and domesticated by humans, all have undergone changes, especially in seed size, that distinguish wild from domesticated. Increased seed size is the most recognizable trait separating wild from domesticated legumes because it is readily determined and because the seeds are the best-preserved legume structures in most archaeological sites. In some legume species plant form changes from vining to erect, but entire plants are seldom preserved in archaeological sites.

In the following review of the origin, history, and migrations of some of the important cultivated food grain legumes, the foregoing processes of human-plant interactions and biological characteristics of legumes should be kept in mind. In particular, so pervasive is the dietary-agricultural combination of cereal with legume that the similarities in diets and processes of domestication obscure the differences. One such difference is the cereal grain–legume combination itself. That is, has legume domestication coincided with cereal domestication in time and place in each of the regions where the combination is found? Or, instead, have cereals and legumes been first domesticated at different times and in somewhat different places so that their dietary combinations have not been as long-standing as they might initially appear?

Food Grain Legumes Native to the Americas

The New World genus *Phaseolus* includes the five bean species domesticated in pre-Columbian times: common beans (*P. vulgaris*), lima and sieva beans (*P. lunatus*), teparies (*P. acutifolius*), scarlet runner beans (*P. coccineus*), and polyanthus beans (*P. polyanthus*). Cultivated varieties of the common bean (*P. vulgaris*) are known archaeologically from Chile to the northern United States. The vulgaris and lunatus beans are the most important in human nutrition; other phaseolus bean species were of more limited distribution and are not included in the following discussion.

RADIOCARBON DATING

Samples of crop plant remains in early and even later levels of archaeological sites in the Americas are often so small that there is insufficient material to be dated by standard (or indirect) radiocarbon methods (^{14}C) that measure the emission of beta particles. Consequently, most of the dates for such samples published before the late 1980s are based on associated organic remains such as charcoal or wood but not on the remains of the actual crop plant samples. With increasing recognition of the extent to which seeds and other small objects may be displaced within archaeological deposits, direct dates on small samples (one-fourth of a bean seed, for example) by Accelerator Mass Spectrometry (AMS) have become essential for use in reconstructing the pathways of early agriculture and domestication.

BEANS IN AMERICAN ARCHAEOLOGY

Phaseolus bean remains are seldom abundant in American archaeological sites. Prior to the introduction of the AMS dating method, there had not been sufficient *Phaseolus* material for dating by radiocarbon methods. Hence, the dates published before 1999 for the earliest appearance of beans (e.g., Kaplan, Lynch, and Smith 1973) in the archaeological record have been based on radiocarbon dates of spatially associated materials. With the availability of AMS dating techniques it has been possible to test and, where necessary, to correct the dates previously reported for beans in American archaeological sites and to provide data relevant to studies of the origins and history of agriculture in the Americas. The following comparison of AMS dates for beans and maize in prehistoric Mexico are revealing for the history of these traditional and complementary components of the traditional Mexican diet.

In south-central Mexico carbonized seeds of the domesticated common bean (*Phaseolus vulgaris*) dated by AMS appear by 2,098 ± 81 YBP[1] (Kaplan and Lynch 1999) in the valley of Oaxaca. A set of AMS dates on maize cobs from the archaeological site of Guilá Naquitz in the Oaxaca Valley of

Mexico averages 5,412 ± 33 YBP (Benz 2001). Southeast of Mexico City in a prehistorically inhabited cave located in the Tehuacán Valley, the earliest date for the appearance of *P. vulgaris* is a single pod fragment AMS dated to 2,285 ± 60 YBP. The size of this pod fragment and the weak tendency toward twisting are traits characteristic of domesticates. Common bean seeds become abundant in the remains of this Tehuacán cave about fifteen hundred years ago, approximately twenty-four hundred years after the earliest maize. In northeastern Mexico in the state of Tamaulipas the earliest AMS dates for firmly identified *P. vulgaris* pods in two prehistorically inhabited caves (the Ocampo Caves) are 1,285 ± 55 YBP and 1,016 ± 60 YBP (Kaplan and Lynch 1999). A series of AMS dates on plant remains from the Ocampo Caves (Smith 1997) shows maize to have been present by about 4,000 YBP.

The result of botanical analyses and the AMS dates of the abundant desiccated prehistoric plant remains from inhabited sites in these three regions show that maize was being cultivated approximately two thousand to three thousand years prior to beans. The earliest beans recovered from these sites are comparable with cultivated bean varieties and probably had been introduced from other regions where they had been domesticated earlier. But the dates do show that there was a substantial period in which, contrary to the historic unity of maize and beans in the New World Indian diet, maize served as the mainstay of the diet without the presence of beans.

HISTORY AND PROTEIN STRUCTURE

As much as archaeological remains and radiocarbon dating add to an understanding of the history and migrations of any crop, plant genetics, especially molecular genetics, often adds even more. For example, Paul Gepts (1988, 215–41) has studied variation in the molecular structure of phaseolin, which is the storage protein of *Phaseolus* beans, and has applied the results to understanding the origin and dispersal of northeastern U.S. varieties of *P. vulgaris*. The majority of the cultivated common bean varieties of the northeastern states in the historic period have a so-called T phaseolin type, which is the most frequent type in Western Europe and the part of the Andes south of Colombia but not in the Mexico–Central America region. In contrast, in Mesoamerica and the adjacent southwestern United States, the traditional bean varieties are predominantly of the so-called S type. The archaeological record of crop plants in the northeastern United States is limited because of poor conditions for preservation—humid soils and no sheltered cave deposits—but those beans that have been found (Kaplan 1970), although carbonized, are recognizable as a southwestern U.S. variety and are therefore probably of the S phaseolin type (the phaseolin of carbonized samples cannot be characterized as S or T).

However, traditional bean varieties cultivated in the northeastern United States are of the T or Andean phaseolin type. Evidently the bean varieties that are characteristic of the historic period in the northeastern United States are mostly South American in origin (Gepts 1988, 215–41). Many of these reached the northeastern United States by way of sailing ships directly from Peruvian and Chilean ports during the late eighteenth and early nineteenth centuries or from England and France, which had been cultivating Andean varieties since receiving them from South America in the sixteenth century and later.

The lima and sieva beans were recognized by Carl Linnaeus as belonging to the same species, which he called *Phaseolus lunatus* to describe the lunar shape of the seeds of some varieties. The small seeded or sieva types are natives of Mexico and Central America. These are distinct from the large-seeded South American lima beans but can be crossed with them and for this reason are still considered to be of the same species. The sievas appear in the archaeological records of Mexico about twelve hundred years ago and do not occur in the known records of Andean archeology. Seeds of the South American group have been found in Guitarrero Cave, the same Andean cave as the earliest common beans of South America and have been AMS radiocarbon dated to 3,495±50 YBP (Kaplan and Lynch 1999). It seems clear that the two groups were domesticated independently.

On the desert southern coast of Peru, pods of the large-seeded lima group dating to 5,616± years ago—in the Preceramic period—were well preserved by the arid conditions (Kaplan and Lynch 1999). Seeds and pods are so abundant in some of the coastal sites that they must have represented a major part of the diet. Ancient Peruvians even included depictions of beans in their imaginative painted ceramics and woven textiles. In the Mochica culture (AD 100–800), painted pottery depicts running messengers each carrying a small bag decorated with pictures of lima beans (*pallares*). Rafael Larco Hoyle (1943) concluded that the lima beans, painted with parallel lines, broken lines, points, and circles, were ideograms. Some of the beans that Larco Hoyle believed to be painted were certainly renderings of naturally variegated seed coats. Other depictions show stick-limbed bean warriors rushing to the attack. Textiles from Paracas, an earlier coastal site, are rich in bean depictions.

The Near Eastern Pulses

The origins and domestication of pulses in the Near East have been the focus of extensive research by plant geneticists and by archaeologists seeking to understand the foundations of agriculture in this region. It is in the Near East where the major crops of the ancient cultures of the Sumerians, Babylonians, Greeks, Romans, and other civilizations of the Mediterranean Basin and Europe and Britain originated. Zohary (1989b, 358–63) has presented both genetic and archaeological evidence for the simultaneous or near-simultaneous domestication in the Near East of emmer wheat (*Triticum turgidum* ssp. *dicoccum*); barley (*Hordeum vulgare*); and einkorn wheat (*T. monococcum*) "hand in hand with the introduction into cultivation of five companion plants": pea (*Pisum sativum*), lentil (*Lens culinaris*), chickpea (*Cicer arietinum*), bitter vetch (*Vicia ervilia*), and flax (*Linum usitatissimum*). Kislev (1985) presented evidence that the broad bean, or fava bean (*Vicia faba*), may be among these earliest domesticates.

THE CLASSICAL TEXTS

Papyrus texts, murals, inscriptions, and archaeological remains from Egypt are rich sources of information on food (Darby, Ghalioungui, and Grivetti 1977) and medicinal herb use (Manniche 1989) in pharonic times. Rameses II spoke of barley and beans in immense quantities, and Rameses III offered to the Nile god 11,998 jars of shelled beans. The term "bean meal" (medicinal bean meal), so commonly encountered in the medical papyri, could apply to *Vicia faba,* to other legumes, or to the Egyptian bean (*Nelumbo nucifera,* the sacred lotus), all of which have been found in tombs. Fava beans were avoided by priests and others; the reasons for this are not clear. The avoidance of favas by Pythagoras, who was trained by Egyptians, is well known, and it may have been that he shared with them a belief that beans "were produced from the same matter as man" (Darby, Ghalioungui, and Grivetti 1977, 683). Other ancient writers on the taboo gave other reasons, such as an act of self-denial by priests of a variety of foods including lentils.

More recently, favism, a genetically determined sensitivity (red blood cells deficient in glucose-6-phosphate dehydrogenase) to chemical components of the broad bean has been implicated as a possible explanation for avoidance of this food (Sokolov 1984; for a counterargument, see Simoons 1998).

In ancient Greece pulses were evidently grown in quantity, judging from a passage in the *Illiad* in which there is a description of beans (probably the broad bean) and chickpeas being cast upon the threshing floor (Isager and Skydsgaard 1992, 42), evidently for removal of the dried pods. Small quantities would have been cleaned by hand.

THE BROAD BEAN

Ladizinsky (1975) investigated the genetic relationships among the broad bean and its wild relatives in the genus *Vicia*. He concluded that none of the populations of these related wild species collected in Israel can be considered the ancestor of the fava bean. Differences in the crossability as well as in chromosome form and number separate the broad bean from these relatives, as do differences in ranges of seed size, presence of tendrils, and epidermal hairs on the pods. Ladizinsky, however, was careful to note that these characters may have evolved under domestication.

Zohary and Hopf (2000, 114) point to the late appearance of substantial amounts of charred, large-seeded broad bean remains by the third millennium BC in the Iberian Peninsula, Europe north of the Alps, the Aegean region, and the Mediterranean Basin. The broad bean seeds in some of these Neolithic and Bronze Age sites are larger than the wild species and may well be the cultivated *V. faba*. Some seeds identified as *V. faba* from sites dating to the seventh through fifth millennia, especially at a site in Israel, are abundant and in the size range of the wild relatives, but their form is like that of the small-seeded cultivated type, which lends uncertainty to the determination of whether they are from wild gathered plants or from early cultivated plants.

The dates for the introduction of the broad bean into China are not secure—perhaps the second century BC or later—but it has become an important crop in "many mountainous, remote or rainy parts of China at the present time, especially in western China" (E. N. Anderson, cited by Simoons 1991, 75). The earliest introduction of broad beans into North America appears to have taken place when Captain Bartholomew Gosnold, who explored the coast of New England in 1602, planted them on the Elizabeth Islands off the south shore of Massachusetts (Hedrick 1919, 594). Less than thirty years later, records (Pulsifer 1861, 24) of the provisioning and outfitting of the supply ship for New Plymouth list "benes" (and "pease") along with other seeds to be sent to the Massachusetts colony.

LENTIL

Lens culinaris (synonym *L. esculenta*), the cultivated lentil, is a widely grown species. Archaeological evidence shows that small seeds of it or its relatives were gathered by 13,000–9,500 YBP in Greece (Hansen 1992) and from several prefarming sites in the Near East by 11,200–9,500 YBP. By the end of the eighth millennium BC, still in the prepottery Neolithic period, charred lentil seeds in the size range of the wild types are present in archaeological sites in the Near East along with cultivated barley and emmer wheat.

Lentils accompanied the earliest spread of agriculture from the Near East to southeastern Europe (Zohary and Hopf 2000, 98–99). Lentil cultivation by historic times was important and well established in the Near East, North Africa, France, and Spain (Hedrick 1919, 331) and had been introduced into most of the subtropical and warm temperate regions of the world (Duke 1981, 111), but evidently not to China, as the crop is not mentioned by Simoons (1991). The Indian subcontinent's production of about 38 percent of the world's lentils and little export (Singh and Singh 1992) make this crop among the most important dietary pulses there, where food grain legumes are an especially important source of protein.

Traditionally, two subspecies are recognized on the basis of seed size: *L. culinaris* ssp. *Microsperma,* which are small-seeded, and *L. culinaris* ssp. *Macrosperma,* which are large-seeded. The large-seeded form is grown in the Mediterranean Basin, Africa, and Asia Minor. The small-seeded form is grown in western and southwestern Asia, especially India (Duke 1981, 110–13).

Ladizinsky (1987) has maintained that gathering of wild lentils, and perhaps other grain legumes such as the pea and chickpea, prior to their cultivation could have resulted in reduced or lost seed dormancy. Dormancy is a genetically controlled factor (or at least partly so) that is favorable to wild plants but not to cultivated ones. The loss of dormancy is of primary importance in the domestication of legumes. Seeds that have the dormancy genotype are not suitable for cultivation because they do not germinate promptly after planting. In contrast, for wild growing plants dormancy allows seeds to wait in the soil for the return of appropriate environmental conditions.

The hypothetical loss of dormancy, argued Ladizinsky (1987), was an evolutionary pathway different from that of the cereal grains for which dormancy of seeds is not a barrier to domestication. His views have been disputed by Zohary (1989a) and by Blumler (1991), who maintained that the pathway of domestication in cereals and legumes were similar and that legume cultivation followed upon the beginning of cereal cultivation.

PEA

Pisum sativum, the field or garden pea, is one of the founder crops of Near Eastern agriculture. It is adapted to the cool winter season of the Mediterranean climate and as a result could be extended to northern Europe (especially Russia) and to the cooler regions of North America. The field pea is extensively grown for use of the dried seed, whole or split, for human and livestock consumption. The dried field pea cooked into a thick broth or pudding has often been referred to as a food of primary importance for the European peasantry of the Middle Ages (Simpson and Ogorzaly 1995, 213). The garden pea has higher sugar content and is widely grown as a green vegetable for human consumption. The garden pea is evidently a relatively late introduction to the human diet at least in Europe, having first been mentioned in a sixteenth-century herbal (Hedrick 1919, 442). The edible pod pea is a type of garden pea having minimal development of the tough parchment layer of the pod. Smartt (1990, 178) notes that peas are relatively free of toxic compounds and antimetabolites.

Zohary (1989b, 363–64) reports that similarities in chromosome structure between cultivated peas and *Pisum humile* populations in Turkey and the Golan Heights point to populations of humile having a particular chromosomal configuration as the direct ancestral stock of cultivated peas.

Peas are present in the early Neolithic preceramic farming villages (7500–6000 BC) of the Near East and are present in large amounts with cultivated wheats and barleys by 5850–5600 BC. They appear to be associated with the spread of Neolithic agriculture into Europe, again in association with wheat and barley (Zohary and Hopf 1988, 96–98). Not until somewhat later (4400–4200 BC) in central Germany are carbonized pea seeds with intact seed coats found. These show the smooth surface characteristic of the domestic crop. From eastern Europe and Switzerland come pea remains from late Neolithic or Bronze Age sites (Zohary and Hopf 1988, 97–98).

The date at which the pea entered China is not known, but along with the broad bean it was known as *hu-tou* or Persian bean, which suggests that it was obtained by way of the Silk Road in historic times (Simoons 1991, 74–75). Chinese restaurants in the West seasonally offer pea vine dishes.

The chickling pea or grass pea, *Lathyrus sativus,* is a minor crop in the Mediterranean Basin, North Africa, the Middle East, and India. It has been documented archaeologically in parts of this broad region since Neolithic times (Zohary and Hopf 1988, 109–10). In India it is a weedy growth in cereal grain fields and is the cheapest pulse available (Purseglove 1968, 278). During times of famine it has been consumed in significant amounts even though, as noted previously, its consumption has caused a paralysis of the limb joints (Aykroyd and Doughty 1964, 119).

CHICKPEA

Chickpeas (*Cicer arietinum*), also called Bengal gram, gram, or garbanzos, like lentils are a cool-season food grain legume that originated in the Near East. Two types of chickpeas are cultivated. The large-seeded type, rounded and pale cream in color, is grown in the Mediterranean Basin, the Near East, Mexico, and South America. The small, irregularly shaped seed type is grown primarily in East Asia, Ethiopia, Iran, and Afghanistan and makes up about 85–90 percent of the world chickpea crop (Hawtin et al. 1980, 613–14).

C. reticulatum (= *C. arietinum* subspecies *reticulatum*), a species that is genetically close to *C. arietinum* and is regarded as its wild ancestor, is found in present-day Turkey. Small charred chickpea seeds in the size range of *C. reticulatum* seeds were present in prepottery levels of archaeological sites dating to 7500–6800 BC in Turkey and northern Syria. The Turkish and Syrian sites from which these seeds were recovered are located within the range of the wild species, so the seeds might well have been gathered from wild stands rather than cultivated. By the end of the seventh millennium BC, larger chickpea seeds were found in sites north of Damascus and in Jericho (prepottery Neolithic B), both of which are far from the range of the wild species. These are probably cultivated forms of the chickpea (Zohary and Hopf 2000, 109–10). With other legumes (lentils and peas) and the cereal grains (emmer wheat and barley), chickpeas are among the earliest agricultural plants in the Near East. By the late Neolithic period, about 3500 BC, domesticated chickpeas had reached Greece, and by 2250–1750 BC they were present in early agricultural sites of the Indian subcontinent (Zohary and Hopf 2000, 111).

The Asiatic and African Pulses

The genus *Vigna,* closely allied to the genus *Phaseolus,* comprises six cultivated species. One of these is the cowpea (*V. unguiculata* subspecies *unguiculata*), which is West African in origin and is the most important and widely cultivated member of the genus (Steele and Mehra 1980, 393), especially in Africa (Purseglove 1968, 322) and Southeast Asia (Herklots 1972, 261). The cowpea (black-eyed pea) is undoubtedly ancient in West Africa, but the recovery and analysis of archaeological plant remains in sub-Saharan Africa is in its early stages, and there is as yet scant archaeological evidence of early agriculture in tropical Africa. However, a few charred seed remains of cowpea from a site in northern Burkina Faso in the southern part of the Sahel have been recovered from excavated levels dating to about AD 935, and Arabic sources describe the cultivation and use of beans, including the cowpea in Mali and Mauritania from the middle of the ninth century AD onward (Kahlheber 1999).

The cowpea appears in the Mediterranean Basin in classical times (Zohary and Hopf 2000, 93). A plant mentioned in Sumerian records about 2350 BC under the name of *lu-ub-sar* (Arabic *lobia*) may have been a reference to the cowpea (Herklots 1972, 261). The earliest mention of cowpeas in the Indian subcontinent is said to be from about 150 BC. They are noted in a medical treatise of the first or second century AD. They were prohibited from use in an Aryan religious ceremony, which further suggests that the cowpea was foreign to India and was introduced about two thousand years ago (Steele and Mehra 1980, 398–99).

The historical and archaeological dates available at the present time serve to document the early distribution of the cowpea but do not tell much about the beginning of cultivation of this important legume. The green pods are widely used as a vegetable throughout the tropics, in Southeast Asia, and in China. The fresh or dried young leaves and shoots are an important vegetable in tropical Africa.

Vigna unguiculata subspecies *sesquipedalis* is the yard-long or asparagus bean, probably a native of India, and is known for its strikingly long pods that are important as green vegetables in India, Southeast Asia, and China (Purseglove 1968, 321–24). Another subspecies (ssp. *cylindrica*), the catjang, is used for fodder as well as for human nutrition in the form of its seeds and green pods, primarily in India (Duke 1981, 298–99).

The remaining cultivated *Vigna* species are Asiatic in origin and are widely cultivated in that continent, being distributed on the basis of their differing adaptation to climatic zones and palatability (Jain and Mehra 1980, 459, 464). *Vigna radiata*, the mung bean or green gram, is well known in the West as the most important source of bean sprouts. It is the most widely grown of this group of Asiatic pulses and has been introduced into eastern and central Africa, the West Indies, and the southern United States. The mung bean, identified archaeologically in India from levels dating from 1660 to 1440 BC (Simoons 1991, 83, 96) is believed, based on good literary-historical evidence, to have entered China in AD 1011 or 1012 during a period of increased trade with India (Anderson 1988, 77).

Vigna mungo, the black gram, is closely related to *V. radiata* but is not as palatable (Smartt 1990, 173). *Vigna umbellata,* the rice bean, is closely related to *V. angularis* (the adzuki bean), which is red-coated and much grown in Japan and Korea and to a lesser extent in northern China. All of the six cultivated vignas are grown in tropical and subtropical regions; the adzuki is also grown in temperate and subtemperate regions (Jain and Mehra 1980, 460–61). According to Jain and Mehra (1980, 466), the widespread cultivation of pulses in Asia—especially in India—is the result of their nutritional contribution within the particular cultural and religious lives of the people and their contribution to maintaining soil fertility.

Conclusion

Throughout the world in the most populous regions and in some of the most and least industrialized places, legumes accompany cereal grains as primary diet components. So pervasive is the combination of these complementary food resources that they are often assumed to have been combined since the very beginnings of agriculture. Indeed, in the Near East legumes and cereal grains characteristic of the region are present in preagricultural archaeological periods, at the beginnings of agriculture, and throughout recorded history. There is as yet insufficient data from preagricultural and early agricultural sites in China to conclude that the same pattern existed there. In archaeological sites on the dry coastal lands of Peru, beans are abundant in the remains of complex agricultural societies prior to the presence of maize. In the highland agricultural societies of central Mexico, maize is present long before beans begin to appear in the archaeological record. It may be that new investigations of early archaeological sites, for example in lowland regions of Mexico or west-central Mexico, will show that maize and beans were domesticated in the same region and the same time, thus resembling the circumstance in the Near East. Currently available evidence, however, suggests that maize was an important crop at least two thousand years before beans were utilized.

Regardless of the differences in the sequence of the establishment of the legume and cereal grain diet, it is remarkable that so many different societies would select the same two plant families from the existing arrays of botanical diversity in so many different regions.

Afterword

Predicting future patterns of legume consumption is less certain than reconstructing historical patterns for many reasons, among which are the influence of global economics and the diversity and regional particularity of human dietary culture. For a historical illustration of the latter, consider data gathered by Aykroyd and Doughty (1964) of the London School of Hygiene and Tropical Medicine. They reported legume consumption in the 1960s to be higher in the more prosperous northern region of Italy than in the less prosperous southern region. Similarly, in India, Japan, and Colombia legume consumption was higher among upper-income groups than among lower-income groups. Yet in Venezuela and the United States, legume consumption varied inversely with income.

Figures from the United Nations Food and Agriculture Organization (FAO) for India show a substantial decline in the supply (a rough approximation of consumption) of pulses per capita from a range of 17.2–23 kilograms (kg) per year in the early 1960s to 12.9–11.3 kg per year in the early 1990s. In Mexico the supply of dry beans declined from a range of 13.7–18.4 kg per year in the early 1960s to a range of 10.9–13.6 kg per year in the first five years of the 1990s. Similar data were obtained for most of the developing countries of Africa: the highest year of the 1990s is lower than the lowest year of the 1960s. These data are typical for developing countries dependent on a cereal grain and legume diet, and recent FAO data suggest that the decline in the supply of pulses or dry beans per capita per year has continued in many of the same developing countries.

There are a variety of political (interstate and civil wars), agricultural, economic, and climatic reasons for this decline. This downward trend, however, does not necessarily mean that the protein supply or protein quality for all population segments of any particular country has lessened, if there have been substitutes of animal for plant proteins. Because FAO reports are for countries as a whole, disproportionate changes in dietary patterns resulting from the disproportionate population growth of economic classes or religious-cultural population segments (especially the largely vegetarian Hindus of India) may not be apparent. However, we may still ask whether the downward trend in the supply of pulses per capita in developing countries and the upward trend in population mean that eventually the long-established, traditional cereal-legume diets are to be lost. Probably not, or not entirely, but the proportion of protein derived from pulses appears to be in steady decline.

Do these opposing trends suggest that the seed meal or other products of soybeans, which are higher yielding than other pulses, will replace or significantly supplement the indigenous pulses in diets of developing countries? There is no clear or consistent answer to this question, but as yet such a substitution does not seem broadly to be the case. Mexico, with a declining consumption of its traditional dry beans, has a minuscule (less than 0.0 kg per capita year per) supply of soybeans for food but an increasing consumption of meat, much of which is imported from the United States. A sample of several developing countries in Africa (Angola, Benin, Botswana) shows the annual consumption of soybeans to be less than 0.2 kg per capita per year. Where soy consumption is low it has not been part of the traditional diet. Soy consumption is highest in industrialized, technologically developed Japan and the Republic of Korea (supply per capita per year of 7.53 kg and 8.10 kg, respectively) because of its central role in the traditional diet of these countries.

What is the future of pulses as components of traditional diets in meeting the requirements of the human population, especially the poor? The answer depends on several factors. One set of factors lies in the fundamental biology of the legume plant and the ability of science and agronomy to alter the adaptability of the crop to marginal agricultural areas, to increase disease resistance, or to increase productivity of the plant while increasing or maintaining acceptable levels of protein percentage and quality. Other factors include the economics of protein supply and the competition for land with high-yielding strains of cereal grains. On the human side, dietary choices and, perhaps above all, the rate of human population growth will continue to affect the demand for pulses.

Note

1. YBP means "years before present time" and is used to indicate age in radiocarbon years. Present time is calendar year AD 1950. Since 1950, nuclear testing has added radioactive carbon to the atmosphere, which requires a correction in calculating radiocarbon data.

References

Anderson, E. N. 1988. *The Food of China.* New Haven, CT: Yale University Press.

Aykroyd, W. R., and J. Doughty. 1964. *Legumes in Human Nutrition.* Rome: Food and Agriculture Organization of the United Nations.

Benz, B. F. 2001. "Archaeological Evidence of Teosinte Domestication from Guilá Naquitz, Oaxaca." *Proceedings of the National Academy of Science* 98: 2104–6.

Blumler. M. A. 1991. "Modeling the Origin of Legume Domestication and Cultivation." *Economic Botany* 45: 243–50.

Darby, W. J., P. Ghalioungui, and L. Grivetti. 1977. *Food: The Gift of Osiris,* Vol. 2. London: Academic Press.

Duke, J. A. 1981. *Handbook of Legumes of World Economic Importance.* New York: Plenum.

Fagan, B. M. 1995. *People of the Earth,* 8th ed. New York: HarperCollins.

FAO (Food and Agriculture Organization of the United Nations). Rome. Statistics available on FAOSTAT at http://faostat.fao.org.

Gepts, P. A. 1988. "Phaseolin As an Evolutionary Marker." In P. A. Gepts, ed., *Genetic Resources of Phaseolus Beans,* 215–41. Dordrecht, Netherlands: Springer.

Hansen, J. 1992. "Franchthi Cave and the Beginnings of Agriculture in Greece and the Aegean." In *Préhistoire de L'agriculture: Nouvelles Approches Experimentales et Ethnographiques.* Monographie du CRA numéro 6.cd. Paris: CNRS.

Hawtin, G. C., K. B. Singh, and M. C. Saxena. 1980. "Some Recent Developments in the Understanding and Improvement of Cicer and Lens." In R. J. Summerfield and A. H. Bunting, eds., *Advances in Legume Science,* 613–23. Richmond, Surrey, UK: Royal Botanic Gardens, Kew.

Hedrick, U. P. 1919. *Sturtevant's Notes on Edible Plants.* New York Agricultural Experiment Station, 27th Annual Report, Vol. 2(2). Albany: New York State Department of Agriculture.

Herklots, G. A. C. 1972. *Vegetables in South-East Asia.* London: Allen & Unwin.

Isager, I., and J. E. Skydsgaard. 1992. *Ancient Greek Agriculture.* Routledge: New York.

Isely, D. 1982. "Leguminosae and *Homo sapiens.*" *Economic Botany* 36: 46–70.

Jain, H. K., and K. L. Mehra. 1980. "Evolution, Adaptation, Relationships, and Uses of the Species of *Vigna* Cultivated in India." In R. J. Summerfield and A. H. Bunting, eds., *Advances in Legume Science,* 459–68. Richmond, Surrey, UK: Royal Botanic Gardens, Kew.

Kahlheber, S. 1999. "Archaeobotanical Remains of Crops and Woody Plants from Medieval Saouga, Burkina Faso." In Marijke van der Veen, ed., *The Exploitation of Plant Resources in Ancient Africa,* 89–100. New York: Kluwer Academic.

Kaplan, L. 1970. "Plant Remains from the Blain Site." In Olaf H. Prufer and Orrin C. Shane III, eds., *Blain Village and the Fort Ancient Tradition in Ohio,* 227–31. Kent, OH: Kent State University Press.

Kaplan, L., and T. F. Lynch. 1999. "*Phaseolus* (Fabaceae) in Archaeology: AMS Radiocarbon Dates and Their Significance for Pre-Columbian Agriculture." *Economic Botany* 53: 261–72.

Kaplan, L., T. F. Lynch, and C. E. Smith Jr. 1973. "Early Cultivated Beans (*Phaseolus vulgaris*) from an Intermontane Peruvian Valley." *Science* 179: 76–77.

Kislev, M. E. 1985. "Early Neolithic Horsebean from Yiftah'el, Israel." *Science* 228: 319–20.

Ladizinsky, G. 1975. "On the Origin of the Broad Bean, *Vicia faba* L." *Israel Journal of Botany* 24: 80–88.

———. 1987. "Pulse Domestication before Cultivation." *Economic Botany* 41: 60–65.

Larco Hoyle, R. 1943. "La Escritura Mochica Sobre Pallares." *Revista Geográfica Americana* 20: 1–36. Buenos Aires.

Manniche, L. 1989. *An Ancient Egyptian Herbal.* Austin: University of Texas Press.

Pulsifer, D., ed. 1861. *Records of the Colony of New Plymouth in New England, 1623–1682,* Vol 1. Boston: Commonwealth of Massachusetts.

Purseglove, L. W. 1968. *Tropical Crops, Dicotyledons,* Vol. 1. New York: Wiley.

Simoons, F. J. 1991. *Food in China, a Cultural and Historical Inquiry.* Boca Raton, FL: CRC.

———. 1998. *Plants of Life, Plants of Death.* Madison: University of Wisconsin Press.

Simpson, B. B., and M. C. Ogorzaly. 1995. *Economic Botany: Plants in Our World.* New York: McGraw-Hill.

Singh, U., and B. Singh. 1992. "Tropical Grain Legumes As Important Human Foods." *Economic Botany* 46: 310–21.

Smartt, J. 1990. *Grain Legumes: Evolution and Genetic Resources.* Cambridge: Cambridge University Press.

Smith, B. D. 1997. "The Initial Domestication of *Cucurbita Pepo* in the Americas 10,000 Years Ago." *Science* 276: 932–34.

Sokolov, R. 1984. "Broad Bean Universe." *Natural History* 93(12) (December): 84–87.

Stahl, A. B. 1984. "Hominid Dietary Selection before Fire." *Current Anthropology* 25: 151–68.

Steele, W. M., and K. L. Mehra. 1980. "Structure, Evolution and Adaptation to Farming Systems and Environment in *Vigna.*" In R. J. Summerfield and A. H. Bunting, eds., *Advances in Legume Science,* 393–404. Richmond, Surrey, UK: Royal Botanic Gardens, Kew.

Zohary, D. 1989a. "Pulse Domestication and Cereal Domestication: How Different Are They?" *Economic Botany* 43: 31–34.

———. 1989b. "Domestication of the Southwest Asian Neolithic Crop Assemblage of Cereals, Pulses, and Flax: The Evidence from Living Plants." In D. R. Harris and G. C. Hillman, eds., *Foraging and Farming, the Evolution of Plant Exploitation,* 358–73. London: Unwin Hyman.

Zohary, D., and M. Hopf. 1988. *Domestication of Plants in the Old World,* Oxford: Oxford University Press.

———. 2000. *Domestication of Plants in the Old World,* 3rd ed. Oxford: Oxford University Press.

2

Early Uses of Soybean in Chinese History

H. T. HUANG

Ancient Records of Soybeans

The ancient character for *shu*, soybean, is found on four bronze vessels of the early Zhou period,[1] indicating that the plant was already of some importance by about 1000 BC.[2] This view is supported by the fact that soybean is mentioned in seven poems in the *Shijing* (*Book of Odes*), a collection of folk songs and ceremonial odes that dates from the eleventh to the seventh centuries BC.

Two of the poems are of particular interest to us. The first poem, Mao Heng 154,[3] *Qiyue* ("Seventh Month"), contains the lines

> In the sixth month we eat wild plums and grapes,
> In the seventh month we boil mallows and soybeans (*shu*). (sixth stanza, lines 1–2)

The quotation indicates that soybeans were boiled before they were eaten. In line 4 of the seventh stanza, we see the phrase "Paddy and hemp, soybean (*shu*) and wheat," which groups soybean with the cultivated grains—paddy rice, hemp seed, and wheat[4]—suggesting that soybean was itself a cultivated plant. The second poem is Mao Heng 186, *Baiju* ("White Colt"). It contains the lines

> Unsullied the white colt
> Eating the young shoots of my stackyard,[5] (first stanza, lines 1–2),

and the lines

> Unsullied the white colt
> Eating the soy leaves (*huo*) of my stackyard. (second stanza, lines 1–2)

The character *shu* (soybean) is not found in this poem. Instead, we see the character *huo,* which denotes specifically the soybean leaf. Thus, the lines taken together suggest that soy seedlings and leaves were grown as vegetables and that their value as animal feed was known.

Soybean was traditionally considered one of the staple grains of ancient China. Collectively the staple grains were known as *wugu* (five grains), a term that was first seen in the *Analects of Confucius, Lunyu,* of the fifth century BC (Legge 1861, 335). According to the *Zhouli* (*Rites of the Zhou*), a work based on material from the Warring States period (480 BC to 221 BC), five grains were cultivated in Yuzhou and Bingzhou, two of the nine provinces of the early Zhou Kingdom. The commentary by Zheng Xuan in the second century AD indicates that the five grains were panicum millet, setaria millet, rice, soybean, and wheat (see *Zhouli* 3rd C. BC, ch. 8 [Zhi Fang Shi], 344–45).[6] In the *Liji* (*The Record of Rites*), circa 50 BC, soybean was one of the five grains mentioned in the *Yueling* ("Monthly Ordinance") chapter (*Liji* 1st C. BC, ch. 6, 257, 272, 284–85, 296), the others being panicum millet, setaria millet, hemp, and wheat. In neither book is there any indication of how the soybean was cooked.

Cooking of Soybeans

Nevertheless, based on the way the other grains, such as millets and rice, were commonly treated, we may assume that soybeans were boiled and then steamed to give cooked granules or *dou fan.* The term *dou* had crept into the vocabulary as synonymous with *shu* by the time of the Warring States. In fact, the *Zanguoce* (*Records of the Warring States*), circa first century BC, tells us that in the Han state "the terrain is hilly and steep. Of the staple grains grown, the principal crop is soybean rather than wheat. What the people consume are mostly cooked soybean granules (*dou fan*) and soybean leaf soup (*huo geng*)" (*Zanguoce,* ch. 8, cited in Li Changnian 1958, 38).[7] The result of cooking soybeans in this way was not entirely satisfactory. For a long time cooked soybean was considered a coarse and inferior food. The *Xunzi* (*Book of Master Xun*), circa third century BC, compared millet and rice to the meat of livestock but soybean and soy leaf to bran and fermentation dregs (*Xunzi* 3rd C. BC, ch. 4, 58). In the famous "Contract between a Servant and His Master," a document dated at 59 BC, one of the hardships the employee was supposed to accept was "to eat only cooked soybean (*fan dou*), and drink only water." Upon hearing this and other indignities that were to be inflicted on him under the terms of the contract, the poor man broke down and wept (*Tongyue* 59 BC, 233).

Similarly, wheat did not give rise to a palatable *mai fan* when cooked in this way. Thus, millets and rice were regarded as superior grains, and wheat and soybean were regarded as inferior grains. This attitude is summed up in a statement in the *Lunheng* (*Discourse Weighed in the Balance*), circa AD 83: "The flavor of rice and the millets is sweet and appealing. Soybean and wheat are, however, coarse. Yet they can also assuage hunger. Those who eat soybean and wheat grumble only that they are coarse and lacking in sweetness. They never complain that their stomachs remain empty and hungry" (Wang Chong AD 82, ch. 8, 86). It was understood that soybean and wheat were eaten in the form of cooked granules, that is as *dou fan* and *mai fan*.

Another reason that soybean was held in low esteem by the ancient Chinese was that the prolonged eating of it as a cooked grain could be hazardous to one's health. The *Yangsheng lun* (*Discourse on Nurturing Life*) of Xi Kang, circa AD 260, says that "ingestion of soybean makes one feel heavy" (*douling renzhong*) (cited in Li Changnian 1958, 61). This may be interpreted to mean that soybean made one feel permanently bloated. The same sentiment is expressed in the *Bowuzhi* (*Record of the Investigation of Things*) by Zhang Hua, circa AD 290: "after eating soybeans for three years, the abdomen would feel heavy [bloated]. One's movement would be impaired" (Zhang Hua AD 290, ch. 4, 6b).

Soybean, however, could be made more palatable by prolonged cooking in water to give a *dou zhou*, a soy congee or gruel. The product was presumably extremely thin and smooth, since in the pre-Han literature the ingestion of *douzhou* is depicted as *chuo shu*, or sipping soybean. The *Liji* (*Record of Rites*) talks about *chuoshu yinshui*, sipping soybean and drinking water (*Liji* 1st C. BC, ch. 4, 179). The same expression is seen in the *Xunzi* (3rd C. BC, ch. 17, 336) and the *Yantie lun* (*Discourse on Salt and Iron*) (Huan Kuan 1st C. BC, ch. 6, segment 25, 89). *Chuo* is an unusual word in the food lexicon; it is halfway between *eat* and *drink*. But to make soybean congee to this degree of consistency was an onerous and time-consuming task. This fact was recorded in the *History of the Jin Dynasty* (AD 265 to AD 420) in the "Biography of Shi Chong," who lamented that soybean was extremely difficult to cook (*dou zhinan zhu*) (cited in Li Changnian 1958, 64).

Soybean As a Food Resource

In view of these difficulties, one may wonder how the soybean ever attained the status of one of the five staple grains of the realm. To the ancient Chinese, however, "the chief virtue of the soybean was that it produced good crops even on poor land, that it did not deplete the soil, and that it guaranteed good yields even in poor years, so that it made a useful famine crop" (Bray 1984, 514). Actually, apart from the immature beans, which can be eaten directly as a vegetable, the raw, mature beans as harvested and stored suffer from three serious defects when cooked as food.[8] These are:

1. The soy proteins are difficult to digest. The beans contain proteins, such as trypsin inhibitor, that suppress the action of proteases in the human digestive system. Unless they are thoroughly cooked to inactivate the inhibitors, the other proteins would be poorly digested and would give rise to growth inhibition and pancreatic hypertrophy.
2. The carbohydrate component contains raffinose and stachyose, two alpha-galactosides that are not hydrolyzed by human digestive enzymes. They pass into the colon, where they are metabolized by anaerobic bacteria, and lead to the generation of gas and flatulence.
3. The beans produce an unpleasant beany flavor when processed due to the oxidation of polyunsaturated oils by lipoxidase. In the intact bean the enzyme is separated from its substrate, but the two can easily come into contact when the structure of the bean is damaged.

For these reasons soybean was difficult to cook by boiling and steaming without prior processing. To circumvent these difficulties, the ancient Chinese expended a great deal of effort to find ways of converting soybeans into processed foods that are wholesome, attractive, easily digestible, and nutritious.

Fermentation

The first and perhaps earliest approach the ancient Chinese employed was fermentation, that is, to expose cooked beans to microbial action. This was the technology developed to convert cooked rice, millets, or wheat to a fungal culture known as *qu,* which had been used successfully for turning grains into alcoholic drinks. The first product from this approach was *shi* (also pronounced *chi*), a fermented soy relish. It is among the foods stored in pottery jars and listed in bamboo slips discovered at Han Tomb No. 1

at Mawangdui (Hunansheng Bowuguan 1973, 1:127).[9] The earliest reference to *shi* is found in the *Chuci* (*Songs of the Chu Kingdom*), third century BC, where it is called *daku* (great bitterness) (Qu Yuan et al. 3rd C. BC, 161).[10] In spite of this connotation, *shi*, presumably in an improved nonbitter form, was quickly accepted as a supplemental food. By the latter part of the Earlier Han period, *shi* had become a major commodity in the economy of the realm. The "Economic Affairs" chapter (*Huozhi Liezhuan*) of the *Shiji*, or *Records of the Historian*, circa 90 BC, refers to "thousand jars of saccharifying mold ferment and salty *shi*" as articles of commerce (Sima Qian and Sima Tan 90 BC, ch. 129, 3274).[11] The *History of the Earlier Han Dynasty* (*Qian Hanshu*), circa AD 100, tells us that two of the seven wealthiest merchants of the realm had made their fortunes by trading in *shi* (Ban Gu and Ban Zhao AD 100, ch. 61, 3694).

The *Shiming* (*Expositor of Names*), a second-century AD work, defines *shi* as something delectable and highly desirable (Liu Xi 2nd C. AD, ch. 13). The *Shuowen Jiezi* (*Analytical Dictionary of Characters*), AD 121, says that *shi* is prepared by incubating soybean with salt (Xu Shen AD 121, 149). Neither statement tells us how *shi* was actually made. For that information we have to rely on a later work, the *Qimin Yaoshu* (*Important Arts for the People's Welfare*), AD 544, that describes the preparation of *shi* as a two-step process:

1. Aerobic Mold Growth. The soybeans were boiled, cooled, and exposed to air until they were covered with a luxuriant growth of mold myceliae.
2. Anaerobic Digestion. The wet molded beans were salted and incubated anaerobically. In time, the beans would be partially digested by the mold enzymes present to give *shi*.[12] (Jia Sixie AD 544, ch. 72)

Indications are that *shi* (fermented soy relish) was already considered a culinary necessity of daily living during the Earlier Han period (202 BC to AD 9). For example, when Liu An, the prince of Huainan, was exiled for fomenting rebellion (in 173 BC) against his brother the Han emperor Wendi, the prince and his retinue were nevertheless provided with such necessities of life as "firewood, rice, salt, *shi* and cooking utensils" (Sima Qian and Sima Tan 90 BC, ch. 118, 3079). *Shi* was also used as a drug. It is listed as a medication in the *Wupu Bencao* (*Wu's Pharmaceutical Natural History*), circa AD 240, where it is said to benefit a person's *qi* (Wu Pu AD 240, 84).[13]

In the *shi* process, very little water was present during the anaerobic digestion (step 2). The soybean components were only partially digested. The structure and shape of the soybean remained intact. If the digestion had been allowed to proceed further through the addition of more water to the system, the bean would have disintegrated, and the product would have become a paste known as *jiang*, which was the principal condiment of China from the Han until the middle of the Song dynasty (ca. 200 BC to AD 1100). In antiquity, *jiang* used to denote a savory paste prepared from meat or fish such as *yujiang* and *roujiang*. But by the start of the Han dynasty, the word *jiang* had undergone a subtle change in meaning. It was increasingly used to denote the fermented paste obtained from soybeans. Since then, unless it was stated otherwise, *jiang* was to mean *doujiang*, just as the character *dou* was to mean soybean.

The earliest literary reference to *jiang* as a fermented soy paste is found in the *Jijiupian* (*The Handy Primer*), circa 40 BC. It lists "*Wuyi yan shi xi zuo jiang*" (fetid elm seed, salty fermented soy relish, pickles, vinegar, and *jiang*) as articles of food (Shi You 40 BC, 31, cited in Li Changnian 1958, 61). The commentary says that soybean and wheat flour are mixed to produce *jiang*. This is a sketchy but reasonable statement of how *jiang* was made. In the process for making *shi*, the addition of wheat flour to the boiled beans would enhance mold growth in step 1 and hence enhance the enzyme activity available for digestion in step 2. Thus, the process for making *jiang* is simply the process for making *shi* in which flour is mixed with soybean and more water is provided in the digestion step.

In the *Wushier Bingfang* (*Prescriptions for Fifty-two Ailments*), circa 200 BC, there is a recipe in which dregs from the *shujiang* were used as a salve to treat hemorrhoids (recipe 143, translated in Harper 1982, 412). The *Lunheng* (*Discourse Weighed in the Balance*) states that there is a taboo against making *doujiang* when thunder is heard, that is, after the arrival of spring rains (Wang Chong AD 82, ch. 23, 226). The preferred time for making *jiang* is the first month to give farmers employment when it is too cold to work in the field. The *Simin Yueling* (*Ordinances for the Four Peoples*), circa AD 160, also advises the making of fermented soy paste from soybean or soy groats in the first month (Cui Shi AD 160, 1st month).[14] These references indicate that *jiang* was an established article of food by the middle of the Han dynasty.

Sprouting

The second approach that the ancient Chinese used to process soybeans was sprouting. This was the technology that had been applied successfully to grains to produce *nie* (malted grain), an agent for making malt sugar as well as alcoholic drinks. The earliest reference to soybean sprout is found in the *Shennong Bencaojing* (*The Pharmacopoeia of the Heavenly Husbandman*), a work based on Zhou and Chin material but probably compiled toward the end of the Han dynasty, circa AD 200. The item on sprouted soybean is as follows: "*Dadou huangjuan* (Yellow curls from the Soybean). The flavor is sweet and mild. It is used to treat numbness in the joints, muscle and knee" (*Shennong Bencaojing* AD 200, 337).

The *Wupu Bencao* (*Wu's Pharmaceutical Natural History*), circa AD 240, explains that *dadou huangjuan* was simply the young sprout obtained when soybean was allowed to germinate (Wu Pu AD 240, 83). The product was probably first made in the early years of the Han dynasty. It was used mainly as a drug and did not become popular as a food until the Song dynasty (AD 960 to 1279).[15]

Grinding

The third approach that the Chinese used to process soybeans began with grinding the beans on a rotary mill. We have seen that both wheat and soybean were considered as coarse grains in antiquity because they did not cook well as *fan*. But the introduction of the stone rotary mill during the Warring States period (480 BC to 221 BC) quickly changed the culinary status of wheat. When wheat was ground in the mill, it gave rise to wheat flour (*mian*), a food resource that could be turned into a wonderful variety of delicious breads and noodles collectively known as *bing* (Huang 2000, 462–68). This development, which took place during the Han dynasty (206 BC to AD 220), transformed wheat from an inferior grain into a highly desirable superior grain. The success of wheat as a primary crop eventually divided China into two dietary zones: the south, where the primary food is cooked rice (i.e., *lishi*, or granule food), and the north, where the primary food is prepared from wheat flour (i.e., *mianshi*, or flour food).

Once the grinding of wheat in the rotary mill had become commonplace, it was only a matter of time before someone applied the same technology to soybean. Unfortunately in this case the product turned out to be flakes rather than flour.[16] But the matter did not end there. It stands to reason that someone would have tried to cook the flakes in water, perhaps to make soybean congee. He or she would have noticed that when the milled flakes were mixed with water, part of the bean solids would merge into the liquid to give a milky emulsion. This would have led the observer to grind the beans in the presence of water, and voilà, soymilk was born.

The raw milk, however, would still suffer from the same defects associated with the raw bean. It would still contain protease inhibitors, flatus-causing oligosaccharides, and lipoxidase. For this reason, I think, soymilk was not immediately consumed as a food and did not become a part of the Chinese diet until the eighteenth or nineteenth century, when it was discovered that prolonged heating of the milk made it palatable and easily digestible.

Soymilk was probably invented during the earlier Han dynasty (202 BC to AD 9). It is likely that manipulation of the raw soymilk produced a bean curd prototype shortly thereafter. This may be why legend has it that the Liu An invented *doufu* (bean curd) during the earlier Han dynasty. The key steps in the *doufu* process are depicted in a mural in a later Han tomb in Mixian, Henan Province (Henan Wenwu Yanjiusuo 1993, 128, 132–33, plate 34).[17] However, one key step, heating of the raw milk, is missing from the mural. The process as shown in the mural is therefore incomplete. The process was not perfected until the late Tang dynasty (AD 618 to 906), when *doufu* became a commercial product.[18] Today, as it gains acceptance among modern consumers who are increasingly aware of the healthful effect of soy proteins, *doufu* has become one of the most significant gifts to the world from the Chinese food system (see the essay by Tan in this volume).

Summary

From the early Zhou dynasty to the end of the Han dynasty (1000 BC to AD 220), soybean was first cooked as a grain to make *fan* (cooked granules) and *zhou* (congee or gruel). The result was not entirely satisfactory, and the Chinese investigated other ways of turning the soybean into palatable and nutritious foods.

The first approach they used was fermentation, which gave them *shi* (fermented soy relish) followed by *jiang* (fermented soy paste). Both products were quickly accepted as desirable articles of food. The second approach was to sprout the beans. The sprouted bean found immediate use as a medication, but it did not become popular as a food until the Song dynasty (AD 960 to 1279). The third approach was to grind the beans in water to give a soymilk. A prototype bean curd or *doufu* was probably made from the milk during the Han dynasty, but the early process was unreliable. Further developments eventually led to the making of *doufu* as a commercial product at the end of the Tang dynasty (AD 900 to 1000) and beyond.

Notes

1. Hu Daojing (1963) points out that the three elongated dots at the lower half of the character for *shu* pictographically represent the root's bulging nodules caused by *Bradyrhizobia.*

2. Although in dealing with Chinese texts the dating notation adopted in Joseph Needham's *Science and Civilisation in China*—in which BC years are preceded by a minus sign (–) and AD years by a plus sign (+)—makes good sense, this article uses the conventional Western notations for the sake of consistency within this volume.

3. The numbering follows the order of the poems collated by Mao Heng, which is the traditional form of the *Shijing* handed down to posterity. For text and translation of the *Shijing,* see Karlgren (1974); for translation only, see Waley (1937). The lines cited in the text are translations by Waley with minor modifications by the author.

4. In this line "paddy rice" is a translation of *he,* a word denoting cereals or grains in general. Since hemp, millets, soybean, and wheat have been mentioned earlier in the poem, it would make sense to render *he* as "paddy rice."

5. Here "stackyard" is a translation of *chang,* a word denoting a piece of flat level ground used for storing stalks of grain. When not in use as a stackyard, it could be used as a vegetable garden.

6. For a discussion of this issue, see Huang (2000, 19–22).

7. A similar passage occurs in the *Shiji* (*Records of the Historian*), ch. 70, Biography No. 10 of Zhang Yi, cited in Li Changnian (1958, 48), in which cooked soybean granule is written as *fan shu.*

8. See Huang (2000, 293) for further details.

9. See also Huang (2000, 336).

10. Presumably bitter peptides were produced in the hydrolysis of the proteins during the early process of making *shi.* These peptides were avoided when the process was refined.

11. For further discussion, see Huang (2000, 336).

12. See translation of recipes in Huang (2000, 338–40).

13. In Chinese medicine *qi* is the motive force that animates life. It is immaterial yet essential to all human functions.

14. Cf. Huang (2000, 347).

15. See Huang (2000, 296–98) for further information on the history of bean sprouts.

16. When raw soybean is ground, the cell structure is ruptured. Yet because of its high fat content, the matrix of protein, fat, and carbohydrate can still stick together to give a viscous mess. The result is a spongy flake.

17. See also Huang (2000, 305–14, 331–33).

18. For discussion on the origin and history of *doufu,* see Huang (2000, 299–333).

References

MODERN PUBLICATIONS

Bray, Francesca. 1984. *Science and Civilisation in China,* Vol. 6, Pt. 2, *Agriculture.* Cambridge: Cambridge University Press.

Harper, Donald. 1982. *Wushier Bingfang, Translation and Prolegomena.* Ann Arbor, MI: University Microfilms International.

Henan Wenwu Yanjiusuo [Henan Provincial Institute of Archaeology]. 1993. *Mixian Dahuting Hanmu* [*Han Tombs at Dahuting, Mixian, Henan*]. Beijing: Wenwu.

Hsu Cho-yun. 1980. *Han Agriculture.* Seattle: University of Washington Press.

Hu Daojing. 1963. "Shishupian" ["Discourse on the Character *Shu* (Soybean)"]. *Zhonghua Wenshi Luncun* [*Essays on Chinese Literature and History,* a journal from Classics Press in Shanghai] 3: 111–19.

Huang, H. T. 2000. *Science and Civilisation in China,* Vol. 6, Pt. 5, *Fermentations and Food Science.* Cambridge: Cambridge University Press.

Hunansheng Bowuguan [Hunan Provincial Museum]. 1973. *Han Tomb No. 1 at Mawangdui, near Changsha,* Pt. 1. Beijing: Wenwu.

Karlgren, Bernhard, trans. 1974. *The Book of Odes, Text, Transcription and Translation.* Stockholm: Museum of Far Eastern Antiquities.

Legge, James, trans. 1861. *Confucian Analects, the Great Learning and the Doctrine of the Mean.* Hong Kong and London: Trubner.

Li Changnian, ed. 1958. *Doulei Shangpian* [Legumes, Pt. 1]. Chinese Agricultural Heritage Series, No. 4. Beijing: Zhonghua.

Needham, Joseph. 1954. *Science and Civilisation in China,* Vol. 1. Cambridge: Cambridge University Press.

Waley, Arthur, trans. 1937. *The Book of Songs* [Translation of the *Shijing*]. London: Allen and Unwin.

CHINESE CLASSICS

Ban Gu and Ban Zhao. Circa AD 100. *Qian Hanshu* [*The History of the Earlier Han Dynasty*]. Reprinted in 1962. Beijing: Zhonghua.

Confucius and Disciples. 5th C. BC. *Lunyu* [*Confucian Analects*]. Translated by James Legge. 1971 [1861]. Mineola, NY: Dover.

Cui Shi. Circa AD 160. *Simin Yueling* [*Ordinances for the Four Peoples*]. Translated in Hsu Cho-yun, *Han Agriculture,* 215–28.

Fang Qiao et al. Circa 646. *Jinshu* [*History of the Jin Dynasty*]. Cited in Li Changnian, *Doulei Shangpian,* 64.

Huan Kuan. 1st century BC. *Yantie Lun* [*Discourse on Salt and Iron*]. Reprinted 1990. Shanghai: Classics Press.

Jia Sixie. AD 544. *Qimin Yaoshu* [*Important Arts for the People's Welfare*]. Edited by Miao Qiyu. 1982. Beijing: Agricultural Press.

Liji [*Record of Rites*]. 1st century BC. In *Liji Jinzhu Jinxi,* edited by Wang Mengou. Taipei: Commercial Press, 1984.

Liu Xi. 2nd C. AD. *Shiming* [*Expositor of Names*]. In *Hanwei Congshu.* Cited in Li Changnian, *Doulei Shangpian,* 57.

Qu Yuan et al. 3rd C. BC. *Chuci* [*Elegies of the Chu State*]. Rendered in modern Chinese by Fu Xiren. Taipei: Sanmin, 1976.

Shennong Bencaojing [*The Pharmacopoeia of the Heavenly Husbandman*]. Circa AD 200. Compilers unknown. Edited by Cao Yuanyu. Shanghai: S&T Press, 1987.

Shi You. Circa 40 BC. *Jijiupian* [*The Handy Primer*]. Cited in Li Changnian, *Doulei Shangpian,* 51.

Sima Qian and Sima Tan. Circa 90 BC. *Shiji* [*Records of the Historian*]. Reprinted in 1959. Beijing: Zhonghua.

Tongyue [Contract with a Servant]. 59 BC. Reproduced in many editions. Translated in Hsu Cho-yun, *Han Agriculture,* 231–34.

Wang Chong. AD 82. *Lunheng* [*Discourses Weighed in the Balance*]. Reprinted in 1990. Shanghai: Classics Press.

Wu Pu. Circa AD 240. *Wupu Bencao* [*Wu's Pharmaceutical Natural History*]. Edited by Shang Zhijun. Beijing: Renmin Weisheng, 1987.

Wushier Bingfang [*Prescriptions for Fifty-two Ailments*]. Circa 200 BC. Compiler unknown, discovered at Han tomb No. 3 at Mawangdui. Translated by Donald Harper.

Xi Kang. Circa AD 260. *Yangsheng Lun* [*Discourse on Nurturing Life*]. Cited in Li Changnian, *Doulei Shangpian,* 61.

Xunzi [*The Book of Master Xun*]. 3rd C. BC. Edited by Xiong Gongzhe. Taipei: Commercial Press, 1984.

Xu Shen. AD 121. *Shuowen Jiezi* [*Analytical Dictionary of Characters*]. Reprinted in 1963. Beijing: Zhonghua.

Zanguoce [*Record of the Warring States*]. 3rd C. BC. Author unknown. Cited in Li Changnian, *Doulei Shangpian,* 3.

Zhang Hua. Circa AD 290. *Bowuzhi* [*Record of the Investigation of Things*]. Cited in Li Changnian, *Doulei Shangpian,* 62.

Zhouli [*Rites of the Zhou*]. Circa 3rd C. BC. Author unknown. Edited by Lin Yin in *Zhouli Jinzhu Jinxi.* Beijing: Shumu Wenxian, 1985.

3

Fermented Beans and Western Taste

SIDNEY W. MINTZ

Introduction

The complex organic process known to the layperson as fermentation has both historical and culinary implications for the intersection of several categories of living things.[1] By this means certain species within a broad grouping or taxon of plant life become edible or more suitable for human consumption. For the nonscientist who knows that leavened bread, wine, vinegar, pickles, cheeses, and other such foods are fermented, fermentation is a process that changes the chemistry and also the taste of the substance that is acted upon. He or she may also know that fermentation is brought about by living microorganisms.[2]

People who are used to eating a fermented food and like its taste, odor, and texture obviously experience no discomfort when eating it. However, at times the difference between being fermented and being spoiled may be the mote in the viewer's eye (or on the taster's tongue, to mix metaphors). Fermented bean curd is a good example, but an equally good one is Roquefort cheese. Yet which is fermented and which is rotten may depend on whether a person has been raised to eat one or the other. Both are considered delicious by some people but spoiled, inedible, or worse by others. Hence, these two foods illuminate the power of culture and social learning to shape perception.

The deliberate application of fermentation is a fine example of human inventive genius. Equally and uniquely human is the operation of culturally conventionalized taste patterns, which serve to set sharply apart what is appetizing, mouth-watering, or finger-lickin' good from what is putrid or disgusting. Globally, it appears that human beings willingly eat just about everything that will not kill them and—it turns out—many things that will. But for any particular food, only some human beings do so readily. People must learn to eat most of the things they come to like most. This cultural patterning is why (at least for the anthropologist) not only legumes such as fermented bean curd but also products such as Roquefort cheese are all related to the theme of this essay.

The plants with which we are concerned fall solely within the botanical family of legumes (*Fabaceae* or *Leguminosae*), as described by Kaplan in the opening contribution to this volume. One of the chief families within the plant kingdom that provide human food, the *Fabaceae* include the tamarind (*Tamarindus indica*), carob or St. John's bread (*Ceratonia siliqua*), lentils, vetches, the yam bean or jícama (*Pachyrrhizus erosus, P. Tuberosus*), many other species of beans and peas (e.g., the genus *Phaseolus*, genus *Vigna*), and numerous useful forage plants, such as alfalfa, as well as plants having known medical uses.

Some species of *Fabaceae* have contributed for millennia to the nutrition of our species.[3] But beans in particular stand out because they are such a common human food, and among the beans the soybean is of course of special importance here. Beans have a reputation, not entirely deserved, for their capacity to produce flatulence, to cause illness, and in some rare cases even to kill. The soybean is particularly indigestible; it contains no starch, only peculiar oligopolysaccharides that the human gut cannot digest. Even so, humans learned millennia ago that the chemistry of soybeans and other legumes could be transformed by fermentation.

The first deliberate experiments with fermentation may have been undertaken to make foods that were poisonous (or potentially so) into edible foods by neutralizing the toxins they contain or by converting them into different forms.[4] We know that many fermented foods may be safely eaten that, in their original state, were toxic or highly indigestible. In some cases the greater preservability or shelf life of the fermented substance may have been an unexpected beneficial accompaniment to the fermentation itself.[5] With some fermented foods, however, preservability was probably the aim of the fermentation, as in the case of at least some dairy foods. Fermentation also often adds to the nutritive value and the sensory (tactile, gustatory, olfactory) attractiveness of the edible product.[6]

The global distribution of fermentation practices in the production of human foods makes plain that it is an ancient and basic building block for the diets of our species. Campbell-Platt (2003) suggests that something like one-third of all of the food eaten on earth today has been treated by some kind of fermentation. The number of foods and drinks that it has helped to process (and thereby to define as edible) is staggering. Among them are meat, fish, cereals, rhizomes such as potatoes and taro, fresh vegetables, dairy products, alcoholic beverages, and legumes. Indeed, it is difficult to think of substances that have not been subjected to fermentation for food-related purposes. Fermentation is so vital in the evolution of human diet that it merits detailed documentation in all its cultural and biochemical variety, particularly as the energy efficiency with which foods are produced becomes an ever more important factor in global nutritional security.[7]

Using fermentation to modify foods beneficially was probably invented independently many times. It would be difficult to document the use of fermentation before the invention of agriculture and the domestication of animals, but some authorities (cf., for example, Aaronson 2000, 314; Miller and Wetterstrom 2000, 1225–26) wonder whether its use may have eased the transition from hunting and gathering to agriculture. Surely it was mastered (perhaps later than other means of preservation, such as sun-drying and salting) once sedentary populations, living primarily by farming, arose. Evidence of fermented beverage making in China has been dated by McGovern et al. (2004) to "the seventh millennium before Christ" and for Iran to circa 6000 BC.[8] Ancient food fermentation in other regions has also been documented (see, for example, Miller and Wetterstrom 2000; Sabban 2000).

Different foods benefit from one rather than another fermentation process and from the biochemical actions of different microorganisms. For the processing of some products, two different fermentations are better than one. As knowledge grew, people exercised more care in isolating and then introducing living organisms that could achieve the results they desired more swiftly or efficiently. They learned eventually to develop so-called single-activity enzymes from fungi, using these for some fermentations (Royse 2003, 2:84). The ferment that was eventually developed for processing soybeans no doubt grew out of earlier processes developed for fermenting cereals (Huang 2000, 154–55, 335).[9] If that predecessor did play a role in the fermentation of soybeans (as Huang proposes and as seems probable), it would have been after their domestication, circa 1000 BC.[10]

Soybeans provide the best example—and perhaps the best clue—as to why world legume history has often involved fermentation processing.

"The soybean is protected from pests by a number of chemicals that range from unpleasant to fairly poisonous, and is thus more or less inedible when raw.[11] Nor is it good food if roasted or otherwise cooked in high, dry heat, for the proteins and other compounds bind into indigestible complexes" (Anderson 1988, 122–23).[12]

In fact, for at least some centuries young soybeans have been quite edible nonetheless. But its chemical composition probably does explain why the domesticated soybean was not a highly desired food in ancient China. Like Anderson, Huang points out that the soybean had some serious drawbacks as a regular food, due both to some of the proteins and indigestible carbohydrate elements it contains and to its beany flavor (see Huang, this volume, and Huang 2000). But soy was nonetheless important to Chinese agriculture because it produced well in poor soil without further degrading it and was a vital fallback food in times of famine.

Although soybeans look like the legume most improved as human food by fermentation, the other main fermented legumes are all beans, too: black gram, Bengal gram, and mung beans (Reddy, Pierson, and Salunkhe 1986, 1). One other commonly fermented legume is the peanut or groundnut, *Arachis hypogaea*. But among these, only the soybean is subjected to substantial fermentation processing. The nonsoybean cases of fermented beans may be evidence of the borrowing of one part of the fermentation process to deal with challenges similar to, but rather less serious than, those that the soybean posed.[13]

The discussion of fermented legumes that follows is divided into three parts: (1) the distribution of fermented legumes in the indigenous systems of those who use them today, that is, the roles they play in local food systems; (2) hypotheses about the near-total absence of fermented legumes in Western cuisines and food traditions;[14] and (3) the possible future for fermented legumes in Western cuisines.

The Distribution of Fermented Legumes in Local Food Systems

Probably the most important fermented legume foods in the world, in terms of their roles in particular cuisines, are soy sauce (Chinese *jiang you*, Japanese shoyu) in China, Japan, Korea and elsewhere; miso and *natto* in Japan; *tempe* (cake made from boiled soybeans, also known as *tempeh*) and *oncom* (cake made from pressed peanuts or soy pulp) in Indonesia; *jiang* (*chiang*) and *shi* (*shih*) in China; and perhaps *papads* and *idli* in India. Probably only *tempe* is important enough in main courses to be considered a basic ingredient. (On fermented legumes in Africa, see the article by Osborn in this volume.)[15]

So commonplace that it sometimes fails to receive the attention it definitely deserves, soy sauce is the most widespread fermented legume product on earth. It has a complex history (Huang 2000, 358–74) and entered into European culinary practice in the seventeenth century. But because soy sauce and its uses are well known in the West, I will not deal with it at length here.

Far less well known in the West, miso is a crucially important soy flavoring in Japanese cuisine, the more fundamental of its two grand soup categories. Elizabeth Andoh has described the place of miso in Japanese cooking: "Unless it is specified that the soup is not miso soup, it's presumed that it is. In the context of a more elaborate meal, this would be the final course. [Misoshiru] is the most common, the default mode, of serving miso, and it also helps to define a Japanese meal" (Andoh, in Grodinsky 2000, 41). Andoh likens regional differences among misos to those that Europeans invoke when dealing with cheeses or wines.[16]

Miso's development as a flavor and color source is a good illustration of the way a culinary culture can magnify small differences within a narrow range in one sphere of life, thereby making such differences culturally conventional. Superficially similar to the way Americans mark differences among beers, say, or Frenchmen among breads, the Japanese subdivided miso into many distinguishable marked categories. The differences among them may seem trivial or too small to be registered sensorially by the outsider, but not so to the native.[17] Miso is used above all as a basis for soup, but it is also important in flavoring many other foods, and the range of miso variation, although perceived as extremely narrow by non-Japanese, is importantly broad from the perspective of Japanese culinary culture. In spite of Andoh's persuasive descriptions, however, and even though miso soup is now globally commonplace, it is unlikely that its culturally specific variety will ever penetrate Western cuisines in force because the perceived differences for non-Japanese are too small.[18] Although the use of miso as a flavoring for roasting food is now fashionable, the differences among misos have not registered among Western diners, or at least not yet.

Natto is even less likely to become commonplace outside Japan. It is composed of soybeans, briefly fermented with *Bacillus natto,* and served either in miso soup, on top of rice, or in *aemono* (salad). Although Hosking (1996) speaks warmly of *natto,* its texture and taste often meet with dislike among foreigners. This is reminiscent of the first reactions of some eaters to such foods as okra, where differences in appearance, texture, and viscosity may block out any appreciation of the substance's taste as such.

Tempe and *oncom* receive thorough treatment in Sidharta's essay in this volume and need not be discussed at any length here. *Tempe* is of great importance in Indonesian cuisine, both as a versatile ingredient that can be imaginatively flavored and as a highly nutritional source of protein and vegetable oils. Of all fermented legume products, it probably comes closest to what Westerners might call a main dish or main dish ingredient. It is more than a flavoring, although it is usually eaten as a side dish or mixed with other foods. *Oncom* is more clearly defined as a snack food; it is made of fermented pressed peanut cake or soy pulp, at times processed with cassava meal or tapioca, served boiled with other ingredients, or deep-fried. In Indonesia its consumption is outweighed by that of *tempe*.

Chinese *jiang* (*chiang*) and *shih* (*shi*) are ancestral to miso and to *natto*. *Jiang*, which is a paste, is very important in China, but also—under different names—in Korea, Indonesia, and the Philippines (Ang, Liu, and Huang 1999, 173–74). It serves as an all-purpose flavoring and sauce ingredient. *Shih* (fermented soybeans) are also used in Chinese cuisine, although they are of less importance than *jiang*.[19]

Finally, two quite different Indian foods based on fermented legumes, *papads* and *idli*, bear mention. Lovers of Indian food may have eaten *papadams*, which are similar to *papads* (except that they expand rapidly when deep-fried) (Ebine 1986). Both breads are made from the flour of *Vigna mungo* (black gram bean), which is slightly fermented before cooking. These breadstuffs or pancakes are eaten with regular meals. *Idli* is also made from black gram flour. It is primarily (but not only) a breakfast food.[20] Some cereal flour (wheat or maize, for example) or flour from another legume may be added to the bean flour used for *papads* or *idli*, but both are based on fermented legumes.[21]

The Absence of Fermented Legumes from Western Food History

The near-total absence of fermented legumes from Western food systems strikes me as curious, given both the abundance of domesticated legumes and the rich tradition of fermentation.[22] A large number of legumes figure in Western cuisines today, including peanuts, lentils, and a great many beans and peas, such as chickpeas, black-eyed peas, lima beans, string beans, and frijoles,[23] and knowledge of fermentation is ancient in Western food processing, whether of cereals, vegetables, meat or dairy products, or wine and beer. When we recall General Charles de Gaulle's complaint about ruling a country with 125 named cheeses, the Scottish liking for variety in single-malt scotches, or the rather remarkable history of European vegetable pickles and pickled meats, then the lack of fermented legumes in Western culinary traditions seems slightly puzzling at least.

For whatever reasons, legumes and fermentation were apparently not conjoined early in the West, and they have not been brought together in practice. With the exception of soy sauce, which was of course a borrowed food, I have not been able to identify any fermented legume product in any Western cooking tradition.[24] In a volume devoted in its entirety to fermented legumes (Reddy, Pierson, and Salunkhe 1986), the contributors review and describe such local specialties as *tempe* (*tempeh*) in Indonesia, *idli* in India, and miso in Japan, but the book is primarily about foods from the non-Western world. Hesseltine and Wang (1986, 326–35), in their *Indigenous Fermented Food of Non-Western Origin,* list nine and one-half pages of named fermented legume products (see also Aaronson 2000). Although these authors do not say as much, the only fermented legume food widely used and known in the West remains soy sauce.[25]

We might begin to think through the difference by noting that the histories of fermentation in these two grand areas have been significantly different. Cereal fermentation has long been typical of both East and West. But in an earlier period the East fermented legumes as well as cereals, and the West did not. That distinction is still largely true. Why should the West have ignored or bypassed legume fermentation? The best student of food fermentation in Asia tackles the question by formulating a persuasive hypothesis, which may help to explain the origins of fermented legumes in China. Reflecting on the uniqueness of what he calls the "mould ferment" to the Far East as early as the Neolithic, he writes:

> It seems to us that the discovery of the mould ferment (chhü or chiu yao) in the Neolithic period is the result of the happy conjunction of three factors, firstly, the nature of the ancient cereals cultivated by the Chinese, that is, rice and millets, secondly, the development of steaming as a preferred method for cooking such cereals, and thirdly, the kinds of fungal spores that were present in the environment. . . .
>
> As far as we know, the convergence of these distinctive factors occurred only in China, and in no other civilisation in the ancient world. This explains why the mould ferment was never developed in the early civilisations of the West. (H. T. Huang 2000, 592–93)

Of course, Huang is talking here about a starter based on the fermentation of cereals, not legumes. However, he goes on to speculate that the knowledge gathered in the creation of *chhü* led to insights about the phenomenon of fermentation as a whole, which could later be applied to other foods. "Although the mould ferment was developed originally for making wine, further exploitation of its activities soon paved the way to the production of an array of fermented foods which have helped to shape the character and flavour of the Chinese diet and cuisine. Many of these are still familiar components of the dietary system today. . . . [This involves] processes that do not currently utilise a ferment but may have done so in the past, such as the use of moulded soybeans in the making of fermented soyfoods" (H. T. Huang 2000, 592–93).

Huang's investigations provide a highly detailed account of ancient Chinese science in the sphere of food fermentation technology. His book marks out the remarkable path along which food technologists moved, beginning several millennia ago. In Huang's opinion, there are two principal reasons that fermented legumes did not develop in the West. The first is that beans other than soy, while not uniformly easy to digest, do not pose the serious problems for human food use that soybeans posed. In the case of soybeans, he sees fermentation as the use of a means already known in order to introduce significant chemical change in a different and difficult food. His second point is the absence of knowledge in the West of the mold ferment, which he believes was the secondary adaptation employed to process soybeans.

Huang's argument is certainly persuasive. But I think some of the mystery persists when we recall that the West was never shy about borrowing. We have borrowed plants, animals, foods, cooking methods, whole cuisines, and an infinity of recipes. But if we never figured out how to ferment legumes for ourselves because we had no need to (absent the soybean), we also did not borrow the techniques for fermenting legumes, even after tasting the benefits of those techniques. Hence, it seems to me that in spite of Huang's brilliant deduction, a question remains. The Chinese, who first developed legume fermentation, have continued to capitalize on its fruits. In the West, that initial gap in food preparation was not filled by borrowing or invention. Significantly, in the West soybeans have come to be used almost entirely for different purposes rather than primarily as human food.

Otherwise said, I believe that Huang is right in explaining why the mold ferment never developed in the West and in suggesting it as the ancestor to the fermentation of soybeans. (Soybeans were counted as a grain in ancient China, so important were they to daily diet.) And once the fermentation of soybeans had been mastered and such products as bean curd, dried bean curd, fermented bean curd, and soy sauce had been produced, the role of soybeans—including their fermented products—became even more vital in Chinese culinary life. The writer has wondered whether this importance was not deepened by a relative lack of animal protein in the Chinese countryside. The Buddhist emphasis on vegetarianism may also have played a role in enhancing the importance of soyfoods, as later came to be true in Japan as well.

There was, then, a powerful cultural momentum in favor of soyfoods, fermented products included. I would say that this is a cumulative momentum, built up over time. It was the nature of the soybean that led its growers and consumers in the direction of fermentation, and from this process a cornucopia of special products was born. The tastes for such foods, then, inhabit a social context: a fabric of cultivation, processing, kitchen lore, cuisine and folklore in which people learn from infancy on about the foods they grow to like. Tastes are more commonly acquired in this way, and because the circumstances were different, it has never happened—so far—with soyfoods in the West.

The Future of Fermented Legumes in the West

There remains the question of the future of fermented legumes in the West, and of course the answers must be provisional and contingent (cf. Wood 1986, 251–58; Hesseltine 1986, 303–16; see also Hesseltine and Wang 1983; Stanton 1983).

A new food may be added to a cuisine because it fits neatly into a food category that is already familiar, or because it serves some concrete need within the borrowing cuisine that was not recognized previously, or for other reasons. In the United States, there has been a historic trend toward absorbing much-altered versions of whole cuisines, first through restaurants, then through simplified home cooking, take-out meals, and packaged frozen foods. But I concentrate here on the borrowing of specific items. Borrowed foods may fill a slot in the borrowing cuisine formerly filled by a more traditional substance, as in the use of teriyaki, tamari, or soy sauce in place of catsup, A1, or Worcestershire sauces, for example; of soy chips in place of potato chips; or of green soybeans (*edamame*) or roasted soy nuts in place of peanuts. Borrowed foods may also take on structurally somewhat more surprising positions in the borrowing cuisine, as when soy protein wholly or partly replaces animal protein in soyburgers or soups.[26]

To look at such shifts and replacements analytically, it needs to be kept in mind that what constitutes a meal is quite differently defined in different cultures. Many cuisines have not conceptualized anything that can be called a main course, and not every cuisine has a dessert course. The center or core of the meal, so often seen as consisting of animal protein in Western cuisines, is preponderantly absent in the rest of the world, where the major source of protein may be cereals or beans, where processed sugars and fats may be consumed in lesser quantities and in different forms from the West, and where a meal may be composed of many small dishes rather than what Douglas calls "a single copious dish" (1975, 249).[27] Although the discussion that follows is necessarily brief, only bumping up lightly against some of the details, it matters to look where fermented foods may or may not fit in, both in their cultures of origin and in the West.[28] At the same time, it is important to stress that fermented soy products are but one segment of soyfoods and serve for the most part as flavors or tastes rather than as basic foods.

We know that modification of culturally defined dietary patterns can be difficult to bring about. But people do change their eating behavior, at times swiftly and radically, as, for instance, in today's enormous popularity of raw fish across the United States, a fashion barely three decades old and hardly to have been confidently predicted (Mintz 2001, 283). It is at least possible, as Pimentel and Giampietro (1994) predict, that Americans will become big eaters of vegetable protein in place of meat during the next half century. If so, a role for fermented legumes in Western food habits may develop.

Their acceptance, however, will depend importantly on how they are described, marketed, and prepared as foods. At this time, and except for soy sauce and miso only, hardly any fermented legume product is being introduced to Americans or Europeans, even in ethnic restaurants.[29] Perhaps we can get a glimpse of the promise of fermented legumes by looking at what has happened during the last two decades with such once-exotic products as soy sauce, balsamic vinegar, coriander, and fresh ginger. Like tropical fruits once barely known in the West such as mango, papaya, and soursop or *guanábana* (*Annona muricata*), these other food flavorings or spices are now becoming almost prosaic in North American recipes. It may be more difficult to move soy products such as dried bean curd into the Western taste mainstream and more difficult yet with fermented legumes. But what

I would call an elemental overview of American food habits may enable us to better see what is possible.

In earlier work, I tried to classify the traditional agrarian diet, using a tripartite schema of complex carbohydrate, legume, and flavor fringe (Mintz 1985, 1998, 2001). I want to elaborate that classification by examining the niches, or taste spaces, into which new elements might enter in the future. This is not a matter of identifying new ethnic cuisines or dishes. It has to do instead with the organization of taste in American cooking and with looking at the way new tastes have been threaded into U.S. food habits. For example, the recent history of capsicums (*Capsicum* spp., so-called peppers, sweet and hot) throws some light on innovation.

Only since World War II has American taste moved away from the idea that sharp or penetrating tastes—borne by such foods as garlic or anchovies—are foreign and alien to what used to be called plain, decent American food. In the last three decades or so, the capsicums, and particularly the piquant varieties, have moved out of the ethnic category and into the American category, partly through the growing popularity of ethnic cuisines (such as Mexican and Thai) but also as added elements in dishes already familiar.

The making over of foreign foods into Americanized additions is not in itself new, as we know from the histories of such things as bagels, pizza, and pasta (once known as spaghetti). In the case of condiments and flavors, this shift toward more taste is particularly noticeable, as the relevant shelves in any supermarket prove. The explosion of mustards, pickled (actually, fermented) cocktail vegetables, barbecue sauces, and salsas is good evidence of such change (as well as, no doubt, of affluence).

It is uncertain whether the same process can be expected to happen with fermented legumes, which stand out particularly for their strong tastes, but the popularity of miso soup (*misoshiru*) may be a straw in the wind. With respect to other fermented soy products, a couple of possibilities come to mind. Chinese food enthusiasts who have been able to taste fermented soybean paste (Chinese *furu,* Cantonese *fu yu,* Japanese *nyu-fu* or *fu-nyu*), as it is sometimes used to flavor Chinese stir-fried vegetables such as water spinach (*Ipomoea aquatica,* Chinese *kongxin cai,* Malay *kangkong*) and watercress, can decide for themselves whether that distinctive taste could be transferred to stir-fried broccoli, celery, or cauliflower. Again, although its strong taste may not win universal approval, miso is now beginning to be used as a dressing for broiled fish in the United States, even outside the pricey Japanese restaurants where it was first introduced. Occasionally miso is also used as an ingredient in a salad dressing or dip, as is soybean paste.

Somewhat in contrast to miso, the future of *okara* in the West might be bright because its more neutral taste enables it to serve as a vehicle for other flavors. I have largely omitted *okara*—the pulp or lees of soybeans after curd is made from them—from the previous discussion since it is usually eaten unfermented. But when *okara* is slightly fermented the taste deepens, and some experimental spreads made from it are being marketed in the West. The use of exotic spreads in the West has been uneven but encouraging: hummus today, *tapenade* tomorrow, *caponata* next Tuesday. The rise in the American liking for sharp-tasting flavors embodied in sour, piquant, or oily substances, daubed on dried breadstuffs and served with alcoholic drinks, may one day provide a broad entry for *okara*-based spreads.

My purpose here has been to describe a series of savory foods whose tastes might prove appealing to Western palates but are unknown for the most part in Western cooking and eating practices. While their future is uncertain in the West, they are different, healthy, and tasty enough to merit serious consideration. Europeans and Americans have become fully accustomed to experimentation in the sphere of food. What is needed now is the will and imagination to make these very ancient foods worth trying. Surely Asian culinary genius has much more to teach us.

Notes

1. I am deeply grateful to Dr. H. T. Huang for precious advice and criticism. His careful readings saved me from making many serious mistakes. I also thank Jackie Mintz for valuable assistance with the organization of this essay and Dr. Eric Mintz for providing several important references about which I knew nothing. Professor C. B. Tan and Dr. Christine Du Bois made invaluable suggestions and corrections. Any remaining deficiencies are my responsibility alone.

2. The agents of fermentation are a variety of microorganisms. They include many species of molds, yeasts, and bacteria, acting through their enzymes. In some cases the term "fermentation" has also been applied to processes in which the enzymes are present in situ in the substrate, as in the production of fermented fish sauce or tea. For the chemist or industrial microbiologist, the term "fermentation" covers a wide range of specific and different chemical actions too varied and complex to be examined in detail here. See, for example, Stanbury, Whitaker, and Hall (1995, ch. 1).

3. Reddy, Pierson, and Salunkhe (1986, 1) suggest that as much as 20 percent of total world protein consumption comes in the form of legumes. Davidson (1999, 447) accepts a much lower figure. How much legumes contribute to global protein

consumption is not entirely clear. Whatever the correct figure, however, only a modest portion of legume production is transformed into fermented food.

4. The rhizome called cassava or manioc in South America (*M. esculenta*, also called *Manihot utilissima*) contains the cyanogenic glucoside linamarin, a deadly poison. It can be removed in several ways, one of which, fermentation, has diffused to Africa, where *gari* is a popular food in Nigeria (cf. Campbell-Platt 1987, 74).

5. I am unable to discuss at length the growing importance of fermentation in relation to weaning foods. Because the weaned infant is particularly vulnerable to pathogens, a number of researchers have begun to look at fermented foods, including legumes, as potential replacements for other foods during weaning. For cases based on fermented legumes, see, for example, Tetteh, Sefa-Dedeh, Phillips, and Beuchat (2004); Kiers, Meijer, Nout, Rombouts, Nabuurs, and Van der Meulen (2003); and Osundahunsi and Aworh (2002).

6. Aaronson (2000, 327) writes: "Fermentation preserves perishable food at low cost, salvages unusable or waste materials as human or animal food, reduces cooking time and use of fuel, and enhances the nutritional value of food by predigestion into smaller molecules that are more easily assimilated. Sometimes, but not always, fermentation increases the concentration of B vitamins and protein in food and destroys toxic, undesirable, or antidigestive components of raw food. Moreover, fermentation can add positive antibiotic compounds that destroy harmful organisms, and the acids and alcohol produced by fermentation protect against microbial reinfection and improve the appearance, texture, consistency, and flavor of food. In addition, fermented foods often stimulate the appetite."

7. "There is no method of producing protein," writes Steinkraus (2003, 512), "that can compete with microbial cells." Steinkraus notes that some bacteria can double their cell mass in twenty minutes. Fungi, particularly mushrooms (which can grow on substrates such as straw and cellulose that are inedible for humans), promise to become a much more important human food in the future.

8. McGovern and his co-workers (2004, 17593) provide a precise analysis of "ancient organics absorbed into pottery jars from the early Neolithic village of Jiahu" (Henan), dating to the seventh millennium before Christ, to establish solid evidence for the prehistoric mastery of the fermentation of beverages in China. The "refinements in beverage production took place over the ensuing 5,000 years," they write, "including the development of a special saccharification (amylolysis) fermentation system in which fungi break down the polysaccharides in rice and millet." In this connection, see also my endnote 9.

In a different essay, Michel, McGovern, and Badler (1992) discuss the evidence for beer making (probably from barley) in Lower Mesopotamia during the late fourth millennium BC. Steinkraus (1983, v) states that saccharomyces were recognized and being cultivated as brewer's yeast in Mesopotamia by 6000 BC.

9. Huang (2000, 154–55) indicates that the fermentation of grain to make an alcoholic beverage involves two separate processes, saccharification and fermentation, and explains that the traditional Chinese method required the incubation of cooked grain "in the presence of water with a microbial preparation called chhü, which contains a mixture of fungal enzymes, spores and myceliae and yeast cells." During incubation the enzymes hydrolyze the starch from the grain, the spores germinate, and the myceliae proliferate to produce more amylases. These yeasts grow in number and ferment the sugars generated in situ to alcohol.

10. It may be useful to point out here that the famous "five grains" of China (Huang 2000, 19–28; Davidson 1999, 305) included soybeans, not a cereal of course but a legume.

11. The intense need for cooking and processing that Anderson suggests applies only to mature soybeans; young soybeans are much easier to prepare and have been eaten in Asia for centuries. Since the publication of Anderson's work, steamed *edamame* (young green-vegetable soybeans) have become a common substitute for peanuts and similar accompaniments to alcoholic beverages in Japanese restaurants in the United States. Consumer opinions of young whole soybeans have been improving quite noticeably in the West.

12. The digestive problems posed by soybeans are concisely summarized in H. T. Huang's essay in this volume.

13. Huang points out that black gram, mung, and other beans "are treated with a leaven that probably contains lactic acid bacteria (and/or yeast). The process is similar to raising a bread dough for baking. No chemical change occurs in the protein or the complex carbohydrates of these beans. In the latter [soybeans] proteins as well as the carbohydrates are degraded, which changes the nutritive and physical properties of the product" (personal communication with the author, 2005).

14. In the balance of this essay, such words and phrases as "the West," "Western," "the non-Western world," etc., will appear with some frequency. I am aware of the dangers that this usage entails. However, to make my point requires this risky glossing-over of important issues.

15. Many lesser-known fermented legumes are omitted from discussion. A thorough discussion of many of these products (plus recipes) is provided by Shurtleff and Aoyagi (1983). Here I refer only briefly to *okara,* the dregs of soy processing, after soymilk and soy curd have been removed. In Japan, unfermented *okara* is used as a human food flavoring and as animal feed. While it had a secure place in the diet of rural Japan and is a richly nutritive food, it lacks the status of fresh bean curd, even among Asians. Yet in a fermented state *okara* is the basis for the Chinese food *meitauza* (Reddy, Pierson, and Salunkhe 1986, 228–29). I am indebted to Eugene Anderson for reminding me that I did not deal here with "stinking bean curd" (Anderson 1988, 124), surely one of the most unpopular of all fermented soybean products, even among the Chinese themselves who produce and eat it.

I have eaten this food, and it is so remarkable that it deserves a separate essay, I think.

16. I do not have a copy of Andoh's original remarks, but Grodinsky has reported on them in some detail (Grodinsky 2000). Andoh (2005) is an outstanding student of Japanese cuisine and an excellent practical scholar of miso. Shurtleff and Aoyagi's 1983 work and the chapter on fermented legumes in their online book (2007) offer rich accounts of miso.

17. Mark Bittman, *New York Times,* January 15, 2005, D1, quoting a Tokyo chef, Ms. Kumiko Kano: "In Japan," she said, "the idea of focusing on a small aspect of something and then exploding it into many possibilities is an appealing notion, in both life and aesthetics. Working in a limited set and not letting it inhibit you but allowing it to take you to another level is part of the pleasure. Think about using just ink and paper instead of the whole palette of colors and media in painting; in the same way, the limits of cooking with plants force me to be more creative, to explode, almost into infinity, all of the possibilities."

18. To be sure, this has not interfered with the North American vogue for single-malt scotches, but that is a different segment of appetite and of the art of being fashionable.

19. Professor Tan has pointed out to me that *shih* paste is drier, saltier, and darker than *doujiang* (*jiang*) and perhaps visually less appetizing. Nonetheless, he writes, it is commonly used for cooking certain dishes (personal communication with the author, 2005).

20. There is considerable interest in the U.S. middle class in new (or old) cereals: spelt and even quinoa and buckwheat (which are not true cereals). Also relevant, perhaps, is the current vogue among college-age adolescents for eating breakfast cereals at any time of the day. These interests seem to have arisen during the rise (and now apparent decline) of the low-carb movement.

21. Some fermented legume products also contain cereals. Cereals play a role in many soy sauces and, in Africa and Asia, in other fermented legume products. Whether this has to do primarily with the organoleptic characteristics of the final food or whether it is somehow associated with the salutary complementarity of legume and cereal is not clear.

22. We might observe at the start that only someone familiar with both cuisines would be likely to notice that difference. Much the same might be said of the striking importance of dairy products in the West and their equally glaring absence in the Far (but not Near) East.

23. Many such legumes were borrowed: a whole host of New World beans, *jícama,* and the peanut, among others.

24. It is remarkable to discover, however, that soy sauce entered into European taste as a flavoring agent as early as the seventeenth century. Products such as Vegemite and Marmite, associated with the United Kingdom, Australia, and New Zealand, are spreads made from yeast extract (yeasts are important in some

fermentations), but they are not fermented products and have nothing to do with legumes.

25. It is probably worth mentioning in this connection that in 1973 Kikkoman opened a soy sauce factory in the United States, its first such adventure outside Japan and a somewhat startling addition to American food production. In 1998 Americans consumed forty million gallons of soy sauce, an important exception to my assertion about the history of fermented legumes in the West.

26. Progresso's Chickarina soup—a vaguely Italian product—has tiny meatballs partly fashioned from soy protein. Trader Joe's vegetarian meatballs are also made in part from soy protein.

27. Of course, all of these patterns are changing more rapidly today than at any time in recent history. But we cannot treat changing differences as if the patterns that preceded them did not exist.

28. Such foods may serve in many different ways. Reddy, Pierson, and Salunkhe (1986, 1) list as possibilities their function as a main course, a flavoring agent, a soup base, or "to add color to the food and change physical state of the substrate." We might add as desserts, as snacks, and as ingredients in main courses without exhausting the possibilities. Only by some attention to the functions of each such food is it possible to determine what it brings to that cuisine.

29. Fermented bean curd paste, as employed in sauces for stir-fried vegetables or to flavor ground pork or other dishes, is matter-of-factly eaten by people of different cultures in restaurants where these items do not appear on the English-language menus.

References

Aaronson, Sheldon. 2000. "Fungi." In K. Kiple and K. Ornelas, eds., *The Cambridge World History of Food,* Vol. 1, 313–35. Cambridge: Cambridge University Press.

Anderson, Eugene. 1988. *Food in China.* New Haven, CT: Yale University Press.

Andoh, Elizabeth. 2005. *Washoku.* Berkeley: Ten Speed.

Ang, Catharina Y. W., KeShun Liu, and Yao-Wen Huang. 1999. *Asian Foods.* Lancaster, PA: Technomic Publishing.

Campbell-Platt, Geoffrey. 1987. *Fermented Foods of the World.* London: Butterworths.

———. 2003. "Fermentation." In S. Katz, ed., *Encyclopedia of Food and Culture,* Vol. 1, 630–31. New York: Scribner.

Davidson, A. 1999. "Legume." In A. Davidson, ed., *The Oxford Companion to Food,* 447–48. Oxford: Oxford University Press.

Douglas, Mary. 1975. "Deciphering a Meal." In Mary Douglas, *Implicit Meanings,* 249–75. London: Routledge and Ralph.

Ebine, H. 1986. "Miso." In N. R. Reddy, M. D. Pierson, and D. K. Salunkhe, eds., *Legume-Based Fermented Foods,* 47–68. Boca Raton, FL: CRC.

Grodinsky, Peggy. 2000. *Exploring Japanese Food Culture.* New York: Japan Society.

Hesseltine, C. W. 1986. "Future of Fermented Foods." In C. W. Hesseltine and Hwa L. Wang, eds., *Indigenous Fermented Food of Non-Western Origin,* 303–16. Mycologia Memoir No. 11. Berlin: J. Cramer.

Hesseltine, C. W., and Hwa L. Wang. 1983. "Contributions of the Western World to Knowledge of Indigenous Fermented Foods of the Orient." In Keith Steinkraus, ed., *Handbook of Indigenous Fermented Foods,* Vol. 9, 607–22. Microbiology Series. New York: Marcel Dekker.

Hesseltine, C. W., and Hwa L. Wang, eds. 1986. *Indigenous Fermented Food of Non-Western Origin.* Mycologia Memoir No. 11. Berlin: J. Cramer.

Hosking, Richard. 1996. *A Dictionary of Japanese Food.* Rutland, VT: Charles E. Tuttle.

Huang, H. T. 2000. *Fermentations and Food Science,* Vol. 6, Pt. 5, *Biology and Technology,* of *Science and Civilisation in China.* Cambridge: Cambridge University Press.

Kiers, J. L., J. C. Meijer, M. J. Nout, F. M. Rombouts, M. J. Nabuurs, and L. Van der Meulen. 2003. "Effect of Fermented Soya Beans on Diarrhoea and Feed Efficiency in Weaned Piglets." *Journal of Applied Microbiology* 95(3): 545–52.

McGovern, Patrick E., Juzhong Zhang, Jigen Tang, Zhiquing Zhang, Gretchen R. Hall, Robert A. Moreau, Alberto Nuñez, Eric D. Butrym, Michael P. Richards, Chen-shan Wang, Guangsheng Cheng, Zhijun Zhao, and Changsui Wang. 2004. "Fermented Beverages of Pre- and Proto-historic China." *Proceedings of the National Academy of Sciences* 101(51) (December 21): 17593–98.

Michel, Rudolph H., Patrick E. McGovern, and Virginia R. Badler. 1992. "Chemical Evidence for Ancient Beer." *Nature* 360 (November 50): 24.

Miller, Naomi F., and Wilma Wetterstrom. 2000. "The Beginnings of Agriculture: The Ancient Near East and North Africa." In K. Kiple and K. Ornelas, eds., *The Cambridge World History of Food,* Vol. 2, 1123–39. Cambridge: Cambridge University Press.

Mintz, Sidney W. 1985. "The Anthropology of Food: Core and Fringe in Diet." *India International Centre Quarterly* 12(2): 193–204.

———. 1998. "Core, Fringe and Legume: Agrarian Societies and the Concept of the Meal." In *The Fifth Symposium on Chinese Dietary Culture,* 377–85. Taipei, Taiwan: Foundation of Chinese Dietary Culture.

———. 2001. "Concluding Commentary." In David Y. H. Wu and Tan Chee-beng, eds., *Changing Chinese Foodways in Asia,* 271–86. Hong Kong: Chinese University Press.

Mintz, Sidney W., and D. Schlettwein-Gsell. 2001. "Food Patterns in Agrarian Societies: The Core-Fringe-Legume Hypothesis." *Gastronomica* 1(3): 41–52.

Osundahunsi, O. F., and O. C. Aworh. 2002. "A Preliminary Study on the Use of Tempe-Based Formula As a Weaning Diet in Nigeria." *Plant Foods and Human Nutrition* 57(3–4): 365–76.

Pimentel, David, and Mario Giampietro. 1994. "Food, Land, Population and the U.S. Economy." Executive summary of a full report by the same title. Washington, DC: Carrying Capacity Network.

Reddy, N. R., M. D. Pierson, and D. K. Salunkhe, eds. 1986. *Legume-Based Fermented Foods.* Boca Raton, FL: CRC.

Royse, Daniel J. 2003. "Fungi." In S. Katz, ed., *Encyclopedia of Food and Culture,* Vol. 2, 84–89. New York: Scribner.

Sabban, F. 2000. "China." In K. Kiple and K. Ornelas, eds., *The Cambridge World History of Food,* Vol. 2, 1165–75. Cambridge: Cambridge University Press.

Shurtleff, W., and Akiko Aoyagi. 1975. *The Book of Tofu.* Berkeley: Ten Speed.

———. 1983. *The Book of Miso.* Berkeley: Ten Speed.

———. 2007. *History of Soybeans and Soyfoods, Past, Present, and Future.* http://www.soyinfocenter.com/HSS/history.php.

Stanbury, Peter F., Allan Whitaker, and Stephen J. Hall. 1995. *Principles of Fermentation Technology.* New York: Elsevier.

Stanton, W. R. 1983. "New Uses for Traditional Food Fermentations." In Keith Steinkraus, ed., *Handbook of Indigenous Fermented Foods,* Vol. 9, 633–36. Microbiology Series. New York: Marcel Dekker.

Steinkraus, Keith, ed. 1983. *Handbook of Indigenous Fermented Foods,* Vol. 9. Microbiology Series. New York: Marcel Dekker.

———. 2003. "Microorganisms." In S. Katz, ed., *Encyclopedia of Food and Culture,* Vol. 2, 507–13. New York: Scribner.

Tetteh, G. L., S. K. Sefa-Dedeh, R. D. Phillips, and L. R. Beuchat. 2004. "Survival and Growth of Acid-Adapted and Unadapted Shigella Flexneri in a Traditional Fermented Ghanaian Weaning Food As Affected by Fortification with Cowpea." *International Journal of Food Microbiology* 90(2): 189–95.

Wood, B. J. B. 1986. "Introduction of New Fermented Foods into Western Culture." In C. W. Hesseltine and Hwa L. Wang, eds., *Indigenous Fermented Food of Non-Western Origin,* 251–58. Mycologia Memoir No. 11. Berlin: J. Cramer.

4

Genetically Engineered Soy

CHRISTINE M. DU BOIS AND
IVAN SERGIO FREIRE DE SOUSA

Introduction

Soybeans are unquestionably an ancient crop yet are also on the cutting edge of the promise, potential peril, and seemingly endless controversy surrounding new agricultural biotechnologies.[1] Roundup Ready soy, introduced commercially in 1996, was one of the first commercially successful genetically engineered (GE) crops. Soy is now the plant with the largest percentage of its agriculture given over to GE varieties (more than half of world soy production in 2005).[2] It is also the crop that occupies by far the largest number of GE hectares worldwide: nearly 60 percent of all such hectares in 2006. The next closest contender is maize, which occupied only 25 percent of GE-cultivated area in that year (ISAAA 2006).

This preeminence makes soy one of the central crops in numerous fierce social debates over GE agriculture. Questions about the healthfulness of GE crops and their effects on natural environments have fueled political struggles over when and how to regulate them. These struggles have been played out not only within societies but also among them in international trade disputes. The financial profits that GE crops offer have led to their own set of fights: corporate battles over intellectual property rights in genetic research and production and struggles between farmers and big companies over farmers' historic practice of saving and planting seeds. Last and most importantly, GE crops figure prominently in moral and practical debates over the extent to which new technologies could help feed the world's approximately 850 million hungry poor (FAO 2005).

Roundup Ready soy, a creation of the Monsanto Company, has been genetically modified to survive application of the herbicide Roundup (also a Monsanto product but now off-patent and sold by other companies as well). Roundup, whose chemical name is glyphosate, is quite lethal to plants yet essentially nontoxic to vertebrates.[3] It is quickly broken down into harmless substances within the larger environment (USDA 2002). Monsanto scientists conferred on soybeans the ability to survive dousings of glyphosate by inserting into the beans a gene from a bacterium that naturally evades Roundup's toxicity.

Glyphosate tolerance in crops is a trait that farmers find very practical because they can spray an entire field at once with glyphosate, killing all weeds without killing their crop. The use of other more toxic herbicides is reduced, and farmer workloads are somewhat eased. Although this trait has no direct benefit to consumers, its benefit to farmers has made it a commercial blockbuster. In 2006 in the United States, the world's largest soy-producing country, 89 percent of soy acreage was glyphosate-tolerant (USDA 2006). In Argentina—also a major soy producer—virtually all of the soy acreage was glyphosate-tolerant (SAGPyA 2006; GE Information Service 2006). Such enthusiastic adoption of GE soy may be furthered by Monsanto's recent development of Roundup RReady2Yield soybeans. In this second generation of Roundup Ready soy, glophosate tolerance was inserted using newer GE technologies that permit higher crop yields.

Brazil was slower to adopt GE soy but is now catching up with its two chief rivals; its area planted with GE soy increased 88 percent in 2005 (James 2005). This area represented 40.2 percent of the total Brazilian soy harvest and turned that country into the third-largest producer of all GE crops in the world (after the United States and Argentina). The seed companies' expectation is that the Brazilian area planted in glyphosate-tolerant soy will increase another 34 percent or more for the 2006–2007 harvest (IBGE 2006).

Glyphosate-tolerant soybeans are vastly more economically important at present than other forms of GE soybeans, but GE soy with other traits will likely become prominent in the coming decade. Auguring this possibility, in August 2007 the Brazilian government struck a deal with the German chemical company BASF to develop their own GE soy, resistant to the herbicide imazapyr, to compete with Roundup Ready. On a different tack, Dupont has GE varieties of soy whose oil is more heat stable than typical soy oil; the new oil works well for frying even when it has not been hydrogenated.[4] Use of this oil could decrease human consumption of the dangerous trans fats that form during hydrogenation (Health Canada 2000). As interest in reducing the trans fats in restaurant and processed foods increases, cultivation of these beans is expected to increase as well. The recommendation by the United Nation's World Health Organization in 2006 that governments phase out trans fats may accelerate this process.

Current work on sequencing the soy genome should facilitate more genetic engineering (Food Navigator 2006), and other GE soybeans can also be expected to be commercial successes. The GE nematode-resistant soybeans that various companies and research groups have worked to create could become lucrative, since nematode parasites are the worst pest facing U.S. soy farmers and are a significant problem in South America as well (NSRL 1999; Monsanto 2004; Pioneer Hi-Bred 2005). The improved-taste soybeans that Dupont has worked to develop could also be quite profitable (Lambrecht 2001, 71–72).

Health Concerns

Genetic engineering thus holds out the promise of crafting foods that improve human health as well as farmer livelihoods. Yet the presence of GE soy in so many people's diets, albeit in small amounts (see this volume's introduction), has caused serious concern in some quarters. Anti-GE activists fear allergic reactions or unknown health effects of GE products. They have communicated these fears to the general public to varying degrees in different countries.

Before these worries can be responsibly addressed, three clarifications about GE soy in human diets need to be made. First, refined oil made from contemporary herbicide-tolerant GE soybeans contains no detectable level of the GE protein that nutrition activists worry about (Pauli, Liniger, and Zimmermann 1998).[5] The purification of the refined oil should also eliminate any effects of potentially unknown changes to the soy plant and what its altered DNA produces (Eric Flamm, U.S. Food and Drug Administration research specialist in the Office of the Commissioner, personal communication with Christine Du Bois, 2005). A food made with oil from glyphosate-tolerant soybeans should therefore not pose any hypothesized GE health threat to the consumer (although arguably cultivation of that soy could threaten the environment). For the present at least, the ingredient "soybean oil" on a food label need not cause concern about genetic engineering, since refined oil from GE soy is identical to oil from ordinary soy.

The exception to this generalization comes from the new varieties of GE soy whose oil compositions have been altered through biotechnology. As noted above, Dupont has developed soybeans that have been genetically engineered to produce heart-healthy oil. Such oils are different from ordinary soy oil in a positive way. They are generally easy to analyze to determine their fat composition and so are unlikely to have surprise molecules within them (Eric Flamm, personal communication with Christine Du Bois, 2005). Moreover, Dupont's genetic modification involved inserting a second copy of one of the plant's own genes into itself, reducing the foreignness of the genetic change. The U.S. government does not require GE oils to be labeled as such; instead, the name of the oil includes a descriptive phrase such as, "high oleic acid soybean oil." Based on such phrasing, alert researchers, activists, organizations, and consumers should be able to deduce which foods contain oil whose composition arises in part from genetic engineering.

The second clarification pertains to soy protein rather than the oil, specifically to foods in which soy protein is a major ingredient rather than just a tiny additive. In industrialized countries, such true soyfoods are generally not made with GE soy. Most soyfood companies assiduously avoid GE soy because they know their core buyers would reject it.[6] As the market for soyfoods expands to consumers who are either unaware of or unconcerned about genetic engineering, however, this tendency is shifting. Increasingly, consumers who care about this issue must check labels carefully to ascertain whether the manufacturer actively eschewed GE ingredients by choosing organic soy (or other non-GE soy). Consumers also need to be aware that today, ten years after Roundup Ready soy became available and then pervasive on U.S. farms, even bags of non-GE soy contain trace amounts of glyphosate-tolerant GE material. Some "seed mixing during seed production and handling—at planting, harvest, processing, storage, or transport"—apparently does occur (Mellon and Rissler 2004, 28).

The third clarification is that the vast majority of GE soy protein worldwide is currently fed to animals, and when it does appear in human foods, it usually is in tiny quantities. Still, some consumers wish that they could have foods that are 100 percent free of GE ingredients. They are concerned that GE foods could cause illnesses, especially allergic reactions.

The issue of potential allergic responses to GE foods is complex. On the one hand, as of this writing (February 2008) there is no peer-reviewed, generally accepted scientific evidence proving that any GE food previously or currently on the market has caused allergic reactions in consumers.

GE soy has been on the market for more than ten years, and no allergic disasters have ensued. In fact, in 1995 a program of Pioneer Hi-Bred International that had inserted a gene for a protein from Brazil nuts into soybeans—in order to enhance the nutritional value of the soy for animal feed—was halted when it was found that people allergic to Brazil nuts were also allergic to this GE soy (Nordlee et al. 1996; Nestle 2003, 174–75). Pioneer Hi-Bred abandoned the research because they correctly surmised that on farms, in silos, and during transportation it would be difficult to keep any Brazil nut–enhanced soy for animals fully separate from soy intended for human consumption.

Troubling though this episode may seem, it was useful in that it taught the biotech industry a costly lesson about not using plants containing known allergens for genetic engineering. Profitability, liability, ethics, and public relations issues make this lesson compelling to corporate decision makers. Thus, when anti-GE activists raise fears that genetic engineers will hide peanut proteins inside other foods, they are promoting an unrealistic view of how corporations work. No profit-seeking company would dream of using a powerful allergen such as peanut protein for genetic engineering.

Even when corporations have been rather hasty in releasing a genetically modified crop, so far no proven allergic reactions have resulted. This was shown in the infamous Starlink incident of 2000. Anti-GE activists determined through laboratory testing that certain mass-produced foods accidentally contained traces of Starlink corn. Starlink was a product of the German-French company Aventis that had been approved in the United States for animal consumption only, but the feed corn had apparently sometimes inadvertently been mixed at farms or in silos with food-grade corn. Starlink was eventually shown medically not to cause an allergic reaction in at least one individual who had vociferously (and litigiously) claimed to have suffered from Starlink's presence in his food; in addition, other data suggested that seventeen people making similar claims may not have had allergic reactions either (Sutton, Assa'ad, Steinmetz, and Rothenberg 2003).

The debacle cost Aventis more than $1 billion spent in recalling the corn and in legal fees and a modest legal settlement (Pinstrup-Anderson and Schiøler 2001, 90). The entire biotech industry took note that marketing crops for animals only is an unrealistic and potentially very costly maneuver. They are unlikely to repeat this mistake.

Moreover, biotechnology may actually be used to reduce allergies—for example, to create soybeans that are less allergenic to individuals who are sensitive to ordinary soy (Pollack 2002).[7] There is thus reason to eschew alarmism over the potential allergenic qualities of transgenic crops.

On the other hand, despite these reassuring aspects of the issue, there is still rational room for concern. For one, the mixing of biotech crops not approved for human consumption and those that have officially been deemed safe continues to occur, as the recent discovery of contamination in the United States long-grain rice supply demonstrated. An experimental type of GE rice that Bayer CropScience had field tested and then dropped from its portfolio years earlier somehow became mixed, in small amounts, with ordinary rice or perhaps cross-pollinated with the ordinary rice, thereby giving it the new gene (see Weiss 2006). The debacle has had severe effects on U.S. rice exporters, whose products are being scrutinized and even barred overseas (Heller 2006).

In addition, an Australian study from late 2005 showed, for the first time, that the process of genetic engineering itself could convert a protein that was not an allergen into a protein that could evoke a clear immune response, albeit one elicited under rather artificial conditions (Prescott et al. 2005).[8] Moreover, this unexpected immune response, which took place in laboratory mice, was found to cause the mice to have immune reactions afterward to ordinary proteins that they previously had not been sensitive to (again, under artificial conditions). The finding caused Australia's Commonwealth Scientific and Industrial Research Organization to drop a research project on the development of pest-resistant peas that had already been in progress for several years and had until then been seen as very promising.

There are two ways to look at this series of events, and both are valid. On the one hand, the scientific testing and regulatory system in Australia succeeded in protecting humans from a potentially allergenic food. As the government agency known as Food Safety Australia New Zealand pointed out, the immunologists' study does not "show that the mice [actually] became allergic to the modified protein in food, nor does the study make any conclusions in relation to its relevance in humans. . . . While the significance of the research results for human allergenicity is not clear, the [plant scientists] decided to end the research program. This type of situation is not unique to the development of GMOs [genetically modified organisms]—the development of conventionally bred, non-GM plants have also been terminated when unexpected or adverse effects have been detected" (FSANZ 2005). Thus, we can conclude that so far biotechnological safeguards have worked; in fact, GE crops generally receive far more testing than crops whose genes are modified by conventional breeding.

On the other hand, it is disconcerting that genetic engineering can, as critics had suspected, cause unanticipated and problematic biochemical transformations of food. It is thus possible to conclude that unless all GE foods are very carefully tested, consumers could possibly be in for some troubling surprises in their diets. This conclusion makes an important point, because the safety of most GE crops has not been as rigorously tested as were the peas (although more rigorously tested than ordinary crops). Were the pea engineers simply unlucky that their GE process yielded a very unlikely and unfortunate result? Or have companies and consumers been lucky that up until now, none of the perhaps undertested GE crops have caused any real health problems?

The issue becomes more disconcerting when one considers the next generation of GE crops that are being studied for their potential use as living sources of medicines or industrial chemicals. The preferred crop for these types of applications is corn, but soy is being experimented with for its potential in this area as well. For example, according to the generally antibiotech Union of Concerned Scientists (UCS), between 1996 and 2004 the U.S. Department of Agriculture (USDA) permitted six field trials of such soybeans in the state of Illinois alone. Precisely what the soy had been engineered to produce was "withheld from the public as confidential business information," but it was revealed that one test plot was intended to produce an unspecified polymer (perhaps for the manufacture of plastics) and another an undisclosed antibody (perhaps for medicines) (UCS 2006). There have been no reported adverse effects from these trials, but the prospect that large-scale cultivation of crops producing such chemicals could be coming, with their potential for being inadvertently mixed up with food crops, makes some activists nervous.

GE advocates insist that companies test GE crops carefully for safety and that, to date, GE crops have shown no ill effects on consumers. Anti-GE activists always reply that the testing is inadequate. Like almost everything about agricultural biotechnology, the positions are hotly debated.

The biotech advocates rightly point out that it is important to consider not only the potential harm to human health of GE crops but also their potential benefits. Genetically redesigned foods could be less susceptible to spoilage. Improved oils from GE soy could help protect large numbers of people from heart attacks, enhancing their quality of life and longevity. Soy that was genetically modified to taste better could encourage more consumption of this protein-rich food as a healthier substitute for meat or for harsh protein deprivation in developing countries. Soy that was genetically engineered to grow better in the particular climates, soil conditions, and latitudes where so many of the world's poor live could provide consumers with a new crop to reduce malnutrition.

Other potential and actual GE crops offer similar possibilities for the provision of essential vitamins, minerals, and even vaccines and for the improved agricultural features that such crops could offer to the poor. The most relevant moral question may not be whether creating GE crops is right or wrong but rather how much the risks outweigh the benefits and for whom. The answers must be sought with careful testing on a crop-by-crop and situation-by-situation basis.

Environmental Concerns

GE crops not only have impacts and potential impacts on human health but also affect the natural environments where they are grown. Environmentalists worry that the added genes in these crops could jump to weed plants—gene jumping does occur in nature—possibly creating especially resilient and therefore especially noxious weeds. A troubling example was detected recently when researchers in Oregon discovered that experimental Roundup Ready bentgrass (designed for golf courses) escaped from a test plot in 2003. This bentgrass is now being found growing wild in small quantities near the test plot. There is concern that its very lightweight, easily windblown pollen could enable it to breed with wild relatives, conferring glyphosate tolerance on them (Lafferty 2006; Pollack 2004).

Several caveats must be noted here. First, glyphosate tolerance turns a plant into a superweed only in the sense that it can no longer be killed by glyphosate. It is still susceptible to other herbicides. In the absence of glyphosate, it has no particular survival advantage over other plants. Moreover, the problem with the grass may not be generalizable to soy, since soy is an almost entirely self-pollinating plant, cross-pollinating less than 1 percent of the time because pollination "occurs before the flower opens, and remaining pollen is largely infertile by the time the flower opens and is visited by bees and other insects" (Traynor, Frederick, and Koch 2003, 108, 119). Finally, herbicide tolerance develops naturally in weeds when fields are repeatedly doused with chemicals, whether or not there are GE crops in those fields. Superweeds are thus nothing new and so far have been manageable (Coghlan 2005).

Genes can also jump to non-GE, nonindustrial versions of crops that have been cultivated in many varieties by small farmers all over the world (called landrace varieties). Since landraces are especially numerous in the regions where each crop originated, these regions are called centers of diversity (i.e., genetic diversity). Controversy erupted in 2001 when two California researchers detected GE genes in landraces of corn in Mexico, the heart of that crop's center of diversity. The concerns were that the GE genes had contaminated the gene pool there, could cause the corn to become toxic or allergenic, or could lead to the eventual extinction of some of the landraces. The quality of this research, the actions of the journal that published the work and then retracted it, and the importance of the study's observations (some experts declared that the contamination was both obvious and not worth worrying about) all came under attack (Pringle 2003, 159–83). But the controversy eventually died down.

There is less concern that genes will jump from GE soy to the landraces in China, its center of diversity, since as noted before soy does not easily cross-pollinate. However, the possibility of such jumping does exist. The UCS posits the following scenario, which could conceivably apply to soy whose oil composition had been altered: "a gene changing the oil composition of a crop might move into nearby weedy relatives in which the new oil composition would enable the seeds to survive the winter. Overwintering might allow the plant to become a weed or might intensify weedy properties it already possesses" (UCS 2005). The risk posited here is unlikely in the Western Hemisphere, since soy does not have weedy relatives in the West. But in China soy does have wild relatives, so theoretically GE soy there requires special monitoring.

Anti-GE activists are also concerned that wild creatures that consume GE crops could be damaged or have their life cycles interrupted, upsetting the intricate web of local ecosystems. This worry received extensive attention beginning in 1999 in the controversy over the effects of GE corn on the health of monarch butterfly larvae (Pringle 2003, 121–35, 138–40; Nestle 2003, 189–92; Lambrecht 2001, 77–80; Charles 2001, 243–48; Pinstrup-Andersen and Schiøler 2001, 47–49). The results of numerous studies suggest that while one kind of rarely planted GE corn can indeed be quite toxic to monarchs, most GE corn probably does not disrupt their life cycles.

No known major wildlife problems have ensued from the cultivation of herbicide-tolerant soy. But if nematode-resistant soy were to become a commercial reality, the possibility exists that the antinematode toxins in the plants could work their way through the food chain and kill off beneficial nematodes (for example, those that eat pest insects). It is hoped that government regulatory agencies will require rigorous testing for this risk.

A more subtle effect on wildlife ensues from the growing of Roundup Ready soy. Because Roundup is so effective at killing weeds, wildlife that depend on the presence of those weeds (for example, certain insects and the birds that eat them) are threatened. A field that is very clean may be too clean for the creatures that used to live there (Pringle 2003, 127). The British in particular have been troubled by this problem, which adds to their suspicion of GE crops (Coghlan 2005).[9]

Biotechnology advocates counter these complaints and the activists' campaigns by pointing out the environmental benefits, actual and potential, of GE agriculture. They emphasize the fact that compared to conventional farming, growing GE crops reduces the need for the more toxic kinds of topical herbicides and pesticides.

GE agriculture can also improve crop yields and make low-till or no-till farming more feasible. In a GE–herbicide-tolerant system, the farmer does not need to till the land in order to remove leftover weeds. Tilling loosens the soil and is a major cause of soil erosion worldwide. The no-till farming that is made more possible by certain GE crops, such as Roundup Ready soy, can thus help reduce the grave global problem of loss of topsoil.

The environmental benefits of GE crops can also dovetail with economic benefits to farmers. Farmers and their cooperatives are worried about competitors who manage to lower their production costs. Recently, some have argued (Brookes and Barfoot 2006; Phipps and Park 2001) that GE crops promote cost reduction and higher-quality products, both decisive factors in the generation of competitive advantages in national and international markets. For example, in conjunction with GE-crop cultivation, the prices of herbicides have dropped significantly. It is estimated that lowered herbicide prices provided a cost reduction to Argentine farmers of approximately US$400 million between 1996 and 2000. This is one reason that Brazil, perceiving the competitive advantage of its neighbor, decided to embrace GE soy.

Political and Legal Reactions to GE Foods

The political and legal responses to the advent of GE crops have varied considerably from country to country and among different population segments within countries. Here we briefly sketch the attitudes toward and regulation of GE crops within those nations whose actions have had the most impact on global GE debates.

Although in the United States the GE controversy has barely reached public consciousness, certain companies have nevertheless felt compelled to make their products as GE-free as possible in order to forestall future potential loss of market share. Pressure from Greenpeace persuaded both Gerber and the H. J. Heinz Company to drop GE ingredients from their baby foods (Lagnado 1999), and snack-food maker Frito Lay and the McDonald's Corporation also backed away from GE ingredients (Brasher 2000; Thompson 2000). In the food retailing industry, two leading chains of natural foods stores declared that they would cease carrying private-label products with GE ingredients (Cox 2000), and Genuardi's, the supermarket chain, broke ranks with fellow mainstream grocers to support mandatory labeling of GE ingredients (Knox 2000).[10]

Consumer concern was expressed in the political fight over the USDA's organic standards program. The program, which since 2002 has permitted foods produced according to strict guidelines to be labeled with a USDA "organic" seal, was originally slated to allow GE foods that otherwise met the criteria to bear the seal. After 325,000 consumer and producer comments on the proposed organic standards, including an outcry against this policy, the USDA reversed the decision (Hesman 2000). This means that a food may not have been produced with even a small quantity of GE soy protein and still be deemed organic by U.S. government standards.[11] American consumers who wish to avoid GE soy as much as possible can now conveniently do so by checking for the USDA "organic" seal.

Meanwhile, in Argentina the public has generally been quite accepting of GE agriculture and foods (see Nestle 2003, 237), an attitude that for several years contrasted with that of rival Brazil. However, 2003 and 2004 represented watershed years in Brazil's public discussions and decisions about transgenic plants. Seeking to boost Brazil's agricultural earnings, President Luiz Ignácio Lula da Silva became more favorable to GE crops than the previous government had been. First, in late 2003 an executive Provisional Act legalized GE soybean planting, mainly in the southern part of the country; the act was later renewed. The act has encouraged GE plantings to spread throughout Brazil (Di Ciero 2006).

Then in 2005 the legislature formally legalized the planting of GE crops. This measure was widely viewed as a long-sought victory for biotech industries; the production of GE plants in Brazil had constantly been a source of controversy. Despite the widespread and apparently innocuous use of GE plants in various parts of the world, the Brazilian public has been fearful about the nutritional and environmental safety of these products. (However, because until very recently Brazil's GE bean cultivation has been low, the Brazilian public has not evinced widespread concern about soymilk use in school programs so far; see the Sousa and Vieira essay in this volume.)

To appease the public, the new Brazilian law established biosafety standards to regulate the use of genetic engineering and the release of GE organisms to the environment. It also established mechanisms for inspections of GE organisms and created the National Committee of Biosafety. In addition, to the biotech companies' dismay, Brazil requires that all mass-produced foods containing 1 percent or more of GE ingredients bear a GE label.

In Japan and Europe, governments and populations have also been insistent about exerting regulatory control over their food supplies (on the issue of control, see Nestle 2003). In Europe especially, activists urge adoption of a proactive precautionary principle. By this they aim to halt adoption of technologies whose effects are not yet fully known and, in the judgment of some scientists, may be or may become significantly detrimental. Activists and academics argue that the precautionary principle is especially needed in a political-economic context in which big profit-driven agricultural companies are, in their estimation, inadequately regulated. There is no legal assurance to consumers that the companies' interests and those of the general public now coincide or will in the future (see Nestle 2003). European consumers, for whom the threat of industrially created mad cow disease (BSE) was traumatic, are particularly sensitive on this point.

Beginning in 1996, the same year that GE soy was first commercially cultivated, the campaigns of Greenpeace and other activist organizations in Europe made the population aware of the presence of GE ingredients in their foodstuffs (Charles 2001). The populace balked, and in 2004 the European Union finalized strict rules by which GE foods must bear labels. This labeling makes supermarkets reluctant to stock such products out of fear that consumers will shun them. Hence, according to a 2004 Greenpeace survey of European grocery shelves, "very few [GE] products can be found across Europe's 30 major [supermarket] retailers, nearly all of which have a non-biotech policy for the entire EU or at least in their main European markets" (Smith 2005).

Europeans' reluctance to eat GE foods has had varying effects on other countries. Most troubling was the incident in 2002 when the governments of three African nations threatened with famine—Zimbabwe, Mozambique, and Zambia—rejected U.S. food aid because it came in the form of GE corn. The Africans had taken Europe's precautionary principle to heart and were highly suspicious of GE products. Indeed, Zambia's president declared, "Simply because my people are hungry is not a justification to give them poison" (cited in Pringle 2003, 185). The African governments were also concerned that if any of their people saved the corn to plant rather than simply eating it, their fields might become contaminated, and Europe might refuse agricultural imports from those countries in the future. Eventually Zimbabwe and Mozambique accepted the corn provided that it arrived already milled and could not be planted, but Zambia chose instead to seek food aid from non-GE sources (Pringle 2003, 184–89).

Yet, more recently, the increasing presence of GE soy in Brazil has not affected European demand for Brazilian soybeans. This is true for at least three reasons: the quantities of GE soy in Brazil are still lower than in other major soy-producing countries; most soy is destined for animal feed, not human food; and for some European countries, soy is already produced in certain areas of Brazil according to very specific demands (size of beans, oil and protein content, and so on), to which it is easy to add the non-GE demand. The latter two factors generally also pertain to Europe's imports of soy from the United States (Charles 2001, 255–58).

Some studies have detected the construction of a myth that international markets are refusing GE soybeans and, as a result, are preferring Brazilian soy. The reality, say these studies, is that shifts in soy commerce have reflected diverse situations in logistics, weather, production, and tax structures in both supplying and demanding countries. Brazil has increased its non-GE whole soybean exports to Europe, while the same has happened with Argentina's GE soymeal. Japan continues to be a great soy importer, mainly from the United States (see, for instance, Pereira 2004).

At the same time, the Japanese public has also expressed concern about GE foods. In response, in 2001 the government instituted a labeling requirement for many foods if they contain more than 5 percent GE ingredients, including soyfoods.[12] This requirement and Europe's requirement have been the subject of World Trade Organization disputes. Soy-exporting countries are concerned not only about access to markets in Europe and Japan for GE foodstuffs—a market that is small now but is expected to grow—but also about the example that those nations set for other countries. In fact, numerous countries have enacted some form or other of anti-GE laws of varying levels of strictness (Greenpeace 2001; Nestle 2003, 238).

But the example that China sets may shift global perceptions positively toward GE crops. China grows insect-resistant GE cotton on more than three million hectares and is close to approving GE rice (James 2005, 4, 6).

Development specialists Pinstrup-Andersen and Schiøler explain that "China has made a massive investment in GM [GE] cotton and a number of GM food crops including rice, potatoes, tomatoes, and maize. The aim is to ease the strain put on the environment by irrigation and agrochemical toxins and to achieve a badly needed increase in plant yields. . . . In other countries, the debate on GM crops may continue to go round in circles or things may eventually grind to a halt, but China appears to be moving full-steam ahead" (2001, 100).

Chinese enthusiasm for GE crops is important for the future of soy because China is a major soy importer and consumer (both for animal feed and human food). The Chinese may at some point take an interest in growing currently existing GE soy or in developing their own GE varieties. In addition, if a country with as large a population as China's were to adopt GE rice without ill effects, farmers, consumers, and policymakers worldwide could take this success as an indication that GE crops in general are likely to be safe (James 2005, 4; Monsanto, personal communication, 2004).[13]

India also has an immense population, also grows GE cotton, and recently experienced "by far the largest year-on-year proportional increase [in GE plantings worldwide], with almost a three-fold increase from 500,000 hectares in 2004 to 1.3 million hectares in 2005" (James 2005, 4). Yet India's impact on global perceptions of GE crops is mixed. One of the world's most famous and charismatic antibiotech advocates is Indian activist Vandana Shiva (Stone 2002).

In addition, negative press reports about the effects of GE cotton farming on poor cultivators in India have circulated widely (e.g., Sengupta 2006). Many of these farmers have gone into debt to be able to buy GE seeds and other agricultural inputs, but no agricultural system is foolproof, and in the wrong weather conditions, for example, any crop can fail. Crop failures can drive these farmers ever deeper into debt.

In the view of many Indians and as alleged in the court case brought against Monsanto by the state of Andhra Pradesh, the GE seeds are overpriced as are fertilizers and pesticides the farmers also purchase, although increasingly the pesticides do not work well (Lambrecht 2001, 271–84). To make matters worse, the farmers must deal with rapacious local moneylenders. This complex combination has helped drive an alarming number of such farmers to suicide, more than seventeen thousand of them in 2003 (Sengupta 2006).[14]

The situation has further fueled arguments over the role of GE crops in the developing world. On one side, anti-GE activists contend that corporate control of expensive seeds and other agricultural inputs is the primary cause of the despair in rural India. On the other side, biotech advocates contend that pest invasions and pesticide failures—remediable through the use of GE crops—are the main cause of the suicides (Lambrecht 2001, 271–84).

Intellectual Property

Biotechnology has another controversial dimension. The sale of GE seeds generally requires the farmer to sign a contract that prohibits saving any of the crop for planting the following year. A number of farmers and farmers' groups have objected strenuously to a contractual requirement that they repurchase GE soy seed from wealthy corporations such as Monsanto year after year. In the case of hybrid corn (and other crops), such repurchasing is a biological necessity, as saved hybrid seed will not perform as desired during the following year. But in the case of GE soy, it is merely a profit-driven necessity.

Hence some farmers resent what they see as the usurpation of a traditional practice—often viewed as a natural right—of saving seed. Many farmer and consumer advocates think that this arrangement puts too much power over the food supply in the hands of a few corporate leaders (see GRAIN 1997). Anti-GE activists and some farmers get particularly upset when Monsanto hires detectives to inspect the fields of farmers suspected of planting its GE crops without a contract and without paying Monsanto's so-called technology fee. Monsanto has taken some of these farmers to court, most famously Canadian farmer Percy Schmeiser, who lost his legal battle with Monsanto in 2001 (Charles 2001, 188–89).

The companies, for their part, decry farmers who plant without permission and those who defend them. They argue that most farmers prefer that their neighbors not cheat by avoiding the technology fee: the playing field should be level, with everyone getting the same deal. Besides, the companies contend, the contracts are needed to maintain profits. These seeds are the products of painstaking and very expensive science. Remove the profit, the companies say, and neither funds for future products nor incentives to make them will remain. To this the antibiotech activists reply, "Fine. Good riddance." But some nonindustry advocates for the poor respond in turn that this technology could eventually provide new sources of nutrients for a world that is still malnourished. The technology therefore should not be discarded (e.g., Pinstrup-Andersen and Schiøler 2001).

Biotechnology and the Poor

In reality, concerns about food safety, environmental impacts of GE agriculture, and legal contracts are often remote from the struggles of poor farmers and consumers in developing countries. The one GE crop that has been developed so far with the poor specifically in mind—beta-carotene-enriched Golden Rice—remains limited for the time being in its utility. Because it has only recently been modified to contain significant levels of beta-carotene, much nutritional testing is still needed. The crop also must be adapted to many different local growing environments (see Ruse and Castle 2002, 29–64; Nestle 2003, 139–66; and Raney and Pingali 2007).

What many farmers need—especially those engaged in low-yield agriculture—are ways to increase their productivity (DeVries and Toenniessen 2001). The technical solutions of the Green Revolution have not always worked well in their environments (Paarlberg 2001, 2005).[15] Certainly, the maldistribution of agricultural land and of the food that global agriculture has already successfully produced are problems for the poor (for a discussion of access to food in India, see Stone 2002). But related to these problems is the immediate and pressing difficulty of low income, which the poor experience on a daily basis. For small farmers, low income partly derives from low farm yields (see Bruinsma 2003, 218–20, 227).

Could biotechnology afford them fresh agricultural choices? Biotech analyst Clive James reports that 90 percent of the farmers growing GE crops in 2005 "were resource-poor farmers from developing countries, whose increased incomes from biotech crops contributed to the alleviation of their poverty. In 2005, approximately 7.7 million poor subsistence farmers . . . benefited from biotech crops—the majority in China with 6.4 million, 1 million in India, [and] thousands in South Africa" (James 2005, 5). Of course, these farmers did not control anywhere near 90 percent of the land area devoted to biotech crops, and as the Indian case demonstrates, adoption of GE crops does not necessarily lead to an improved life. Still, many poor farmers have found the new seeds helpful and eagerly plant them year after year (e.g., see Pinstrup-Andersen and Schiøler 2001, 47).

The longer-term question is whether there will be enough investment in developing more seeds from which greater numbers of poor farmers could benefit. The farmers' initial inability to pay for GE seeds—or their acquired inability to continue paying for them due to spiraling debt—could inhibit companies from undertaking the required research and development to create the seeds in the first place. Why develop a product if its targeted purchasers will not be able to afford it?

Complementing private effort is public, nonprofit research in biotechnology, but it remains underfunded and excessively hobbled by intellectual property contracts and disputes (see Stone 2002; DeVries and Toenniessen 2001, 72–74; Pringle 2003, 32–36). The governments of developing countries can also themselves invest in biotechnology, but so far few have been willing or able to do so (see Ruse and Castle 2002, 299–321).

A bright note came in 2005, however, when the nonprofit group Grand Challenges in Global Health (GCGH) granted more than $41 million for pro-poor biotechnology projects. The GCGH is a partnership among the Bill & Melinda Gates Foundation, the Canadian Institutes of Health Research, the Foundation for the U.S. National Institutes of Health, and the Wellcome Trust. The four projects whose funding was announced in 2005 deal with increasing the nutritional value of staple crops in developing countries (bananas, cassava, rice, and sorghum) rather than increasing yields (Bill and Melinda Gates Foundation 2005); both are valuable aims. But it is not clear if this example will set a trend or if developing new varieties of soy useful to poor farmers will figure among the priorities. Despite repeated calls from prominent crop scientists—notably Norman Borlaug, Nobel Peace laureate and "father" of the Green Revolution (Borlaug and Carter 2005)—for pro-poor biotechnology, whether the world community takes on this task in earnest remains to be seen.

Conclusion

The soybean is the most important oilseed crop globally and the world's chief source of vegetable protein. Yet "the soybean, even though known as a miracle crop, is far from perfect. Among the major problems with soybeans are their beany flavor, flatus-producing ability, oxidative and flavor instability, deficiency of sulfur-containing essential amino acids, presence of antinutritional factors, and proneness to attack by such production hazards as diseases, insects, and weeds" (Liu 1997, 478). Some of these deficiencies are not severe compared with those of other plants; for example, soy's amino acid profile, while not quite as good as that of egg or meat, is still remarkably nutritious for a plant. Other deficiencies do not negate the value of soybeans because they can be remedied through human activity. Thus, antinutritional factors are inactivated through proper soy processing, and agricultural problems such as pests and diseases are addressed through the conventional breeding of superior varieties.

But agricultural scientists are aware that more improvements could always be made. Genetic engineering offers the tools for clever, startling changes to the soy plant. These possibilities are exciting to some in society, frightening to others, and ambiguous to many. Debates and struggles have therefore ensued in many arenas, including concerning GE foods and human health, GE crops and the environment, labeling laws, trade patterns, profits, intellectual property, and the needs of the poor. Issues of control, dread, outrage (Nestle 2003), promise, hope, and choice (Pinstrup-Andersen and Schiøler 2001) surround the genetic engineeering of this bean. Because the stakes are high, the issues complex, and the stakeholders so numerous and varied, it seems prudent to follow the advice of Pinstrup-Andersen and Schiøler: "Moving Forward: Handle with Care" (2001, 127).

Notes

1. The authors wish to thank Ted Hymowitz, Larry Buxbaum, and Sidney Mintz for their reading of this manuscript. Any errors are, of course, entirely ours.

2. The terms "GE soy," "GMO soy" (GMO stands for "genetically modified organism"), and "transgenic soy" are interchangeable. The term "biotechnology" is used in this essay to refer to genetic engineering, although "biotechnology" can also refer to certain other modern crop transformations that do not involve direct genetic manipulation.

3. Glyphosate "binds specifically to 5-enol-pyruvylshikimate-3-phosphate synthase (EPSP synthase or EPSPS) . . . which catalyzes the reaction of shikimate 3-phosphate and phosphoenolpyruvate to form 5-enol-pyruvylshikimate-3-phosphate (EPSP) and phosphate. . . . The binding inhibits EPSPS and thus prevents the plant from making aromatic amino acids essential for the synthesis of proteins and some secondary metabolites. The plant will die within days. EPSPS is present in all plants, bacteria, and fungi, but not in animals" (Liu 1997, 494).

4. These varieties are labeled G94-1, G94-19, and G168 (Health Canada 2000). They are different from the heart-healthy soybeans from Monsanto and Dupont discussed in Du Bois's essay in this volume on the United States. The beans discussed there had their fat profiles changed by conventional breeding; their only genetic engineering is for Roundup resistance.

5. If, however, someone were to have a known allergy to the altered protein (a condition not currently seen in relation to herbicide-tolerant soy), he or she would likely prefer to err on the side of caution and avoid oil from the engineered beans, much as individuals allergic to peanut protein avoid products made with peanut oil just in case the oil was inadequately purified.

6. Sometimes a product's soy protein is not genetically modified, yet the company does not trumpet this fact. For example, since 2002 Mead Johnson & Company has used only identity-preserved non-GE soybeans for the protein in its

soy-based infant formula (Enfamil brand), yet this fact has been available only to consumers who call the product hotline and are transferred from the initial customer representative to a specialist in the products division. The information appears nowhere on the label.

7. However, there may be no need for genetic engineering in order to produce soy with low allergenicity. Promising new research has identified two Chinese soybean lines that do not produce the protein responsible for most soy allergies (Joseph, Hymowitz, Schmidt, and Herman 2006). Conventional plant breeders should be able to make good use of these soybean lines since the discoverers intentionally made them publicly available by not patenting them.

8. For detailed scientific debate about whether or not the food-safety testing of Roundup Ready soy has been adequate, see Carman (1999) and FSANZ (2003).

9. For other potential environmental problems associated with GE crops, see the UCS's "Food and Environment," http://www.ucsusa.org/food_and_environment/genetic_engineering/risks-of-genetic-engineering.html.

10. In 2002, the California-based Safeway Company purchased Genuardi's. Safeway's policy on GE foods is that it would be prohibitively expensive to label them since ingredients come from so many different suppliers. The tasks of keeping GE and non-GE ingredients separate and of monitoring the proper production of non-GE foods would noticeably add to costs (Safeway, personal communication with Christine Du Bois, 2005).

11. A nonorganic ingredient is permitted in a food labeled "organic" with the USDA seal only if no organic version of that ingredient is commercially available. Soy and its components are, in fact, commercially available in organic versions, so nonorganic soy should not appear in USDA organic foods. The exception has been lecithin, which generally comes from soy but was not manufactured in organic versions until 2003 (although there were non-GE versions available). Lecithin appears in a wide variety of foods in very tiny quantities. In September 2007 the world's sole organic soy lecithin supplier, Clarkson Soy Products LLC, completed a major expansion of its lecithin-production capacity.

It should be noted that the status of and precise specifications in the rules are in question (see Bain 2005; Warner 2005).

12. But soy sauce is exempt from the labeling requirement, as is soy oil.

13. Some would greet Chinese GE success with skepticism, however, since the Chinese government might or might not be forthright about any ill effects suffered.

14. A great many factors helped drive the suicides, however (see Stone 2005, 214).

15. Many areas of Africa are too dry to benefit from Green Revolution technologies, which require ample water. In addition, in Africa the population density is relatively low, and the transportation system is often poor. These factors make the timely delivery of Green Revolution inputs such as irrigation and fertilizer prohibitively costly or challenging. See Paarlberg (2001).

References

Bain, Ben. 2005. "Purists Battle Processors over Rules for US Organic Foods." *Financial Times* (London), December 31.

Bill and Melinda Gates Foundation. 2005. "Grants—Grand Challenges." http://www.gatesfoundation.org/GlobalHealth/BreakthroughScience/GrandChallenges/Grants/default.htm?showYear=2005.

Borlaug, Norman, and Jimmy Carter. 2005. "Food for Thought." *Wall Street Journal,* October 14, p. A10.

Brasher, Philip. 2000. "U.S. Expected to Reduce Biotech Crop Plantings." *Philadelphia Inquirer,* April 1, pp. C1, C7.

Brookes, G., and P. Barfoot. 2006. "GM Crops: The First Ten Years—Global Socio-Economic and Environmental Impacts." *ISAAA Brief* No. 36. Ithaca, NY: ISAAA.

Bruinsma, Jelle, ed. 2003. *World Agriculture: Towards 2015/2030. An FAO Perspective.* London: Earthscan.

Carman, Judy. 1999. "The Problem with the Safety of Roundup Ready Soybeans." http://members.iinet.net.au/~rabbit/notjcsoy.htm.

Charles, Daniel. 2001. *Lords of the Harvest.* Cambridge, MA: Perseus.

Coghlan, Andy. 2005. "Enter the Superweed." *NewScientist,* August 27, p. 17.

Cox, James. 2000. "Retailers Dropping Bio-foods." *USA Today,* January 4, p. 1A.

DeVries, Joseph, and Gary Toenniessen. 2001. *Securing the Harvest: Biotechnology, Breeding and Seed Systems for African Crops.* New York: CABI Publishing.

Di Ciero, Luciana. 2006. "Brasil É O Terceiro No Plantio De Transgênicos." *Biotech Brasil,* January 13. http://www.biotechbrasil.bio.br/2006/01/13/brasil-e-o-terceiro-no-plantio-de-transgenicos-2/.

FAO (Food and Agriculture Organization of the United Nations). 2005. "Committee on World Food Security." 31st Session, Rome, May 23–26. http://www.fao.org/docrep/meeting/009/J4968e/j4968e00.htm.

Food Navigator. 2006. "Soy Database Provides Access to Genetic Info." October 2. http://www.foodnavigator-usa.com/news/ng.asp?n=70979&m=1FNUO02&c=njwlzjcnteougfh.

FSANZ (Food Standards Australia New Zealand). 2003. "FSANZ Response to Article Entitled 'GE Foods and Human Health Safety Assessments' by Dr. Judy Carman, Spokesperson on GE Food, Public Health Association of Australia." http://www.foodstandards.gov.au/search/?keywords=Judy+Carmen.

———. 2005. "Genetically Modified Peas and Reported Effects in Mice." Fact Sheet, December 2. http://www.foodstandards.gov.au/newsroom/factsheets/factsheets 2005/geneticallymodifiedf3097.cfm.

GE Information Service. 2006. "European Commission Supports Argentina in Monsanto Battle." *GE Information Bulletin* 48 (September). http://www.geinfo.org.nz/092006/05.html.

GRAIN (Genetic Resources Action International). 1997. "Soybean: The Hidden Commodity." *Seedling,* June. http://www.grain.org/seedling/?id=28.

Greenpeace. 2001. "Summary of Global Legislation on GE Foods." http://www.organicconsumers.org/gefood/worldreport.cfm.

Health Canada. 2000. "High Oleic Soybean Lines G94-1, G94-19, and G168." http://www.hc-sc.gc.ca/fn-an/gmf-agm/appro/oleic_soybean-soja_oleique_e.html.

Heller, Lorraine. 2006. "Bayer Petitions for Approval of GM Rice in Contamination Case." September 11. http://www.foodnavigator.com/news/ng.asp?id=70468.

Hesman, Tina. 2000. "Federal Agency Sets Standards for Organic Food; Biotech Products Are Disallowed from Foods That Get Special Seal." *St. Louis Post-Dispatch,* December 21, p. A1.

IBGE (Instituto Brasileiro de Geografia e Estatística). 2006. Statistics available at http://www.sidra.ibge.gov.br/.

ISAAA (International Service for the Acquisition of Agri-Biotech Applications). 2006. http://www.isaaa.org/resources/publications/briefs/35/executivesummary/default.html.

James, Clive. 2005. "Executive Summary Brief 34: Global Status of Commercialized Biotech/GM Crops 2005." Ithaca, NY: ISAAA. http://www.isaaa.org/.

Joseph, Leina M., Theodore Hymowitz, Monica A. Schmidt, and Eliot M. Herman. 2006. "Evaluation of Glycine Germplasm for Nulls of the Immunodominant Allergen P34/Gly m Bd 30k." *Crop Science* 46: 1755–63.

Knox, Andrea. 2000. "Genuardi's Goes against Industry on Food Labeling." *Philadelphia Inquirer,* April 19, pp. C1, C8.

Lafferty, Mike. 2006. "Broken Loose: Escaped Grass Highlights Questions about Genetically Altered Crops." *Columbus Dispatch,* September 5, p. 6D.

Lagnado, Lucette. 1999. "Strained Peace: Gerber Baby Food, Grilled by Green Peace, Plans Swift Overhaul." *Wall Street Journal,* July 30.

Lambrecht, Bill. 2001. *Dinner at the New Gene Café.* New York: Thomas Dunne.

Liu, KeShun. 1997. "Soybean Improvements through Plant Breeding and Genetic Engineering." In KeShun Liu, ed., *Soybeans: Chemistry, Technology, and Utilization,* 478–523. New York: Chapman & Hall.

Mellon, Margaret, and Jane Rissler. 2004. "Gone to Seed: Transgenic Contaminants in the Traditional Seed Supply." http://www.ucsusa.org/food_and_environment/genetic_engineering/gone-to-seed.html.

Monsanto. 2004. "Divergence, Monsanto Collaborate to Develop Nematode-Resistant Soybeans." http://monsanto.mediaroom.com/index.php?s=43&item=151&printable.

Nestle, Marion. 2003. *Safe Food: Bacteria, Biotechnology, and Bioterrorism.* Berkeley: University of California Press.

Nordlee, J. A., S. L. Taylor, J. A. Townsend, et al. 1996. "Identification of a Brazil-Nut Allergen in Transgenic Soybeans." *New England Journal of Medicine* 334: 688–92.

NSRL (National Soybean Research Laboratory). 1999. "Research Uses Biotechnology in Search of Nematode Resistance." *NSRL Bulletin* 6(2) (June). http://www.nsrl.uiuc.edu/news/nsrl_pubs/bulletins/june99/index.html.

Paarlberg, Robert. 2001. "Environmentally Sustainable Agriculture in the 21st Century." Paper presented to the Aspen Institute Congressional Seminar. Queenstown, MD: Aspen Institute.

———. 2005. "From the Green Revolution to the Gene Revolution." *Environment* 47(1) (January/February): 38–40.

Pauli, U., M. Liniger, and A. Zimmermann. 1998. "Detection of DNA in Soybean Oil." *Zeitschrift für Lebensmitteluntersuchung und -Forschung A* 207(4): 264–67. Abstract available at http://www.springerlink.com/index/42EAYJ5287VYEANW.

Pereira, Savio Rafael. 2004. "A Evolução do Complexo Soja e a Questão da Transgenia." *Revista de Política Agrícola.* 13(2) (April/May/June): 26–32. Brasilia: Embrapa/MAPA.

Phipps, R., and J. Park. 2001. "Environmental Benefits of GM Crops: Global & European Perspectives on Their Ability to Reduce Pesticide Use." *Journal of Animal Sciences* 11: 1–18.

Pinstrup-Andersen, Per, and Ebbe Schiøler. 2001. *Seeds of Contention.* Baltimore: Johns Hopkins University Press.

Pioneer Hi-Bred (Dupont). 2005. "Cyst Nematode Resistance." http://www.pioneer.com/pipeline/spec_sheets/soycyst.pdf.

Pollack, Andrew. 2002. "Gene Jugglers Take to Fields for Allergy Vanishing Act." *New York Times,* October 15, p. F2.

———. 2004. "Genes from Engineered Grass Spread for Miles, Study Finds." *New York Times,* September 21, p. A1.

Prescott, Vanessa E., Peter M. Campbell, Andrew Moore, Joerg Mattes, Marc E. Rothenberg, Paul S. Foster, T. J. V. Higgins, and Simon P. Hogan. 2005. "Transgenic Expression of Bean Alpha-Amylase Inhibitor in Peas Results in Altered Structure and Immunogenicity." *Journal of Agricultural Food Chemistry* 53: 9023–30.

Pringle, Peter. 2003. *Food, Inc.: Mendel to Monsanto—The Promises and Perils of the Biotech Harvest.* New York: Simon & Schuster.

Raney, Terri, and Prabhu Pingali. 2007. "Sowing a Gene Revolution." *Scientific American,* September, 104–11.

Ruse, Michael, and David Castle, eds. 2002. *Genetically Modified Foods.* Amherst, NY: Prometheus.

SAGPyA (Secretaria de Agricultura, Ganadería, Pesca y Alimentos, Argentina). 2006. Statistics available at www.sagpya.mecon.gov.ar/.

Sengupta, Somini. 2006. "On India's Despairing Farms, a Plague of Suicide." *New York Times,* September 19, p. A1.

Smith, Jeremy. 2005. "European Shelves Mostly GMO-Free." Reuters, February 3.

Stone, Glenn D. 2002. "Both Sides Now: Fallacies in the Genetic Modification Wars, Implications for Developing Countries, and Anthropological Perspectives." *Current Anthropology* 43(4): 611–30.

———. 2005. "A Science of the Gray: Malthus, Marx, and the Ethics of Study Crop Biotechnology." In Lynn Meskel and Peter Pells, eds., *Embedding Ethics: Shifting Boundaries of the Anthropological Profession,* 197–217. New York: Berg.

Sutton, Steven A., Amal H. Assa'ad, Christine Steinmetz, and Marc E. Rothenberg. 2003. "A Negative, Double-Blind, Placebo-Controlled Challenge to Genetically Modified Corn." *Journal of Allergy and Clinical Immunology* 112(5) (November): 1011–12.

Thompson, Jake. 2000. "Governors Promoting Biotech Food." *Omaha World-Herald,* May 3, p. 1.

Traynor, Patricia L., Robert J. Frederick, and Muffy Koch. 2003. *Biosafety and Risk Assessment in Agricultural Biotechnology.* East Lansing, MI: Agricultural Biotechnology Support Project (ABSP) of Michigan State University. http://www.iia.msu.edu/absp/biosafety_workbook.html.

UCS (Union of Concerned Scientists). 2005. "Risks of Genetic Engineering." http://www.ucsusa.org/food_and_environment/genetic_engineering/risks-of-genetic-engineering.html.

———. 2006. Database at http://go.ucsusa.org/food_and_environment/pharm.

USDA (United States Department of Agriculture). 2002. "2002 Annual Report and 2003, 2004, and 2005 Annual Performance Plans." http://www.ars.usda.gov/aboutus/docs.htm?docid=1800&page=3.

———. 2006. "Press Release: Biotechnology Varieties." http://www.nass.usda.gov/Statistics_by_State/Michigan/Publications/Current_News_Release/pr0646.txt.

Warner, Melanie. 2005. "What Is Organic? Powerful Players Want a Say." *New York Times,* November 1, p. C1.

Weiss, Rick. 2006. "Gene-Altered Profit-Killer: A Slight Taint of Biotech Rice Puts Farmers' Overseas Sales in Peril." *Washington Post,* September 21, D1.

SECTION TWO

Ethnographic Studies of Soy's Acceptance

5

Tofu and Related Products in Chinese Foodways

CHEE-BENG TAN

Introduction

Examination of the production and consumption of tofu (bean curd) in a present-day Chinese village in Fujian, and of the significance of this remarkable vegetable-protein food more generally in Chinese life, can increase understanding of the production and consumption processes as well as highlight what can be learned from the Chinese experience. What follows is concerned primarily with the three main tofu products, namely tofu; *doufujiang*, more commonly known as *doujiang*, which is soymilk; and *doufu hua* (soybean custard), or more commonly *douhua*. However, it should be noted that in the process of making tofu, other products can be made as well, including *doufu pi* (tofu skin) and *zhizhu* (tofu sticks). Moreover, fresh tofu can be further processed to make other foods, including *doufu pao* (small blocks of deep-fried tofu puff); *dong doufu* (frozen tofu); and *doufugan* or *dougan*, or dried tofu (fresh tofu that is extrapressed to partly dehydrate it and is then air dried). Dried tofu can be processed yet again to make *xun doufu* (smoked tofu) or *wuxiang doufu* (five-spiced tofu). Dried tofu can also be soaked in brine and fermented to make *chou doufu*, that is, pungent (usually referred to as smelly) tofu, which Hsu and Hsu (1977, 301) translate as "molded beancurd."[1] Tofu can also be fermented to make another product called *doufuru*, or simply *furu*.[2]

Chinese everywhere consume tofu as part and parcel of their food culture. It is called *doufu* in Putonghua (Standard Chinese or Mandarin), *dauh-fuh* in Cantonese, and *tauhu* in Minnanhua or Hokkien (H).[3] Not only is it eaten regularly at home, but many tofu dishes are sold in restaurants and vended at hawker stalls. Certain areas of settlement are even known for their tofu or for particular tofu dishes or derivatives. In Taipei County, Taiwan, for example, Shenkeng Township's restaurants are so well known for their tofu dishes that Shenkeng Tofu has become a household name in that region and Shenkeng Township a mecca for tourists. In Kuala Lumpur, Malaysia, *rang doufu* (stuffed tofu, locally called *yong tauhu*)[4] at Ampang Road is so famous that even the rich patronize the rather ordinary food shops there. Mention Ampang Yong Tauhu and the locals immediately know what you are referring to.

Regional cuisines in China provide a wide range of palatable tofu foods, and a substantial majority of Chinese people are socialized from infancy to eat tofu dishes and related products. The modern interest in health food as well as beliefs about the health-enhancing, nonfattening, and allegedly even beauty-enhancing qualities of tofu and related products (e.g., soybean custard) help to ensure their continuing significance in Chinese foodways.

Historical Background

The history of tofu is obviously linked to that of the soybean in China, which Huang so ably traces in this volume. Soybeans have turned up in archaeological finds from various late prehistoric and early historic sites (Chang 1976, 13). Indeed, archaeologist Cheng Te-k'un (1980, 7) describes the region in northeastern China, northward from the Liao River valley to the Heilongjiang River, as, in ancient times "the world's foremost producer of soya beans."

By the time of the Han dynasty (206 BC–AD 220), soy was an important crop along with rice and wheat (Wang 1984, 31); indeed, soybeans were found in the famous Han tomb (No. 1) of Mawangdui in Changsha (Wang 1984, 97). Yu (1977, 73) points out that during that dynasty, China produced more millet than other grains, but soybeans and wheat were probably more important to the very poor. In the *Han Shu* (Book of Han, first century AD), written by Ban Gu, it was noted that the poor had only soybeans to chew and water to drink (Yu 1977, 73).

More significant is the *Han Shu*'s mention of the prior invention of *shi* (*chi*), fermented and salted soybean, that becomes darker in its final edible form. It is an inexpensive appetizing food that perhaps originated in the Zhou dynasty in the early third century BC (see Li 1955, 194). However, some scholars are of the opinion that it was first processed a bit later, around 200 BC (Yu 1977, 81). In any case, the famous Chinese *Records of History* (*Shiji*, ca. 90 BC) mentions the sale of *shi* during the former (Western) Han dynasty (Li 1948, 170; cf. Yu 1977, 81).

In the *Qimin Yaoshu*,[5] an early Chinese work (AD 544) by Jia Sixie of the Eastern Wei period on the preparation of processed food and liquor, detailed instructions are given for the preparation of *shi* and *jiang*. A primary difference between *shi* and *jiang* is that the former is made from soybeans alone without the addition of any wheat (Li 1948, 172; Li 1955, 194). *Jiang* is clearly a different kind of soy condiment from *shi*. All of this history suggests that the Chinese were quite familiar with making soy-based sauces and fermented soybeans from an early time, even before they knew how to make tofu. Thus, although the *Qimin Yaoshu* describes how to ferment soybeans (*shi* and *jiang*), there is no mention of making tofu.

For a long time, scholars thought that the process of making tofu was invented by the famous Liu An, grandson of the first Han emperor Liu Bang. Known as the "Lord of Huainan," Liu An (179–122 BC) was not only a politician but also a famous scholar. It was the famous Confucian philosopher Zhu Xi (1130–1200) who mentioned that the Lord of Huainan invented the making of bean curd (Chen 1991, 245). Perhaps because of Zhu Xi's stature, subsequent scholars did not question his claim until the version hardened into history. Furthermore, this version was also cited in the famous *Chinese Materia Medica,* written by the celebrated herbalist Li Shizhen. In English publications such as the popular book by Shurtleff and Aoyagi (1979, 112–13), Liu An is also mentioned as having invented tofu. But in the 1950s the Chinese chemist Yuan Hanqing, after searching the early Chinese sources, pointed out the fallacy of tracing the history of tofu to Liu An (Chen 1991, 245).

In the 1960s the Japanese scholar Shinoda Osamu also made a thorough search of Chinese sources without finding any evidence of the Liu An connection. Osamu found the earliest Chinese record in the work of Tao Gu (903–70), which mentioned tofu that the people referred to as *xiao zaiyang,* or "small mutton" (Shinoda 1971, 41). The name given for bean curd, *doufu,* is the same as today. In other words, tofu was already being consumed in the Tang dynasty, and Tao's description indicates that the Chinese already knew about the value of tofu as a substitute for meat. By the time of the Song dynasty (AD 960–1279), there were many references to tofu (Chen 1991, 245–46).

Because of tofu's perishable nature, however, providing archaeological evidence of its presence is difficult. Thus, while there are references to soybeans in archaeological works, there has been no mention of tofu as part of archaeological findings. However, an important essay by Chinese archaeologist Chen Wenhua (1991) describes the drawings of tofu processing in one of the two Han tombs discovered during 1959–60 in Mixian Dahuting Cun in Henan Province.[6] Tofu processing involves soaking the soybeans, milling them, filtering and cooking the soy milk produced, stirring in the coagulant, and pressing the curd to drain off excess water. The Han tomb drawing shows all of these steps except the cooking of the soymilk. Chen thinks that the mural had depicted various kitchen utensils and that perhaps there was no need of special utensils to cook soymilk, so there was no need to draw this step. More to the point, the drawings cannot be about making liquor or sauce. Chen is certain that they are about making tofu. Thus, while the Liu An story is not accurate, it is not incorrect to say that some early type of tofu was already being made during the Han dynasty although two centuries later than Liu An's time (Chen 1991, 247).

By the time of the Tang dynasty (AD 618–907) tofu was a common product in China, and it was introduced to Japan in the later Tang or early Song dynasty (AD 960–1279) (Huang 2000, 318). By the sixteenth century it had become localized as a Japanese food (Shinoda 1971, 54). Tofu was also introduced to Korea and Vietnam, where today it is an important component of local foodways.[7]

Production and Marketing of Tofu

Today tofu is produced on a small scale or family basis and in big factories, both in China and around the world. The small-scale production of tofu harkens back to the past. This can be seen clearly in the inland Fujian village in Yongchun County where I conducted fieldwork during academic vacation periods in 1989, 1999, and 2001. This is a Chen-surnamed village, which I call Beautiful Jade. It had a population of 1,238 persons in 1998 when I began my research there. There are two families that make tofu, soybean custard, and soymilk for sale to the villagers. In both families a husband-wife team, with children helping, does all of the processing. The description here is based on the observation of Mr. and Mrs. A, who learned the trade from Mrs. A's mother's brother (see figure 1).

First, soak the soybeans for two or three hours to soften them for grinding. Next, put the beans through an electric grinder, adding water while grinding. The ground product is then put into a big wok to cook. It takes about half an hour to cook six *jin* of soybeans (each *jin* being approxi-

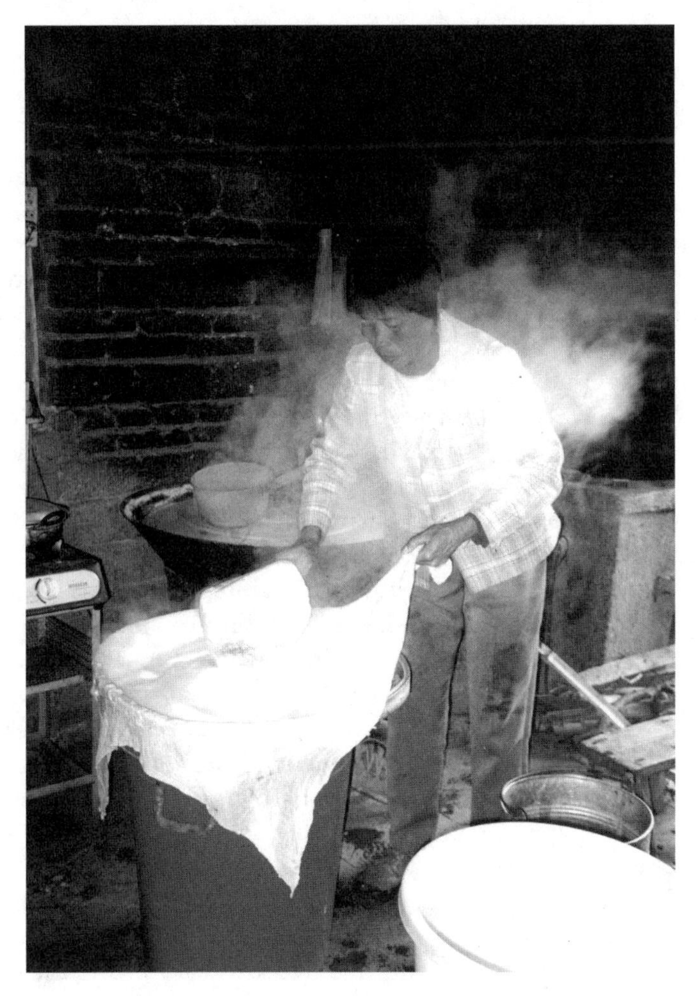

Figure 1. Tofu making in a Yongchun village, Fujian: filtering. (Photo by C. B. Tan, 1999)

mately half a kilogram). The cooked soybean paste is filtered through a cloth to produce the *tau ning* (H), the soymilk, which is collected in a container. The remaining lees are called *tau che* (H), which Mr. and Mrs. A use to feed their three pigs. To make tofu, *chio gou* (H) (gypsum) is added to the soymilk. For six *jin* of soybeans, about one hundred grams of gypsum are added. The measured gypsum is put in a bowl, water is added, and the dissolved gypsum is stirred before being poured into the soymilk. The soymilk is then stirred; after ten minutes it becomes *tau-hu hua* (H), or soybean custard. To further process this into tofu, the soybean custard is put in four wooden trays (called *tau* in Minnan dialect) covered with *tau-hu geng* (H), or tofu cloth.

The semisolidified tofu is wrapped in the tofu cloth and tied. A flat piece of wood is put on top of the tofu in the wooden trays. In addition, a stone weight is placed on top of each wrapped tofu to press out the water. After half an hour, the weights are removed and the wraps opened. A wooden mold, bearing square block impressions, is placed on the newly formed tofu to mark it off into small blocks that can be easily cut. The tofu is now ready for sale. The wooden mold is 28 × 28 cm square and is 13 cm in thickness. Each demarked square measures 7 × 7 cm, the size of a block of tofu sold. Firmer tofu is made by leaving the weights in place longer to dewater the tofu further.

The whole process of making tofu from grinding beans to pressing takes only an hour. For small-scale production as described here one person can handle the job, but it is easier with two. It is thus suitable for cottage industry. Each day Mr. and Mrs. A make tofu from about thirty *jin* (approximately thirty kilograms) of soybeans, but for the Chinese New Year they use more than one hundred *jin*. They buy their beans from a shop in the nearby market town. These are beans from Hunan Province. In the past the villagers planted soybeans but gave it up because of plant diseases.

In 1999 the beans cost 1.50 yuan[8] per *jin*, while gypsum cost .60 yuan per *jin*. Every morning either Mr. A or Mrs. A carried the tofu, soymilk, and soybean custard in containers and baskets on a shoulder pole to sell to villagers door to door. Each piece of bean curd was sold at 0.35 yuan in 1999. Labor-intensive production at low cost yields an inexpensive product.

Thus soymilk, soybean custard, and tofu are made serially, each of the first two being transformable into the next. The invention of this process in ancient China was revolutionary, but once invented it remained essentially the same until the present. The famed Chinese physician Li Shizhen of the Ming dynasty described the making of tofu as follows:

1. Soak the beans (in water).
2. Grind the beans (to give a bean milk).
3. Filter the milk (to remove coarse residues).
4. Cook the milk (to homogeneity).
5. Add *yen lu* (bittern), leaf of *shan fan* (mountain alum),[9] or vinegar to curdle the milk.
6. Collect the curd. (Huang 2000, 303)

This description still holds. The difference today is primarily in mechanization and scale of production. There are sometimes variations in the order of steps, however. In the Beautiful Jade (Fujian) case described above, the product was cooked before filtering. Lin Ming-Teh (1999) also observed this order of steps in a factory in Taiwan: soaking, grinding, cooking, filtering, adding gypsum, and pressing. However, in the case of the Gao Village described below, the soymilk is filtered before cooking. Thus, it appears that it does not matter whether the milk is cooked or filtered first.

The availability of electricity in the modern industrial era has made tofu production quite easy unlike in the preindustrial era, when the life of a tofu maker was considered very tough because the beans had to be ground by manual labor for hours. The arduous life of making tofu without the use of electricity is described by Mobo Gao, speaking of her mother in pre-1978 Gao Village in Jiangxi Province:

> My mother used to make tofu once every month as a kind of business. She would grind soya beans first with water on a family mill, then she would use a cloth net to extract the liquid. The liquid would then be heated in a huge wok with baked gypsum until it boiled. It would then be left to cool until it became jelly-like. Finally my mother would put the jelly into a cloth which would be placed under a mill stone, and had the water squeezed out until she had solid tofu. She would have to spend several hours in the evening grinding the soya beans. Then she would spend the whole of the next day finishing the rest of the work. It was an agonizing process for a woman with bound feet. When other villagers came to get some tofu, they would give my mother the amount of soya beans required to make the same amount of tofu. All my mother would get in return for her labor was enough raw materials for the next load of tofu as well as the soya bean residue, which was good for the family pigs. (Gao 1999, 56)

Gao describes the production and consumption of tofu in a region where the poor villagers planted soybeans. In such a region tofu is an important source of protein, and apparently all families knew how to make it. Gao (1999, 56) describes how when one household made tofu, others would either borrow some pieces or would give some soybeans in exchange for equivalent pieces of tofu. Those who borrowed would return the same amount of tofu when they themselves made it. In this way not all households needed to make tofu every day.

While the soybean is a cheap source of protein and "yields more usable protein per acre than other common cultivated plants" (Simoons 1991, 71), it is not a staple food like rice. The Gao villagers eventually allocated more land for rice planting, as rice could be planted twice a year and its "unit yield in terms of quantity is much higher than the soya bean yield or [that of] any other crop" (Gao 1999, 57). This was during the Mao Zedong era when villagers did not have access to modern farming techniques that might have increased soy yields.

In the post-Mao period, many Gao villagers migrated to coastal cities to work. The money they sent back to the village, along with the emergence of sideline production and entrepreneurship among farmers, led to commercialization of many goods. Villagers now go to the markets more often to buy things. They no longer make their tofu; instead, they buy it (Gao 1999, 58). Here we see that in China, as people move away from a subsistence farm economy, tofu becomes a market commodity.

The process of making tofu in modern factories (cf. Lin 1999) is surprisingly quite similar to what I have described. When Professor Sidney Mintz and I did research on tofu consumption in Hong Kong in 1999, we visited a tofu factory that employed thirty workers. While the process of making tofu was mechanized, the soaking of beans and the final pressing to dewater were still manual. As in the family production described above, soymilk and soybean custard were produced, too.

Also as in the family production, the leavings were not wasted: they were sent to the mainland for fish feed. In the 1960s, Osgood (1975, 393) reported that the leavings from the small family factory that he studied in Hong Kong were used to feed pigs, as in the Fujian village described above. Interesting research in Japan and China reveals that silkworms raised partly on soybean dregs can produce bright, good-quality silk (Matsubara 1993; Wu, Xu, Miao, and Zeng 1996). This new way of using tofu lees could further protect their status from being merely industrial waste. However, due to the complicated technical facilities needed for this method and therefore its higher cost, this approach to silk production has not yet been applied commercially.[10]

Traditional tofu production can remain a small-scale, small-town enterprise, as I observed in a small coastal community called Bintulu in Sarawak, Malaysia, in 2000. A little Chinese shop there sold soymilk and soybean custard, both warm and iced. The shopkeeper made these soyfoods herself. The simple way of producing tofu can also be observed in Vietnam. My observation of a tofu-making, Vietnamese husband-wife couple in Hanoi in 2003 suggests that family-based production in Vietnam accords with that of Beautiful Jade in rural Fujian. However, the Hanoi tofu was tubular in shape, and the couple claimed that Vietnamese tofu is better than Chinese tofu because no gypsum is used. The couple explained that instead, they add some "overnight soy juice" to cause coagulation (for more details on Vietnamese tofu production, see the essay by Can Van Nguyen in this volume).

Tofu production is basically an urban phenomenon, where there is a sufficient concentration of consumers to make its manufacture profitable. Hence, in Malaysia I have not come across tofu production in truly rural areas, even where there are Chinese. Tofu sold in rural village shops is bought from towns, while soymilk and soybean custard are generally sold only in towns. The situation in China is special, as the rural population (in Fujian, for example) tends to be concentrated and quite big, and tofu production has been one of the few ways in the post-Mao era for people in the less prosperous interior regions to earn cash. As we have seen, even in soybean-producing areas, tofu has become a market commodity rather than a homemade product for family consumption. In rural communities such as Beautiful Jade or a Dong community in Longsheng, Guangxi, that I observed in May 2001, one or two local families make tofu for sale to fellow villagers.

Tofu of different sizes and types, along with related products, is sold in morning wet markets all over urban China. In some urban centers there are still peddlers selling tofu, carrying the products in baskets or containers hung over a shoulder pole. I saw this in Yongchun County's seat and in Chengdu, Sichuan, in 1999. Different provinces and regions of China have their local varieties of this fresh tofu. In Kunming, for example, it is common to see tofu sold in big blocks; these are called *ban doufu*. In the wet market of Ganluo County's seat in Sichuan Province, I observed tofu sold in big blocks too, although they were smaller than those I saw in Kunming. However, the smaller blocks of soft and firm tofu are more common everywhere in China and overseas. In areas where soybeans are produced, younger beans called *maodou*[11] or hairy beans (*edamame* in Japanese) are commonly sold too. These are for cooking and eating directly, with relatively minimal processing. In Kunming at a morning market on May 15, 1999, I observed a seller grinding these green beans; the product was sold to make porridge.

The supermarkets of cities such as Hong Kong sell not only locally manufactured tofu and related products but also nicely packaged imported items. In Hong Kong there are attractively packaged soymilk and soybean custard from Japan and Canada. It is very much a globalized market. Even the locally made tofu may be manufactured from beans imported from the United States or Canada. In fact, Hong Kong manufacturers prefer the larger soybeans from the United States and Canada over those from China. Lin Ming-Teh (1999, 25) reports the same preference at the tofu factory he visited in Taiwan.

China used to be the largest producer of soybeans; in the early twentieth century, Manchuria alone accounted for 90 percent of the world's soybean exports (Wolff 2001, 246). The plentiful Manchurian beans allowed soyfoods to become widely consumed by all classes in Japan (Wolff 2001, 248). Today, however, the United States is the world's largest producer (Shurtleff and Aoyagi 1979, 3; Du Bois and Mintz 2002), while in South America, Argentina and Brazil have also emerged as major growers (figure 2) (Lindsay 2004; Rohter 2003; Sousa and Vieira in this volume).

Soybeans are of course still produced in various parts of China, especially in the northeast. It is common to see soybean plants in rural Sichuan as well. In a Yi village near Ganluo that I visited in August 1999, I saw soybeans planted between rice plots, enabling farmers to make full use of the available land. Soy's nitrogen-fixing abilities make it an excellent choice for crop rotations (Simoons 1991, 71). Nevertheless, China today depends on imports of soybeans to meet its rapidly growing demand. China

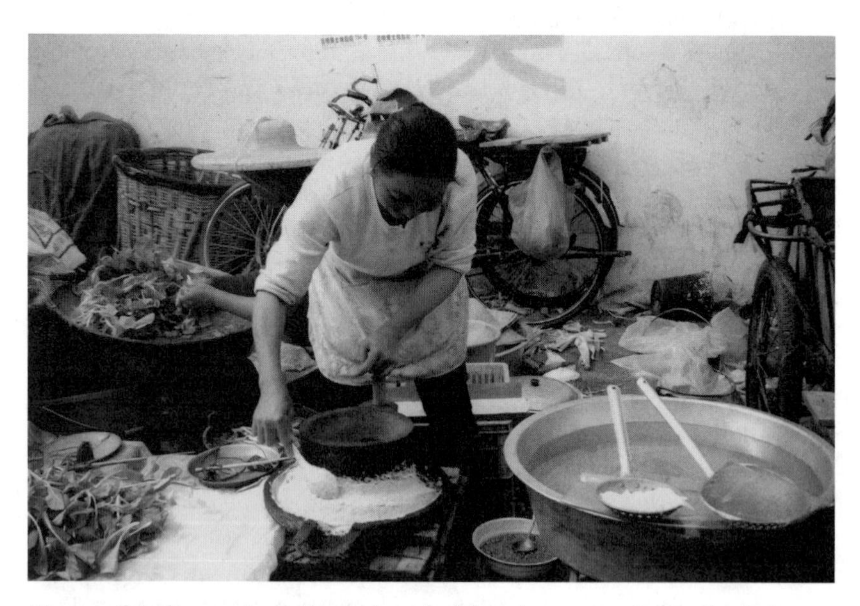

Figure 2. Grinding unripe soybeans (*maodou*) for sale at a morning market in Kunming, Yunnan. (Photo by C. B. Tan, 1999)

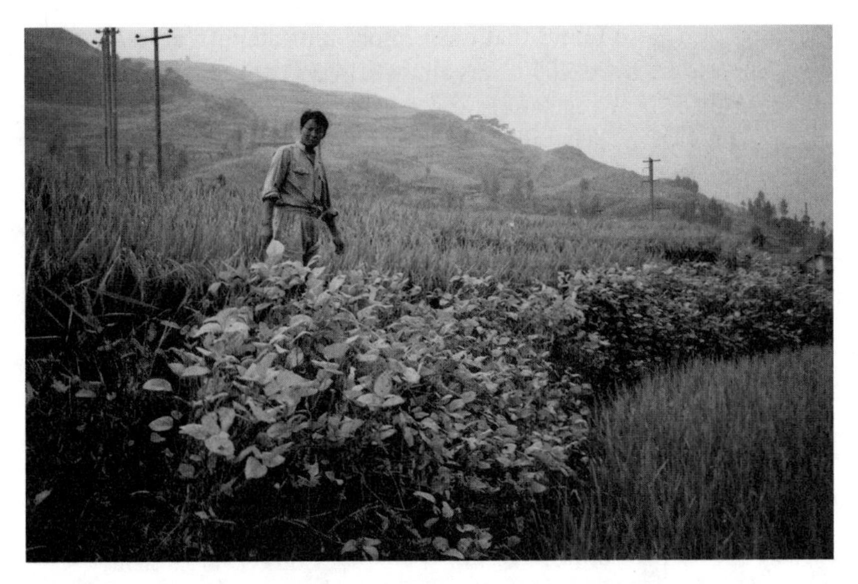

Figure 3. Soybean plants in between rice plots in a village in Ganluo County, Sichuan. (Photo by C. B. Tan, 1999)

imported 14.5 million metric tons of soybeans in 2002 (Bloomberg 2003, 6) and 20.7 million tons in 2003 (Tuan, Fang, and Cao 2004). Although shifts in Chinese trade policies disrupted such imports somewhat in 2004, China is expected to continue importing ever-growing quantities of soy for quite some time (figure 3) (Tuan, Fang, and Cao 2004).

Consumption: Tofu and Chinese Foodways

Tofu is an inseparable part of Chinese foodways, as essential as pork, chicken, and various kinds of vegetables. Tofu is part of the primary diet of ordinary Chinese, who are socialized from infancy to eat tofu and related products. The Chinese grow up acquiring a good knowledge of tofu dishes and related soyfoods.

Hence, Anderson and Anderson (1977, 328) aptly point out that rice, tofu, and cabbage or mustard leaves (which may be pickled) make up the ordinary person's household food in South China. Similarly, Mintz and Tan (2001, 121) found in their Hong Kong research that home was where tofu was eaten regularly. This suggests the significance of home and socialization in Chinese tofu consumption. In the same study, Mintz and

Tan (2001, 121) also found that most informants ate tofu at least once a week but seldom by itself;[12] it was almost always cooked with meat (usually pork or fish) or vegetables, and was also used to make soup. These findings fit with my general knowledge of Chinese foodways in Malaysia and Singapore as well.

A very simple way of cooking tofu is with bean sprouts. The sprouts may be from green peas or soybeans, but the latter are larger and coarser. This is a common home dish among ordinary Chinese Malaysians, and it is obviously a healthy one. Mely Tan (2002, 169) reports that this is a common dish in Indonesia too, although there instead of tofu the bean sprouts may be stir-fried with *tempe,* fermented soybean cake.

A unique feature of tofu is its ability to absorb juice from the meat and vegetables that it is cooked with, and it can be combined almost endlessly with other foods. This enables people to make all kinds of dishes, and over time each region of China has produced its special tofu recipes. The long history of tofu consumption in China and the country's great regional diversity have enabled China to develop hundreds and perhaps thousands of such recipes. Even the Qing scholar Yuan Mei (1984) listed nine vegetarian tofu dishes in his small but famous recipe book. Today's Chinese cookbooks list many tofu dishes (e.g., Liang 2002; Lin Haiyin 1971, 171–215).

Some tofu dishes known throughout China are reproduced or imitated by restaurants. An example is Wensi Doufu, a vegetarian dish invented by the monk Wen Si in Yangzhou of Jiangsu (for a recipe, see Zhou 1986, 82). A more widely known example is Mapo tofu. Originating in Sichuan, it is now available in Chinese restaurants all over the world but is often adapted to suit particular types of Chinese tastes. In Hong Kong, for example, the Chinese generally do not eat hot peppery foods, and so the Mapo tofu in most restaurants there is really not hot and certainly not numbingly hot as is the case with Sichuan foods. To those who are used to the authentic Sichuan style, it falls short.

Thus, certain standard Chinese tofu dishes have become globalized as they have spread to different Chinese centers worldwide. At the same time these dishes have been adapted in accordance with the tastes of differing migrant groups of Chinese. This makes marketing space for the selling of authenticity. Even in Hong Kong, there are specialist Sichuan restaurants that sell authentic Mapo tofu. This is also a good example of global homogenization and global differentiation, to use Goody's terms (Goody 1998, 166), even within Chinese food. There is also local adaptation through the influence of non-Chinese foodways and ingredients. Thus, tofu recipes are always part of a regional diet, being "the food of a community" and hence part of a "genuine cuisine" (Mintz 1996, 96).

Among Chinese overseas, *rang doufu* (stuffed tofu), usually tofu stuffed with fish meat, is linked with the Hakka[13] identity. *Rang doufu* is a very popular food in ordinary Chinese restaurants and at food stalls in Malaysia, where tofu is not only stuffed with minced fish meat but also with long chili, slices of bitter gourd, and eggplant. In Taiwan, *rang doufu* is also associated with the Hakka. In fact, in Mainland China the Hakka are known for their *rang doufu* too, even though it is also made by other Chinese (Zhen 1990, 128). But although the association of *rang doufu* with the Hakka has its origins in China, the linkage is more pronounced in Southeast Asia and in Taiwan. In these places, where different Chinese groups coexist in the same towns, people strongly associate this food with the Hakka in particular.

The migration of Chinese overseas helped to spread the eating of tofu worldwide. Chinese in Malaysia and Singapore, for example, have both traditional and locally innovated Chinese dishes, many of which use tofu. Even the fire pot style of eating that is popular during winter in northern China (Hsu and Hsu 1977, 310) is very common in many Chinese restaurants in these tropical countries. Called *man-lo*[14] (Hokkien for *menlu*) in Malaysia and Singapore, this kind of eating involves diners sitting around a table that has a gas stove in the center. As the pot containing clear soup boils, diners put into it raw meat (usually chicken and seafood), vegetables, eggs, tofu, and, toward the end of a meal when the soup has become very tasty, noodles. As the cooked food is consumed, new batches of meat and vegetables are added. This can go on until everyone is satisfied. What is interesting here is that tofu is an essential item for a fire pot, both in northern China as reported by Hsu and Hsu (ibid.) and in these tropical countries. Perhaps tofu is favored because it absorbs appealing flavors from the soup.

In Southeast Asia, Chinese migrants also influenced the cooking styles and recipes of the local non-Chinese populations. In fact, the Malay-Indonesian word *tauhu* is derived from the Hokkien term for tofu, as is *taugeh* for bean sprouts that, as already noted, ordinary people often cook with tofu. There is a very popular tofu snack shared by all Malaysians including indigenous Malays. Fried firm tofu cut into two pieces is stuffed with shredded raw cucumber and boiled bean sprouts. Some homemade chili sauce is put into the stuffed tofu, and this delicious item is prized by Malaysians, who like spicy food. Another popular Malay dish that makes use of tofu is *lontong*. This is of Javanese origin and thus is especially popular among the Malays of Javanese descent. *Lontong* is rice wrapped in coconut or banana leaves and then boiled and eaten with a vegetarian curry dish, which contains among other things strips of firm tofu and *tempe*. *Tempe*, fermented soybean cake, is a popular soyfood among the Javanese in Indonesia. Myra Sidharta and I visited a *tempe* factory in Marang in December 2002, and we found that the process of making *tempe* is actually quite simple.[15]

In urban centers in Mainland China, Taiwan, Hong Kong, Macau, Singapore, Malaysia, and many Chinese settlements in the diaspora, soymilk and soybean custard are commonly sold. In Chengdu, Sichuan, in 1999, these products were easily available even at roadside stalls. Mintz and Tan (2001, 122) also found soymilk and soybean custard to be popularly consumed in Hong Kong, although not as much as tofu, which is used in cooking. The soymilk and soybean custard are snack foods. The growing concern for food that is healthful and not fattening is making their consumption popular. Media reports depicting tofu and related products as healthy help to reinforce the association of tofu products with well-being.[16]

In Hong Kong, innovations cater to customers' tastes, with some shop outlets serving flavored soymilks and soybean custards. These products bear appealing names such as ginger juice soymilk, coconut milk *dau-fa* (Cantonese for "soybean custard"), chocolate *dau-fa*, etc. While most Chinese in Hong Kong prefer to buy their tofu fresh at wet markets rather than packaged at the supermarket, bottled soymilk and packaged soybean custard, including imported items, are popular with shoppers; they are convenient for storing in the refrigerator and for eating as snacks at any time. Soybean custard packaged in single portions is also convenient for individual eating, as it can be brought along easily when one is moving about (figure 4).

Overall, both socialization and modern marketing strategies ensure the persistent consumption of tofu and related products in Chinese populations. Wet markets and supermarkets represent both the traditional sale of fresh products and the modern sale of globalized packaged foods. We have also seen that as people move from a subsistence to a commercial economy, tofu becomes a market commodity (i.e., not homemade), and as the local economy becomes more engaged with the global market, consumers also become involved in a globalized market for these products, consuming both local and imported soyfoods.

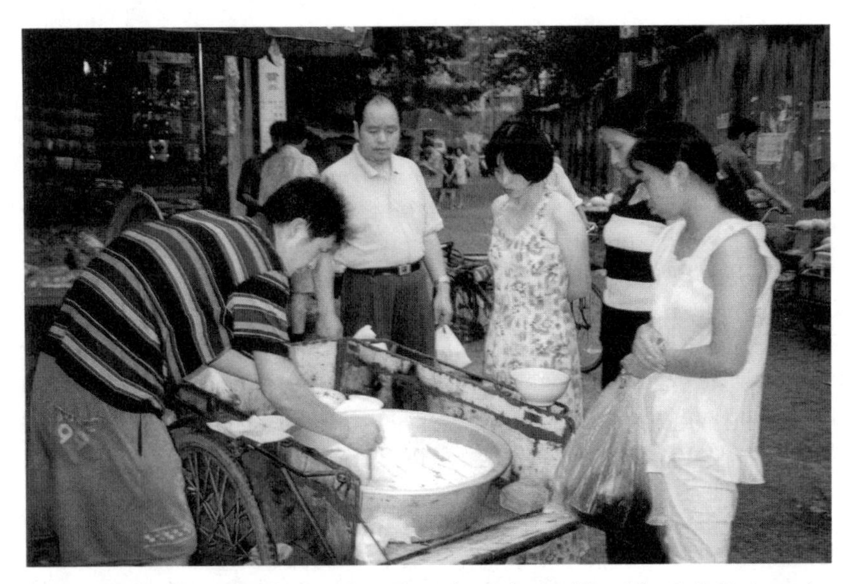

Figure 4. Selling bean curd custard in Chengdu, Sichuan. (Photo by C. B. Tan, 1999)

Tofu's Symbolic Associations

In Beautiful Jade, cooked tofu is one of the food items offered to gods and ancestors. For example, on the Chinese New Year's Eve, the first worship is to the Kitchen God. I observed in February 1999 that all the families in the Half Moon Hill section of the village included in their offerings to the god a plate of fried firm tofu cut into triangles and another plate of the same dish cut into the usual squares. Asked why they offered two plates of tofu in different shapes, I was told that in so doing they were offering two items representing two different dishes instead of just one. For cash-poor villagers, tofu is included as an offering of the same status as fish or meat. However, my observation of Chinese offerings in Malaysia suggest that there at least, tofu by itself does not have special religious significance; it can be included as an offering, but it is not an essential one.

Rather than having any particular religious symbolism, the significance of tofu is that it is an uncomplicated and cheap food for the poor to use in offerings or for the preparation of a simple funeral meal. Among the Baba, who are Malay-speaking Chinese in Melaka, Malaysia, pork rice porridge called *bah-be*[17] (the term is derived from Hokkien) is served on the day of the funeral. This is porridge cooked with lean pork and tofu strips and spiced with soy sauce. It is a simple, delicious, and easily prepared dish that allows mourners and friends to have a quick meal before the funeral procession.

While the Chinese regularly eat tofu, symbolically it remains a cheap food for the poor. This usually keeps tofu from rising to the level of haute cuisine, even though five-star restaurants may have special tofu dishes that are anything but cheap (see the essay by Jianhua Mao in this volume). Thus, when Chinese people prepare food for guests at home, tofu is usually not chosen unless one really has difficulty providing meat dishes. At restaurants, it is usually at the request of guests that the host orders a tofu dish, lest he or she be seen as avoiding the more expensive foods. While tofu is cheap, in places that do not produce soybeans and where tofu is a market commodity, cash-poor people may not even buy tofu and eat it regularly. It is, after all, not a staple.

This association of tofu with the prosaic and inexpensive is not necessarily negative. In Chinese, *doufu guan* (tofu official) refers to an official who is not corrupt, as historically those who were not corrupt did not enrich themselves and therefore could not afford foods fancier than tofu. On the other hand, because tofu is soft and crumbles easily if handled carelessly, linguistically it can symbolize something that has no solid foundation. Hence, projects that are faulty because of corruption can be described as tofu projects.[18] In Chinese there are many idioms involving tofu, referring mainly to its soft texture, to its status as a cheap food, or to the historically tough life of a person who depended on making and selling tofu for a living (see Zhu 1971 on tofu in Mandarin Chinese). Thus, tofu is important not just in Chinese foodways but also in Chinese language and thought.

Conclusion

Tofu was invented in China and remains an important food for the Chinese, both in China and in the diaspora. It has contributed to the diversification of Chinese cuisines, enriching both meat and vegetarian dishes.

Like rice porridge, tofu is important for both rich and poor Chinese. When available, tofu provides essential protein for the poor. Thus, and again like rice porridge, in the context of want it is associated with poverty. There are many unique dishes both for rice porridge and tofu in Chinese foodways. Tofu is particularly significant as it is a protein food, and it can be prepared in multiple ways: fried, steamed, boiled, and cooked via many other techniques besides. In this respect it is also like various kinds of Chinese noodles, which can be cooked in many ways and from which numerous novel dishes can be fashioned. In Southeast Asia, the introduction of Chinese noodles has led to the creation of various Malay and Indian styles of noodles. This is true of tofu too. Thus, rice porridge, noodles, and tofu represent three important Chinese contributions to the globe's diverse foodways.

Today tofu has entered the foodways of many cultures worldwide. Chinese migrants have played important roles in this globalization. These migrants and those from other East Asian societies constitute major tofu consumers wherever they go. The restaurants that they and their descendants run no doubt contribute to the diffusion of tofu dishes to people of different ethnic origins and from many walks of life.

The historic adoption of tofu in Japan added to the diversity of tofu consumption, and Japan, like China, plays a crucial role in popularizing tofu and soy products (especially soy sauce) worldwide. In fact China, Japan, Korea, and Vietnam may be considered the core tofu culture areas, where the greatest number of tofu cuisines are to be found and thus where tofu and related foods have continued to spread worldwide.

The concern with health food and the popularity of vegetarianism among some in North America and Europe have also helped to introduce tofu to non-Asian populations. Medical reports about newly discovered healthful properties of soybeans help to promote tofu and soyfoods both in Asia and in the West.[19] Even McDonald's came up with a Tofu Burger, introduced in the Japanese market (BBC News 2003; Nakamoto and Rahman 2003). But science also brings new controversy, the issue of genetically modified food being a case in point; most American soybeans are genetically modified.[20]

Soymilk has become a nutritious drink able to compete with a whole range of globalized beverages. Soybean custard as a delicious and healthy snack is still generally confined to Chinese and other Asian consumers, but with the advent of modern packaged items in supermarkets and with more reports about soy as a health food, it has great potential to become a globalized snack. Not only restaurants but also supermarkets help to introduce tofu and related products to non-Asian consumers, especially in North America, Europe, Australia, and New Zealand.

The Chinese experience shows that tofu and related products can help make cuisines more diverse and tasteful. This hedonic allure is important for promoting tofu consumption. Chinese experiences in simple tofu production and in myriad ways of cooking it can show people from cultures not familiar with tofu, including those individuals who choose tofu for health or other compelling reasons (e.g., vegetarianism), how to enjoy eating this food.

However, real adoption by populations beyond those of East Asian origins requires localization of tofu recipes into their own foodways. In other words, Chinese ways of eating tofu cannot be copied exactly if tofu is to be accepted as part of another people's cuisine. If tofu is to become a part of South Indian foodways, for example, it has to be cooked in ways acceptable to the Indians, such as in curries. The French in France may enjoy eating tofu in Chinese restaurants, but if it is not localized into their cuisine, it cannot become a part of the usual French diet. We have seen the culinary adaptability of tofu, so culinary indigenization of tofu and related products is clearly quite possible. What hinders it is the lack of tofu dietary exposure, and in this respect Chinese and other East Asian restaurants still play an important role in introducing tofu dishes to nontofu eaters. As for the poor in regions where tofu is not eaten, publicity portraying tofu as a vegetarian meat substitute along with information about how to adapt it to local cuisines (see the essays by Osborn and Du Bois in this volume) should help to make this healthy food more appreciated and accepted.

Notes

1. Smelly tofu is easily available in such cities as Chengdu and Kunming in West China. It is also very common in Taiwan, and in Tam Kang, not far from Taipei, there are a number of smelly tofu stalls. In Hong Kong, the strict laws against pollution make the selling of smelly tofu rather difficult, as sellers may be prosecuted for air pollution (Mintz and Tan 2001, 126). In Southeast Asia smelly tofu is not commonly found.

2. Various parts of China have their own famous brands of *furu,* much as with tofu itself. The technique of making fermented tofu has been extensively described in Chinese. In English, see Huang (2000, 326–28) for a good description.

3. In this essay, Chinese transcription is in Putonghua (Mandarin) unless otherwise specified. Minnanhua transcription is indicated by "H." Minnanhua is the language spoken by the Chinese of southern Fujian origin, and those in Southeast Asia identify themselves as Hokkien (derived from the name Fujian pronounced in Minnanhua). The Hokkien are the largest Chinese speech group in Malaysia, Singapore, and Indonesia.

4. *Rang doufu* is also popularly called *niang doufu. Yong tauhu* is the Cantonese pronunciation of *niang doufu.*

5. For an English summary of how to make fermented soybean as detailed in the *Qimin Yaoshu,* see Li (1948, 171–74).

6. The mural was not reported until 1981, when it was mentioned in a publication compiled by the Henan provincial museum (Chen 1991, 246).

7. The history of tofu, its production, and related products are described and assessed comprehensively by Huang (2000).

8. US$1 is about 8.27 Chinese yuan.

9. This leaf is a thin sheet of mineral.

10. I am grateful to Dr. Ji Dongfeng, director of the Institute of Sericulture, Zhejiang Academy of Agricultural Science, for this information. I also thank Dr. Yang Jian of the College of Humanities & Social Sciences, Nanjing Agricultural University, for helping me get in touch with Dr. Ji.

11. Both the pods and beans are green in color in contrast with fully ripened and sun-dried beans, which are yellowish and are used for making tofu.

12. With proper sauce, tofu by itself can be delicious too. *Liangban doufu,* for example, is cold tofu dipped in a sauce at the time of eating. For the best taste, it is usually boiled in hot water, then dipped in cold water to chill it, and finally flavored with the sauce. I ate a similar dish in Kamakura, Japan, in December 1999. Called *yudofu,* it is tofu in boiled water. Just before it is eaten, it is taken out of the water and flavored with soy sauce. It is quite simple yet elegant and delicious. A more common preparation in Chinese snack shops is the deep-frying of tofu that has been coated with flour. Called *cuipi doufu,* or crispy skin tofu, it is flavored with some sauce for eating. Below the crispy outer coat is white, soft, warm tofu.

13. Hakka is an important Chinese speech group in Malaysia and Taiwan, and in fact there are Hakka Chinese in different parts of the world. Their ancestral homeland is in the eastern Guangdong and western Fujian provinces in China.

14. The final vowel is here an open midback one.

15. With one method of making *tempe,* soybeans are soaked for about six hours and then half-cooked for about half an hour. The skins are next removed in a machine. After this, the beans are put in a huge basket and mixed with a mold starter. They are then laid out on a flat platform or in a tube for thirty-six hours, after which they become *tempe.* See the essay by Myra Sidharta in this volume for more details.

16. For a Chinese physician's analysis of the health properties of soyfoods, including tofu and soymilk, see Li (1999).

17. The final vowel here is a *schwa* (midcentral neutral).

18. For example, Kwan (1999) discussed "tofu" building projects in China. In fact, one can find many items in a Google search in Chinese under *doufu gongcheng* (tofu projects).

19. See, for example, Anonymous (2001) for a report arguing that plant-based estrogens in soy, or phytoestrogens, help to reduce the threat of Alzheimer's disease in postmenopausal women. Soybean is also portrayed as good for the fights against breast cancer and heart disease (Margaret Cheng 1999). Whether true or not, such reports in Hong Kong reinforce the value of eating soyfoods.

20. Although most American soybeans are genetically modified, the soybeans used to make tofu in the United States generally are not. Tofu manufacturers are aware of the controversy surrounding genetically modified products and are careful to protect their market shares. Most genetically modified soybeans in the United States are fed to chickens and pigs. I thank Dr. Christine M. Du Bois for pointing this out to me.

References

Anderson, E. N., Jr., and Marja L. Anderson. 1977. "Modern China: South." In K. C. Chang, ed., *Food in Chinese Culture: Anthropological and Historical Perspectives,* 317–82. New Haven, CT: Yale University Press.

Anonymous. 2001. "Preliminary Soy Studies Suggest Reduction of Alzheimer's Threat in Postmenopausal Women." *Doctor* 2(4): 1. Hong Kong.

BBC News. 2003. "McDonald's Tastes Revival." http://news.bbc.co.uk/2/hi/business/3134325.stm.

Bloomberg. 2003. "Soya Bean Import Surge Blamed for Bottleneck." *South China Morning Post,* June 8, 2003, p. 6.

Chang, K. C. 1976. *Early Chinese Civilization: Anthropological Perspectives.* Cambridge: Harvard University Press.

Chen, Wenhua. 1991. "Doufu Qiyuan yu Heshi" ["When was the Origin of Beancurd?"]. *Nongyue Kaogu* [*Archaeology of Agriculture*] 21: 245–48.

Cheng, Margaret. 1999. "The Great Soybean Phenomenon." *South China Morning Post,* July 16, p. 20.

Cheng, Te-k'un. 1980. *The World of the Chinese: A Struggle for Human Unity.* Hong Kong: Chinese University Press.

Du Bois, Christine M., and Sidney W. Mintz. 2002. "Soy." In S. Katz, ed., *Encyclopedia of Food and Culture,* Vol. 3, 322–26. New York: Scribner.

Gao, Mobo C. F. 1999. *Gao Village: Rural Life in Modern China.* Hong Kong: Hong Kong University Press.

Goody, Jack. 1998. *Food and Love: A Cultural History of East and West.* London: Verso.

Hsu, Vera Y. N., and Francis L. K. Hsu. 1977. "Modern China: North." In K. C. Chang, ed., *Food in Chinese Culture: Anthropological and Historical Perspectives,* 295–316. New Haven, CT: Yale University Press.

Huang, H. T. 2000. *Fermentations and Food Science,* Vol. 6, Pt. 5, *Biology and Biological Technology,* of *Science and Civilisation in China.* Cambridge: Cambridge University Press.

Kwan, Daniel. 1999. "Delegates Attack $93b Waste on 'Tofu' Building Projects." *South China Morning Post,* March 13, 1999, p. 9.

Li, Ch'iao-p'ing. 1948. *The Chemical Arts of Old China.* Easton, PA: Journal of Chemical Education. Original Chinese edition published in 1940; revised Chinese edition published in 1955.

———. 1955. *Zhongguo Huaxue Shi* [*History of Chinese Chemistry*], rev. ed. Taipei: Taiwan Shangwu Yinshuguan.

Li, Jiaxiong. 1999. "Doufu Yangsheng Liaoli" ["Tofu and the Management of Health"]. *Zhongguo Yinshi Wenhua* [*Quarterly of the Foundation of Chinese Dietary Culture*] 5(4): 10–15.

Lin, Haiyin, ed. 1971. *Zhongguo Doufu* [*Tofu in China*]. Taipei: Chun Wenxue Chubanshe.

Lin, Ming-Teh. 1999. "Daxi Doufu Wenhua de Tansuo (Zhong)" [A Study of the Tofu Culture of Daxi: Part 2"]. *Zhongguo Yinshi Wenhua* [*Quarterly of the Foundation of Chinese Dietary Culture*] 5(4): 24–29.

Lindsay, Reed. 2004. "Soya Beans Rescue Argentina, but Many Fear the Long-term Cost." *South China Morning Post,* April 19, p. A11.

Matsubara, Fujiyoshi. 1993. "The Yellow Variation of Silk Produced by Silkworms Fed on an Artificial Diet and Mulberry Leaves." *Nisanshi* [*Journal of Japanese Silkworms*] 62(2): 162–64 [in Japanese].

Mintz, Sidney. 1996. *Tasting Food, Tasting Freedom: Excursion into Eating, Culture, and the Past.* Boston: Beacon.

Mintz, Sidney W., and Chee-Beng Tan. 2001. "Bean-Curd Consumption in Hong Kong." *Ethnology* 40(2): 113–28.

Nakamoto, Michiyo, and Bayan Rahman. 2003. "McDonald's Japan Tries a New Recipe." *Financial Times* (London), August 9, p. 11.

Osgood, Cornelius. 1975. *The Chinese: A Study of a Hong Kong Community.* 3 vols. Tuscon: University of Arizona Press.

Rohter, Larry. 2003. "Soybean Boom Sows Seeds of Discontent in Brazil." *South China Morning Post,* September 23, p. A14.

Shinoda, Osamu. 1971. "Doufu Kao" ["The Study of Tofu"]. In Lin Haiyin, ed., *Zhongguo Doufu* [*Tofu in China*], 39–58. Taipei: Chun Wenxue Chubanshe.

Shurtleff, William, and Akiko Aoyagi. 1979. *The Book of Tofu: Food for Mankind,* Vol. 1, condensed and revised. New York: Ballantine.

Simoons, Frederick J. 1991. *Food in China: A Cultural and Historical Inquiry.* Boca Raton, FL: CRC.

Tan, Mely G. 2002. "Chinese Dietary Culture in Indonesian Urban Society." In David Y. H. Wu and Sidney Cheung, eds., *The Globalization of Chinese Food,* 152–69. Richmond, Surrey, UK: Curzon.

Tuan, Francis C., Cheng Fang, and Zhi Cao. 2004. "Chinese Soybean Imports Expected to Grow Despite Short-term Disruptions." Electronic Outlook Report from the Economic Research Service of the U.S. Department of Agriculture. Washington, DC: USDA. http://www.ers.usda.gov/publications/OCS/Oct04/OCS04J01/.

Wang, Zhongshu. 1984. *Handai Kaoguxue Gaishuo* [*An Outline of Han Archaeology*]. Beijing: Zhonghua Shuji.

Wolff, David. 2001. "Bean There: Toward a Soy-Based History of Northeast Asia." In Thomas Lahusen, ed., *Harbin and Manchuria: Place, Space, and Identity,* 241–52. Durham, NC: Duke University Press.

Wu, Xiaofeng, Xu Junliang, Miao Yungen, and Zeng Shuiyun. 1996. "A Study of Breeding Silkworms on a Diet Consisting of Soybean Dregs." *Journal of Zhejiang Agricultural University* 22(4): 369–72 [in Chinese].

Yu, Ying-Shih. 1977. "Han." In K. C. Chang, ed., *Food in Chinese Culture: Anthropological and Historical Perspectives*, 53–83. New Haven, CT: Yale University Press.

Yuan Mei. 1984 [1792]. *Shuiyuan Shidan* [*Recipes of Suiyuan*]. Annotated by Zhou Sanjin et al. Beijing: Zhongguo Shangye Chubanshe.

Zhen, Shu. 1990. *Jiang Yin Jiang Shi* [*About Drinking and Eating*]. Hong Kong: Zhonghua Shuju.

Zhou, Sanjin, ed. 1986. *Mingcai Xiaoshi* [*Brief History of Famous Dishes*]. Shanghai: Xuelin Chubanshe.

Zhu, Jiefan. 1971. "Zhongguo Yanyuzhi 'Doufu' Juzi Luechao" ["Notes on Tofu Phrases in Chinese Proverbs"]. In Lin Haiyin, ed., *Zhongguo Doufu* [*Tofu in China*], 59–69. Taipei: Chun Wenxue Chubanshe.

6

Tofu Feasts in Sichuan Cuisine

JIANHUA MAO

Translated by Ying Liu and Xiaolu Wang

Introduction

Tofu dishes play a special role in Sichuan cuisine.[1] Local classic texts such as the *Chengdu Tonglan* (*A Survey of Chengdu*, AD 1909) and the *Tiaoding Xinlu* (*New Record of Gastronomy*, printed in the nineteenth century) enumerate seventy-three tofu dishes (Appendix B). Xiong Sizhi (2001), a famous food scholar, writes that the people of Sichuan can make more than two hundred courses with tofu, including the world-famous Mapo tofu.

Such texts describe elaborate dishes worthy of presentation in a grand feast. A host of other dishes popular with people of modest means are cheaper but also delicious and nutritional. They include tofu custard, sweet tofu custard, sour and spicy tofu custard, homestyle tofu custard, guojiang douhua (cross-river tofu custard, so-called because the custard is heated in water), koumo mushroom tofu custard, braised tofu, and boiled tofu. The tofu feast is one important component of Sichuan cuisine. Such a feast is an important part of traditional festivals or family events in which tofu plays a crucial role.

This essay begins with a survey of contemporary tofu dishes, including the flavors and techniques used. It then examines the flowering of a restaurant marketing technique that I call "cultural packaging." Such cultural packaging is presented in its general aspects first and then as it has specifically been applied to tofu dishes. Finally, the conclusion explores the implications of these techniques and trends both for diners and marketers and also explores challenges to the commercialization of Sichuanese tofu dishes in the Chinese and international spheres. As one of the driving factors shaping the 21st century—including soy's fate in this century—Chinese commercialism in new fields must be taken seriously.

A Survey of Contemporary Tofu Dishes and Feasts

One of Sichuan cuisine's features is an abundance of flavors, as proved by the common saying "eating in China, flavor in Sichuan." In some Sichuan cooking schools, twenty-three standard flavors are taught:

Intense aromatic flavors whose formulations include capsicum and the numbing seasoning called fagara:
- homestyle flavor (the most common flavor in Sichuan, consisting mainly of hot chili, Sichuan salt, and thick broad bean sauce)
- fish-fragrant flavor
- strange flavor (*guaiwei,* a mixture of soy sauce, sugar, hot chili, vinegar, and garlic)
- red hot oil (*hongyou*) flavor
- numbing hot (*mala*) flavor
- sour hot (*suanla*) flavor
- burnt chili (*hula*) flavor
- tangerine peel flavor
- numbing (*jiaoma*) flavor (made in part by frying fagara in oil)
- numbing salty (*jiaoyan*) flavor (fried salt mixed with fagara powder)

Other aromatic spice flavors (Here fragrance is emphasized over intensity. Thus, hot chili is not used, although fried salt mixed with fagara may be used.):
- sauce-fragrant flavor
- five-spice flavor
- sweet and savory flavor
- wine sauce flavor
- smoked flavor
- salty and delicious flavor
- mashed garlic flavor
- sesame sauce flavor
- mustard flavor
- salty and sweet flavor

Flavors thought to be savory but not aromatic:
- litchi flavor
- sweet and sour flavor
- ginger juice flavor

Since the early 1990s, chefs of Sichuan cuisine have created novel flavors, among which fermented bean sauce flavor, spicy fermented bean sauce flavor, eggplant flavor, and fruit juice flavor are the most popular. The number of Sichuan flavors that are now popularly recognized has reached twenty-seven. Twenty-four of them are made with aromatic spices, while more than ten make use of chili or fagara (Sichuan's mildly numbing, prickly "pepper"). This listing demonstrates Sichuan cuisine's abundance of flavors. Being spicy and mildly numbing is only one aspect of Sichuan cuisine.

Below I describe some tofu dishes served at two famous restaurants in Chengdu in order to show the usage of flavors and cooking techniques.

TOFU COURSES AT THE CHEN MAPO TOFU RESTAURANT

We studied a branch of the Chen Mapo Tofu Restaurant, an old and well-known Chinese establishment, at Xiyulong Street in Chengdu. Thirty-three tofu dishes are served there and are classifiable into seven types of flavors, with seventeen in the salty and delicious category, accounting for 51.5 percent of the total; ten in the homestyle category, accounting for 30.3 percent; and five in the numbing hot category, accounting for 15.1 percent. Compared to the twenty-seven flavors available in Sichuan cuisine, these seven basic flavors present a relatively limited range. We can conclude from this categorization that in this restaurant, as in others, more flavors could be applied to tofu dishes than currently are.

These dishes have been prepared using a variety of cooking techniques: *du* (stew), *shao* (braise or simmer), *zheng* (steam), *qiang* (quick-fry with hot oil), *zha* (fry with hot oil), *guotie* (fry with little oil in a pan), and *zhu* (boil). In the case of bear paw tofu (see Appendix B), more than one cooking technique is used, as it is first fried and then stewed. Yet despite the variety of these techniques, compared to the multitude of ways that pork and chicken are prepared in Sichuan the range is once again limited. We can conclude that more techniques could be applied to tofu dishes.

We will return to an examination of this restaurant later when we explore the phenomenon of cultural packaging.

A TOFU FEAST IN WENSHU TEMPLE

One approach to tofu is to harmonize the arrangement of various flavors and techniques in cooking tofu dishes. Confronted with the rivalry between restaurants, tofu chefs make great efforts to show off their skills by employing different techniques and by arranging diverse dishes to make tofu feasts.

Wenshu Temple is located in downtown Chengdu and is one of the four biggest Chan temples in China. The attached Green Heaven and Earth

Vegetarian Restaurant is the acknowledged exemplar of Sichuan vegetarian cuisine; the restaurant's tofu feasts are particularly famous. In a tofu feast offered by chief chef Chen Jinqiao, many of the dishes are made of soy; mock fish or fowl is actually tofu but is made to resemble real meat or fish. All the courses in the feast seem simple, yet the arrangement is so artful that the chef's skills appear amazing.

Almost every one of the fifteen courses in this feast is unique to this restaurant, and only three are flavored with chili. It is apparent that tasting savory, instead of simply numbing hot, is a key principle of Sichuan haute cuisine.

In creating attractive tofu for feasts, some chefs attempt to use more ingredients, including expensive meats and seafood, and to add more techniques to the production of fancy courses. This is possible because Chengdu, the "City of Heaven," is abundant in resources.

Since many people in the region are well off, feasting and traveling have been very popular. Indeed, historically the people have been fond of chasing fresh experiences and seeking diversity. According to historical records such as Fu Chongju's *Chengdu Tonglan* (officially published in 1909), Chengdu's people are rather curious about new things. It is therefore quite natural that restaurateurs who know the local people well would also strive to innovate with cultural advertisements and marketing for their restaurants and dishes.

Cultural Packaging of Sichuan's Dishes and Feasts

In order fully to understand trends in tofu feasts in Sichuan Province, we must turn to the general phenomenon of cultural packaging. My research indicates that from the middle of the 1980s to the end of the 1990s, Sichuan's haute cuisine, with the restaurants of Chengdu as typical representatives, moved away from an emphasis on chefs' skills toward an emphasis instead on cultural meanings. Hundreds of years of development had brought Sichuan's cuisine to a climax. Yet in a very competitive climate, restaurants have continually had to come up with innovative dishes, lest they be pushed out of business. Some old and established restaurants in Chengdu, such as the Rongleyuan and Jingchengyuan restaurants, lost market share and were shut down.

In their places have sprung privately owned restaurants run by people from literary circles. Striving to gain renown in the field of cuisine, these new owners not only promote innovative cooking techniques but also evoke aspects of Chinese history and literature (hereafter referred to as cultural packaging) in their restaurants. Some of these newly booming enterprises, including the Chengdu Gongguancai Restaurant, the Baguo Buyi Cuisine Restaurant, the Huangcheng Laoma Restaurant, the Shizilou Restaurant, and the Caigenxiang (Garden Fresh) Restaurant, are now quite famous in China.

In order to compete with haute cuisine rivals elsewhere in China, the owners try to overcome Sichuan cuisine's reputation for being too popularized and ordinary. They attempt to raise the status of the cuisine by relating each item to aspects of Chinese history or literature while also improving the interior decor of the restaurants. For example, pavilions, terraces, and towers are built into the restaurants' limited spaces, and small bridges and paths are created and decorated with different flowers depending on the season. Some restaurants even give prominence to local landmarks and culture by decorating with wheelbarrows, mill wheels, millstones, huge glazed pots, corncobs, or red peppers. Some restaurants favor images of old Sichuan folklore; for example, the owner of the Baguo Buyi restaurant had a large fresco painted depicting the scenery of Chongqing Chaotianmen Dock. This painting, which is under bright lights, is so vivid that customers feel personally on the scene.

In these restaurants, the experiences of *yinren* and *yinqu* have been added to the dining encounter. *Yinren* ("people of the repast")—meaning companions for customers during the meal—are actually waiters and waitresses. Nowadays, waitresses in quaint or rural dress have often replaced traditional waiters. Customers very much appreciate these young women of Sichuan, who are hired because they are beautiful, smart, considerate, and caring. *Yinqu* ("amusements of the repast") refers to activities during a meal such as drinking games, the intoning of couplets, and the singing of *qu,* which is a type of verse. These days some restaurants not only provide traditional entertainment but also create new services, such as giving a special toast in the customers' honor or inviting customers to wash hands in a special ceremony. Since these restaurants emphasize the cultural packaging of dishes, some customers jokingly refer to eating at these restaurants as "eating culture."

Below I detail the cultural packaging of feasts at six restaurants in Chengdu. The first four restaurants do not emphasize tofu particularly; they are included to show the context for the last two restaurants, which do feature tofu prominently.

OLD CHENGDU GONGGUANCAI RESTAURANT

Old Chengdu Gongguancai Restaurant provides the most typical example of the culture of eating. A wooden plaque, the menus, and the restaurant's pamphlets declare: "Chengdu is a famous city of history and culture, where celebrities gathered in the past. These people's homes were called *gongguan* ('residence of high officials'). Usually the hosts were gastronomes versed in cuisine, and they innovated many wonderful dishes. This led to a new school of Sichuan cuisine that stressed culture and was called *gongguancai* ('dishes made in high officials' residence'). This school of cooking developed from the local traditions and the essences of the four famous Chinese cuisines (Sichuan cuisine, Guangdong cuisine, Beijing cuisine, and Jiangsu cuisine)."

This introduction shows the market orientation of the restaurant, which endeavors to create an atmosphere of history and culture, thereby upgrading the reputation of the restaurant and adding cultural value to the courses. All of the courses in Gongguancai Restaurant have stories associated with them. Recognized by the China National Trade Bureau, these well-known Chinese courses and attendant descriptions include:

Terrapin and Fish Soup: Made of tortoise, turtle, and fish by secret techniques imparted by the mystics of Tuojiang River. This dish was originally invented by an ancestor from the Li Gongguan (Li Official Residence) at Kuixinglou Street 43, Chengdu.

Simmered Meat in Sticky Rice Wine: Cooked in ginseng soup. This tender, red-colored dish was invented by Liu Xiang, a local war lord in the 1930s.

Beggar's Fish: Cooked without its sticking to the wok. The fish is very tender, with a special flavor. It was invented by Liu Chongyun, a local army officer under Liu Xiang in the 1930s.

Plain Stewed and Steamed Pork with Rice: Different from traditional steamed foods, this dish includes the flavor of an unseasoned stew. It was introduced by Luo Chengxiang, a top scholar at the end of the Qing dynasty, in the early twentieth century.

Duck with Chinese Herbs and Orange Juice: Made of orange juice, full-grown duck, and a mushroom from the Qinghai plateau known as Chinese caterpillar fungus. This special dish is thick with the aroma of herbs and is very nutritious. It was introduced by Yang Shenxiu, chief secretary of the Sichuan Education Bureau in the 1940s.

In addition, Mr. Li Chaobai, owner of the Gongguancai Restaurant and a former college professor, wrote a poem for his restaurant that mentions the ancient Chinese civilizations of Ba and Shu. This is hung on a wall.

The success of Gongguancai Restaurant is the fruit of such packaging. In fact, we do not know how many of the dishes were really created in

Sichuan, and the diners do not research the origins of what they eat. However, through these stories customers do learn in a general way something about Sichuan's history, culture, and society. The mental stimulation that is offered attracts patrons, who rely on the restaurant's reputation for credibility as well as good food.

BAGUO BUYI RESTAURANT

Baguo Buyi Restaurant was established by He Nong, an outstanding literary figure of the 1990s. This restaurant also demonstrates the success of cultural packaging in the cuisine industry. The restaurant is decorated with characteristics of Chongqing City, and most courses are replete with Chongqing flavors. Several young scholars from famous universities in Chengdu were involved in the restaurant's design and decoration. Wei Minglun, a celebrated playwright, was invited to write an ode for the restaurant's inscription, which reads in part:

> The land of Ba [an ancient kingdom that ruled over present-day Chengdu] is famous for wonderful poetry and wine. Plebeians and mandarins alike enjoyed their lives here. Today restaurants take names like "Imperial capital" or "Dynasty" and compete with each other in luxuries. But here, at this restaurant, the name Baguo Buyi ["common people of Ba in plain clothes"] shows the better motives of your host, who wants to share the bitterness as well as the sweetness of life with people all over the world.
>
> Delicious food and interesting stories prompt people to ask more about these tales. They wonder as they eat, where was the buffalo-herding boy pointing? In whose house did the poet sleep last night? How many guests caroused until morning and then slept in Chang'an with the fragrance of nice wine? Which wandering swordsman was singing the sad song along the River Yi? When the wise lady Zhuo Wenjun was selling wine, what did her counter display look like? Is it true that the great poet Su Shi left the precious recipe behind? Where is the Xishan (West Mountain) relic? . . . They also think: When Song Jiang drank at Xunyanglou Restaurant, he wrote on the wall a poem against the ruling class. That was the beginning of the story of heroic outlaws at the marshes of Mount Liang, who were all compelled by the oppressive government to rebel.[2] . . . Or they imagine Chairman Mao Zedong in his early years as a common person in plain clothes, lingering in a small tavern with a cup instead of the wand [of political power] in his hands—would he have drunk Sichuan liquor? Would he have ordered Hunan hot chili with his wine? . . . National affairs, love among neighbors, thoughts of wisdom—all these happen during the clinking of wine glasses.

> These are more than places for eating. These are where people of ideas and integrity gather; these are the cradles where literature for generations is produced!
>
> . . . Let's appreciate the splendor of tonight. We will not have hunger in this prosperous time; instead, we have a wonderful feast for the millennium. As a saying goes: revolution is to feast. Thus, dining places are highly related to revolution. And indeed, Baguo Buyi is falling over itself in its hurry for reform. . . .
>
> The special situation of the country, the precious quintessence of the country, the profound academic thoughts of the country, the delicious food of the country—all these are good issues discussed at table. Mouth and mind are not opposed to each other; spiritual and material civilizations can exist together in harmony. So sing and play finger-guessing games during the meal; but don't forget duty and responsibility after the feast. . . . My words end with a poem:
>
> Dining will not disappear until humans end;
> So long live the restaurant, long live Sichuan cuisine!
> Everything in the world is secondary, but eating is most important;
> When people are satisfied with a wonderful meal, an excellent piece of writing will follow.

This amusing ode sometimes makes diners think. It is a clear example of cultural productions dealing with food.

LIANZHENTANG CULTURAL COLLECTOR'S RESTAURANT

There are yet more restaurants lifting the banner of culture, among which is the Chengdu Lianzhentang Cultural Collector's Restaurant, which was established in 2001 by Xiong Sizhi, a famous gourmet, food scholar, and expert on folklore. The menu for a feast held by the Sichuan Folklore Association there in 2002 highlights the owner's passion for associating foods with literary works and folk culture:

Savory tea: "Esoterically Made Savory Tea" (tea made in the restaurant's own style)

Appetizers: "Red hot oil Zhuge rutabaga." This is a huge pickled rutabaga with red hot oil. The name alludes to the famous figure of Zhuge Liang in the masterpiece fourteenth-century historical novel of the Ming dynasty, *Romance of the Three Kingdoms.* It was believed that Zhuge Liang encouraged his soldiers to plant this vegetable to supplement the army's food supply.

"Coral Radish." This is a sour dish made from carrot soaked in lemon juice. The soaked carrot is then cut into a coral shape. In the Sichuan dialect, the words for "coral" and "sour" are both pronounced *suan*, giving a further association of this dish with coral.

Cold cuts: "Cry of a Monkey Heard in a Shallop." The recipe's name is derived from one of many well-known poems about China's Three Gorges. The Three Gorges especially inspired the great 8th-century (Tang dynasty) poet Li Bai, who wrote the poem alluded to.

Hot courses: "Bamboo Shoots Facing the Boat." This name is derived from the poem "The Feast" by the famous Tang dynasty poet Du Fu.

"Pork in an Old Jar." This dish is part of the restaurant's party package called "Four Joy Feast"; this package is served for birthdays, promotions, luck and marriage feasts.

"Dried-Simmered Wuchang Fish." Invented in this restaurant, this dish uses a fish that Chairman Mao Zedong wrote a poem about. The poem was popular during the Cultural Revolution.

"Homestyle-Flavored Sea Cucumber"

"Hot Oil on Bean Stem." This is from the restaurant's party package called "Allusive Dishes." It is made with stir-fried soybean sprouts whose tips and roots have been removed. From the province of Shandong, this dish is believed to have originated with the family of Confucius.

"Lantern-Shaped Steamed Pork." This is a reference to traditional Chinese lanterns.

"Sour Hot Hoof Tendon"

"Carp Tail in a Dragon Pool." The dish is from the party package "The Feast of Mount Emei." According to local legend, the carps in the Dragon Pool on Emei Mountain each used to have two tails. The dish is made to resemble this astonishing sight.

"Coming Home on a Horse from a Trip in the Countryside." The dish's name is derived from a Chinese poem. To make it, red sweet potato is peeled, steamed, mashed, and fried, and sugar is added. In the presentation of this sweet snack, decorations are included—pumpkin rind for "mountains," water melon rind for willow trees, and carrots for butterflies. The image of a horse's hoof is made on the sweet potato. The whole dish thus represents coming home on a horse.

"Mashed Chicken with Chef's Special Broth"

Snacks: "Fried Golden Stick of the Monkey King." From the package "Allusive Dishes," this is made from peeled sweet potato that has been steamed and mashed. It is shaped into round sticks and then fried until golden brown. The name refers to the magical stick used by the Monkey King in the famous sixteenth-century novel *Journey to the West,* which was based on older legends.

"Chrysanthemum Porridge." Chrysanthemum is popular in traditional Chinese poetry.

"Rice Ball with Pickled Vegetables"

Green Chili Jiaozi Dumpling (dumpling with meat and vegetable stuffing)

Main Food: Xiao Mao'er, a small bowl of rice shaped like a skull cap, together with two pickled dishes. In Sichuan's dialect, a small bowl of rice is called *xiao mao'er,* or "small skull cap." A small bowl of rice is placed upside down in a bigger bowl to form the shape.

In this feast, many items are named after cultural or historical items, such as "Cry of a Monkey Heard in a Shallop" and "Coming Home from a Trip in the Countryside." Such names are frequently derived from traditional Chinese poems, and the foods themselves are artfully arranged to look like landscapes. The names do not disclose any of the ingredients or cooking techniques used in the courses. Customers know nothing about the dishes without explanation from the waiters and waitresses.

TUTAO VILLAGE (EARTHENWARE VILLAGE)

The Tutao Village restaurant is on Jinluo Road, in the Baiguolin District of Chengdu. The establishment's wall is decorated with coir raincoats, bamboo hats, and portraits of Karl Marx, Friedrich Engels, and Mao Zedong. Quotations from Mao appear as well, creating the atmosphere of the Cultural Revolution of the 1960s. Jokingly, the staff calls the restaurant the Commune Canteen. The owner is referred to as the village head, and the customers are referred to as heroes and heroines. All waiters and waitresses wear green military outfits, as did many civilians during the Cultural Revolution. The wait staff handles food orders in the old style, with the waiters shouting out the customers' orders directly to the cooks.

The menu here has the special title "Analects of Tutao Village," and all the courses have whimsical names that cannot be understood without explanation (provided to the customers by the waiters). The menu includes:

Snakes and Monsters (spicy hot boiled eel, loach fish, bullfrog, duck blood jelly, tofu, and beef)
Become Wealthy Together (boiled cabbage with canned pork)
Red All Over the Country (numbing hot fresh fish)
Red Storm (hot boiled beef or pork)
Not Afraid of Hardship and Death (fried bitter gourd with hog's large intestine)
Bombing an Embassy (braised hog's large intestine in soy sauce)
Young Ox (beef with special marinade)
Chicken Peddler (cold rice noodles)
The Carrot and the Stick (double sautéed pork slices with *guokui*—that is, Sichuan pancake)
Progress with an Open Mind (sautéed meat with bamboo shoots)
Smoking and Burning (long-preserved meat)
Well-Versed in Both Civil and Military Abilities (fried green chili and potato slices)
Budding (fried bean sprouts)
Associating with Evil People (boiled tofu with duck blood jelly)
Living Off Someone (boiled potato)
Rapid Advances in a Career (numbing hot chicken wing and wing tip)

All of these names were once popular terms at the time of the Cultural Revolution. People who lived through this historical period understand the political meanings, social problems, and even ideologies revealed in these names and smile with comprehension at the owner's jokes. In the restaurant, the shouting of orders such as "No. 4 ordered Red All Over the Country" (this is derived from a famous song glorifying Mao) or "No. 1 ordered Bombing an Embassy" are heard frequently, arousing continuous laughter and creating a joyful atmosphere. Presumably people who were traumatized during that era do not go to this restaurant.

The four restaurants described above may seem to have taken us far from our topic of tofu. However, cultural packaging and advertising are quite similar for all dishes within the higher levels of Sichuan restaurant cuisine. With this context in mind, we can now circle back to the present situation of tofu feasts by examining two more feasting contexts.

JIANMEN TOFU

Two hundred kilometers from Chengdu, Jianmen was once a town of strategic military importance, famous since ancient times for its dangerous, mountainous topography. It is also in a region with abundant soybeans. Jianmen tofu, made with spring water and a grindstone, enjoys a good reputation in China. Currently, more than 120 kinds of tofu dishes exist in Jianmen. Many have names containing cultural information, such as:

Three Heroes in the Peach Garden (three kinds of crispy "nuts": shelled peanuts, walnut kernels, and dried bean curd)
Set Fire to Chibi (crispy rice, pork cutlet, and tofu)
Zhangfei Selling Meat (braised pork joints with tofu)
Zhou Yu's Navy (braised fresh fish with tofu)

All of these names derive from the previously mentioned *Romance of the Three Kingdoms*. The references to three heroes, to Zhangfei, and to Zhou Yu all deal with characters in the story, while Chibi refers to a great battle that this historical epic relates.

These courses are common in any Three Kingdom Tofu Feast, a banquet package served in many restaurants. The description for each dish invokes a story from this period in the third century AD. The restaurant links cuisine to historical events and sites such as the kingdom of Shu-Han, which was one of these fabled Three Kingdoms and was located around present-day Chengdu. The marketing thus draws on consumer psychology, endeavoring to gratify diners' curiosity, their pursuit of novelty, and their admiration for the famous. This type of cultural packaging enables Jianmen restaurant owners to succeed in the restaurant industry despite the limited space in their establishments.

CHEN MAPO TOFU FEAST

Our detailing of the cultural packaging of foods in Sichuan Province ends with a detailed examination of the Chen Mapo Tofu Feast. This feast, prepared by the Chen Mapo Tofu Restaurant of the Chengdu Dietary Company, was nominated in 2002 for the Chinese Famous Feast Award, a national honor bestowed by the State Commercial Ministry. The menu and its analysis show that this banquet is of great originality and skill, full of connotations from Chinese folklore.

THE FOUR COLD DISHES:

Shredded chicken in red hot oil and fish-flavored lima beans

Shredded fish in ginger juice with fagara and "jade belts" (partly shelled broad beans with hulls remaining around their middles)
Shredded duck in a thick gravy with shallots and oily snow peas
Strange-flavored shredded rabbit and black soybeans in rice sauce (made with fried sugar cane juice)

HOT DISHES:

An Overlord Saying Farewell to His Concubine (see explanation below)
Specially Steamed Pork with Golden Sand (the "sand" is egg yolk)
Three Fish Leading to Prosperity
Tofu with Palm-like "Ginseng"
Gold Coin Tofu
Bear Paw Tofu
Mapo Tofu
Braised Tofu with Seafood
Silver Needle and Jade Noodle (fine noodles with mung bean)

SNACKS:

Sour and Spicy Tofu Jelly
Golden Gourd Jiaozi (dumpling with meat and vegetable stuffing)

Number symbolism in this tofu feast. The Chinese take a great interest in numbers. To those Chinese who are still superstitious, numbers appear to suggest or even predict fate. For instance, the number 2 is believed to imply "couple," which is lucky, since good things are thought to come in pairs; the number 3 means "more"; the number 4 means "safe and sound" (restful in all seasons);[3] the number 6 suggests that something is "favorable"; the number 8 represents "stability" (the number is pronounced similarly to the Chinese character "fa," which means "rich and flourishing"); the number 9 represents "great" (a number for *yang,* the creative force, at its highest level); and the number 10 represents "perfection" since it is the completion of the numbers from zero to ten.

All numbers involved in the menu of the Chen Mapo tofu feast above are lucky numbers, as the details below demonstrate:

The four cold dishes:
four meats: chicken, duck, fish, and rabbit
four beans: lima beans, broad beans, snow peas, and black soybeans
eight flavors: red hot oil, ginger juice, thick spicy gravy, strange flavor, fish-fragrant, fagara-favored salt, shallot-flavored oil, sweet flavor

Each cold dish is made of two main ingredients: one meat and one vegetable.

The hot dishes. There are nine hot dishes in all. The numbers 1, 3, 5, 7, and 9 are *yang* numbers in the *ying-yang* classification system. The number 9 is, of course, the greatest of this group. Numbers larger than 9 are dependent on zero in the base ten system, and so in this system 9 is the highest yang number. For this reason, in ancient times the number 9 was always related to emperors.[4] Certainly it is an auspicious number.

Note that the third hot dish is "Three Fish Leading to Prosperity." Here three means "more," which is also very lucky.

The snacks. There are two snacks, which evokes the idea of good things going in couples. Each snack is divided into ten small plates, which means "perfection."

The symbolism of auspicious allusions. In Chinese tradition, the seven most important things in daily life are oil, salt, firewood, rice, soy, vinegar, and tea. All but the wood are types of food or drink: the centrality of food to the Chinese way of thinking is evident. But while the common people are satisfied simply with sufficient food (and warm clothes), the wealthy go after refined dishes. The Chinese see good eating as a kind of happiness. Hence elaborate dishes intrinsically convey good fortune.

In addition, in the Chen Mapo Tofu Feast above we see appropriate auspicious symbolism. We will first consider the symbolism associated with the cold meats, then images associated with the beans, and finally symbolism in the hot dishes, including those with tofu.

Concerning the meats in the four cold dishes, we note that the Chinese have long considered chicken and fish to be auspicious. *Ji* (first tone), meaning "chicken," is pronounced almost the same as *ji* (second tone), meaning "lucky" or "favorable." People believe that this poultry is very clever. A quotation from the *Chunqiu Shuojie* (*Explanation on Spring and Autumn*) in the *Taiping Yulan* (*Imperial Encyclopedia of the Taiping Era*), completed in AD 983, states: "The cock is the accumulation of *yang* and the image of the South. Fire and sun are objects of *yang;* hence cocks crow at sunrise. That is the telepathy between things of the same kind" (Li Fang et al. 1968 [AD 10th C.]). This feature of the cock makes it a luck-bearing animal of great importance, which can both drive away devils and bring good fortune.

Fish is also said to be auspicious, since the Chinese character *yu* ("fish") is pronounced the same as *yu* ("to be superabundant"). Among fish, carp is the most positive because *li* (third tone), meaning "carp," is pronounced almost the same as *li* (fourth tone), meaning "profit" or "benefit." In upbeat paintings made to predict "abundance each year," "more than wealth and dignity," and so on, fish can always be seen. In any feast of Chinese cuisine there must be a fish course.

Rabbit is tender and agile. Many people believe that it brings good luck. A somewhat mysterious yet popular idea is that when a snake coils up around a rabbit a lucky thing will happen and that when a person born in the year of the rabbit marries someone born in the year of the snake, the family prospers and becomes wealthy.

Duck is not usually mentioned among common auspicious animals, but the similar poultry of goose and wild goose are very auspicious. The wild goose is an animal with a strict family hierarchy, and a mating pair of wild geese will live together their whole lives. Therefore, wild goose is a good present for an engagement, and domestic goose is often used as a substitute for wild goose. Ducks and geese are also similar in shape; hence, duck can potentially substitute for goose. In any case, duck is perceived to be a healthy food.

All four meats in the cold dishes at the Chen Mapo Tofu Feast thus have multiple positive associations for diners.

With respect to the beans in these cold dishes, we also find rich symbolism. These four supporting ingredients (lima bean, broad bean, black soybean, and snow pea) symbolize the four seasons according to either the times of their production or their colors. Note that when it is fried in oil, the partly shelled broad bean loses its whiteness and presents two colors: the kernel is yellow, and the hull is dark red. The addition of red increases the colors to five. Whether coincidentally or by design, the five colors correspond to China's traditional five basic elements (metal, wood, water, fire, and earth) and five directions (south, north, east, west, and center) (cf. Durkheim and Mauss 1963, 70–77).

As for the hot dishes, except for Mapo tofu, the signature dish of the restaurant, the courses are all named with auspicious Chinese characters. "Specially Steamed Pork with Golden Sand" and "Gold Coin Tofu" are decorated with the character *jin* for "gold," "Silver Needle and Jade Noodle" evoke silver and jade ware, "Bear Paw Tofu" suggests delicacies from the mountains and the similarly appreciated wild meat of venison (even though such ingredients do not actually appear in the recipe), while "Braised Tofu with Seafood" and "Tofu with Palm-like Ginseng" (that is, sea cucumber) refer to expensive seafoods. Conferring ideas of wealth and good fortune, these terms enhance the perceived value of the courses.

"Three Fish Leading to Prosperity" is adapted from the Chinese saying "three sheep lead to prosperity"; Chinese diners tacitly understand the association. The name "Overlord Saying Farewell to His Concubine" comes from the historical story of Xiangyu, King of Chu, and his concubine Yuji. In the opera based on this story, Xiangyu wears a traditional pattern of facial makeup that is copied in the dish. The image is painted so delicately with vegetable dyes that the diner hesitates to even touch it with chopsticks. This dish is actually tofu cooked with turtle and chicken. Turtle is called *wangba* in Sichuan's dialect, *ba* sounds like the *ba* for "overlord," and *ji* for chicken sounds the same as *ji* for "concubine," hence the association of these foods with Xiangyu and his companion. Even the snack of "Golden Gourd Jiaozi" carries with it a meaning: the wish for many descendants, as symbolized by the many gourds the plant produces.

We thus see that this feast brims with novelty and fancy endeavors. Its colors, flavors, and fragrances are carefully arranged so as to impart ideas and stories from Chinese culture in order to enhance the appeal of the foods, including tofu. It fully merits the title "Famous Chinese Feast."

Conclusion and Recommendations

Because of recent development of the Chinese economy, many Chinese are now much better off than before. The conception of appropriate or desirable food has advanced accordingly; the variety of available dietary choices is unprecedented. "Rich people have rich meals while poor people have tofu meals" has been a popular saying among the common people since ancient times. However delicious tofu was, its consumption implied poverty. But nowadays, tofu, a healthy food, has become a favorite choice for many people, rich and poor alike. This fits with Yuan Mei's assertion in his 1792 book of recipes, *Suiyuanshidan* (*Recipes of Sui Garden*), that tofu is more delicious than bird's nest soup when cooked properly. Tofu is suitable for use with any kind of flavor, for it tends to absorb flavors well without altering or overpowering them. The cooking techniques of Sichuan cuisine, abundant in flavors, play a creative role in the preparation of tofu dishes. Nonetheless, there is cause for concern and room for improvement in the development of Sichuanese tofu cuisine. Below I discuss three such areas of concern.

COMPLEX COOKING TECHNIQUES MAY CURB TOFU'S POPULARIZATION

We have noted that tofu dishes, which are cheap and traditionally associated with those who are less well off, are sometimes thought to be too common for upscale feasts. To meet the challenge of overcoming this perception, Sichuan chefs have developed new cooking techniques that have greatly influenced the value and taste of tofu dishes. Different ingredients are now used more often in the dishes, the process of cooking is more complicated, and special cookers are involved. All of these innovations are like double-edged swords, however, and both the advantages and disadvantages of this approach should be taken into consideration.

Elaboration of cuisine can create a problem of timing, since preparing a good tofu feast is a lengthy undertaking. Local customers can book a tofu feast in advance so the restaurant can be fully prepared. However, local customers are quite limited in number, particularly those with higher incomes who seek to thrill their palates. As for tourists from all over the world, many of them can afford a nice feast and hope to have a fabulous meal in a new place. The problem is that they often cannot book the meal in advance, and without sufficient preparation the cooks cannot make perfect dishes. Hence, although these restaurants are famous for their food, tourists cannot enjoy the full range of what they might offer, and this is a great pity for all involved.

Such elaborate feasts are also difficult to popularize among common people. Ordinary people busy with daily jobs cannot afford the various ingredients, complicated processing, and time cost involved in making these dishes at home. They also cannot go to these restaurants; expensive dishes will discourage people of modest means outside the gate. Hence, despite the great development both of tofu dishes and of feasts, most people are only interested in a limited number of dishes. Popular dishes can be counted easily and include sour hot tofu custard, cross-river tofu custard, simmered tofu with dark soybean sauce, Mapo tofu, and boiled tofu.

PROBLEMS WITH THE CULTURAL PACKAGING OF TOFU

Above I surveyed the present situation of Sichuan cuisine, paying much attention to cultural packaging. Undoubtedly, the enhancements made to restaurant environments, the training of waiters, and allusions to the cultural background are of great significance. At the same time, this approach seems to be a dead end for new restaurants. Many recently established restaurants are uniquely decorated with special features, but they struggle to surpass the pioneers. Hence, a seemingly persuasive idea is not always effective at the level of business practice.

Strange names that do not correlate with the dishes themselves create much unexpected trouble for restaurant owners. The dishes are like clowns who attract young spectators at the beginning of their act but lose their appeal after the makeup and costumes have been removed. Sometimes techniques not much relevant to a dish may add value, but such techniques are overused in tofu dishes. Mahjong tofu, in the shape of mahjong tiles, is a good example of such a gimmick. Another is Lohan tofu, which is made in a round shape with nine peas on it. It is said to resemble the head of an Arhat (*lohan*), a Buddhist who has attained enlightenment. In some courses the most important part is a food sculpture of flowers and animals or birds. Most of the consumers' attention is transferred from the tastes and textures of the foods to the appearance of the sculptures. But that is to put the cart before the horse and misdirects the chefs' creativity. Tastes and textures must always be the top priority in order to woo diners to revisit.

Cultural packaging also distracts chefs and diners away from nutritional issues. Tofu is abundant in protein, has little fat, and is cholesterol-free. Nutritionally aware people often honor it as the most valuable treasure for vegetarians and the best partner for nutrition in rice-eating countries. In part because of their nutritional awareness, more and more Europeans and Americans are consuming tofu products today. Tofu is also, of course, an important part of the Japanese diet. Without sacrificing nutritional understanding, the Japanese have applied both traditional and modern cooking techniques to tofu products. But in the case of Sichuan, too often we find that chefs know little about nutrition, focusing instead exclusively on appearance and flavors.

Yet recently I found with joy that a series of books on new classical Sichuan cuisine had been published by the Sichuan People's Press. These books do pay attention to nutrition. For instance, crispy bean curd with pine nuts is introduced with a nutritional description of the tofu that combines modern science with traditional Chinese understandings of health: "Tofu is sweet, its feature being cool. Once in the digestive system, it may be beneficial to *qi*,[5] bringing saliva and clearing away both excess body heat and toxic materials. The protein it contains can be compared to fish, containing eight amino acids necessary to human beings." Because attention is being paid here to nutritional issues, in a general way this description shows a favorable trend in the development of Sichuan cuisine.

We also see that quality cookbooks from outside Mainland China have recently been published in the domestic Chinese market, such as *Vegetarian Food: Tofu,* edited by Xu Rentang (2001) from Taiwan. In this book, the recipes for most dishes are highly detailed and standardized and come with an intensive nutritional analysis, which is certainly a revelation to food scholars on the mainland.

PROBLEMS OF STANDARDIZATION AND INTERNATIONALIZATION OF SICHUAN'S TOFU DISHES

The problems of standardization and internationalization are hard nuts to crack theoretically and practically. The same dish cooked by the same chef in the same restaurant can taste different at different times. Such variability increases when the multiplicity of restaurants is taken into account. For instance, double-sautéed pork slices is a typical Sichuan dish popular in many restaurants, but different restaurants serve this dish with various flavors. Whether the restaurant can make perfect double-sautéed pork slices with excellent fragrance, flavor, and appearance is regarded as a criterion by which to judge the grade of the restaurant. The taste and quality depend largely on long practice.

A deficiency in cookbooks is part of the problem. Commonly, mainland cookbooks use too many vague terms, such as "slow fire" or "30 percent fire." It is not clear how high the flame on a gas stove or oven should be. Other vague words such as "add a little . . . ," "properly," and "50 or 60 percent cooked" are also frequently used without strict standard definitions. If you ask a chef what such a term means, the most probable answer is that one should cook or otherwise prepare the food until it "feels right." This creates a situation in which less-experienced chefs and many ordinary people are embarrassed because they cannot make dishes with quite the right flavors, despite their having followed recipes as strictly as the vague language allowed.

The most important reason for this problem is the lack of standardization for cooking techniques. Merely establishing a chain of Sichuan-style restaurants would not be enough to solve this problem; only a broader standardization of cooking processes can ensure the high quality and expanding popularity of Sichuan cuisine. This process will require time and the collaboration of food scholars, nutritionists, restaurant managers, and chefs. But some standardization is a worthy goal since in the twenty-first century the tourism economy is a key industry at the provincial and national levels, and restaurant management is a crucial part of this industry. More successful restaurants are economically desirable. Moreover, unless this problem is solved, the production of famous Sichuan dishes on a large scale would be hard to realize, impeding the growth of Sichuan cuisine on the world market.

In fact, there are precedents to draw upon. Hong Guangzhu noted in his book *Chinese Tofu* (1987) that "Mapo tofu was born in Sichuan. The Japanese then introduced this dish into Japan and invented canned Mapo tofu. Although the history of its production has not been long, currently it sells well all over the world, according to a Japanese scholar. Export sales per year have reached hundreds of thousands of sacks [one sack equals 250 kilos]. This fact should stimulate the Chinese" to do something (Hong 1987, 129). The Japanese production method that Hong notes involves standardization on a large scale. In addition, some fast-food restaurants in the mainland have currently reached considerable scale in their standardized production. Thus, the standardization and mass production of famous Sichuan cuisine, especially tofu dishes, is not a mere dream.

Yet the internationalization of Sichuan's cuisine, including its tofu dishes, can be surprisingly difficult. Illustrating this point was the picture of the status of Chinese cuisine in the West that food writer Fuchsia Dunlop offered at the Academic Conference on Sichuanese Culinary Culture and the Opening Up of Western Regions in 2001. She focused on Britain, where she has worked as a Chinese restaurant critic for several years. She outlined some common Western stereotypes that have helped to prevent truly authentic Chinese cuisine from enjoying the international acclaim it deserves:

1. "Chinese food is junky and full of artificial additives": Dunlop suggested that the widespread use of monosodium glutamate (MSG) in particular is a great barrier to British appreciation of Chinese food because it is never used in high-class restaurants or domestic kitchens in Britain and is strongly associated with packaged meals and junk food. She also explained that Western consumers are becoming more and more concerned about the use of artificial additives of all kinds in food and that many people blame MSG for unpleasant physical symptoms. We infer from Dunlop's observation that the healthfulness of the tofu in tofu dishes could be cancelled out by the perceived unhealthiness of MSG in the recipes.

2. "Chinese food is exotic to the point of being weird": Dunlop explained that British people these days have a conservative attitude as to what animals, and what parts of animals, they are willing to eat and that many of them are revolted by the idea of eating Chinese delicacies such as chicken's feet, duck's tongues, and sea cucumbers. Tofu dishes that include such ingredients could seem a little frightening.
3. "Chinese food is too oily and rich to eat every day": Dunlop explained that most British people have little or no experience with Chinese domestic cooking. They only know Chinese food from Chinese restaurants, which tend to serve richer dishes with an emphasis on deep-fried foods, including tofu (Dunlop 2001).

Dunlop explained how certain cultural differences, such as the lack of any British concept corresponding to the Chinese *kou gan* (mouth feel), make it difficult for the British to appreciate many of China's predominantly texture foods, such as shark's fin and goose intestines. However, we observe that texture can be important in the West in reactions to tofu: since tofu is often used in the West as a substitute for meat, some Westerners are disappointed with its texture, preferring something that feels like meat as they bite into it. Thus, cultural differences in texture expectations must be taken into account.

Dunlop also pointed out that most British people have no idea how to order a good selection of dishes in a Chinese restaurant and are confused by Chinese restaurant menus. As a result, British diners-out usually order Anglicized set menus, which bear little relation to real Chinese food. She added that almost all so-called Sichuanese restaurants in Britain are run and staffed by Cantonese immigrants, so it is simply impossible to find genuine Sichuanese food. This is true of tofu dishes as well as other Sichuanese specialties.

This information about foreign perceptions of Chinese food indicates that there is a long way to go before Sichuanese cuisine can make its mark internationally. The cuisine clearly needs better marketing of its features. For example, we must work to change the common misconception that Sichuan cuisine is all numbing and excessively hot. Meanwhile, we should introduce nutritional planning into our approach so that in a world environment of increasing heart disease, hypertension, and diabetes, we produce food that is both delicious and genuinely healthy. The old Chinese view that "much oil keeps a dish fresh" needs to be modified in order to avoid greasiness, and the nutritional value of foods such as tofu needs to be emphasized both in recipes and marketing. If we put these recommendations into practice, Sichuan's tofu dishes can come to play a key role in people's health.

For the Chinese, tofu dishes are favorites not only as daily food but also in feasts. For people in other cultural areas, tofu might gain acceptance through the use of local flavors and cooking techniques that are simpler than those of the Sichuan chefs. Color, flavor, techniques, and nutrition should all be taken into consideration as important factors for globalizing tofu.

Notes

1. The unabridged version of this essay was originally published in Chinese in the proceedings of *The 8th Symposium on Chinese Dietary Culture* (Taipei, Taiwan: Foundation of Chinese Dietary Culture, 2004), 337–57. I would like to thank Professor Xiong Sizhi, a famous culinary expert and folklorist in Sichuan, for his explanation of a number of dishes discussed in this essay. The version of the essay published here also benefited from the editorial guidance of Dr. Christine Du Bois and Professor Chee-Beng Tan.

2. See the stories from the famous Ming dynasty Chinese fiction *Shuihu Zhuan,* translated into English as *Outlaws of the Marsh* (Shi and Luo 1980).

3. Among Cantonese speakers, however, the number 4 symbolizes death, as the word in Cantonese is homonymous with the word for death.

4. See, for example, the symbolism for the number 9 in the *Qian Hexagram of Yijing* (*The Book of Change*), originally written in the Western Zhou period (1121–771 BC) and later edited by Confucius.

5. In traditional Chinese medicine, *qi* is the life force.

References

Dunlop, Fuchsia. 2001. "Chuancai Zai Yingguo" ["Sichuan Food in Britain," translated into Chinese by Liu Yaochun]. In Sichuan Sheng Mingren Xiehui [Sichuan Celebrity Association] and the Sichuan Sheng Minsu Xuehui [Sichuan Folklore Association], eds., *Chuancai Wenhua Yanjiu* [*Research into Sichuan Culinary Culture*], 208–18. Chengdu, China: Sichuan University Press.

Durkheim, Emile, and Marcel Mauss. 1963. *Primitive Classification.* Chicago: University of Chicago Press.

Hong, Guangzhu. 1987. *Zhongguo Doufu* [*Chinese Tofu*]. Beijing: China Trade Press.

Li Fang et al. 1968 [AD 10th century]. *Taiping Yulan* [*Imperial Encyclopedia of the Taiping Era*]. Taibei Shi: Taiwan Shang Wu Yin Shu Guan, Minguo 57 [in Chinese].

Shi, Nai'an, and Guanzhong Luo. 1980. *Outlaws of the Marsh.* Translated by Sidney Shapiro. Beijing: Foreign Language Press.

Sichuan Sheng Mingren Xiehui [Sichuan Celebrity Association] and Sichuan Sheng Minsu Xuehui [Sichuan Folklore Association], eds. 2001. *Chuancai Wenhua Yanjiu* [*Research into Sichuan Culinary Culture*]. Chengdu, China: Sichuan University Press.

Xiong, Sizhi, and Li Du. 2001. *Juzhu Zuibei Si Wushu* [*Lifting Chopsticks and Wine Glass, I Miss My Homeland of Shu*]. Chengdu, China: Sichuan People's Press.

Xu, Rentang, ed. 2001. *Su: Doufu* [*Vegetarian Food: Tofu*]. Shenyang: Liaoning Science & Technology Press.

7

Fermented Soybean Products and Japanese Standard Taste

ERINO OZEKI

Standard Taste As a Cultural Model

In many academic fields, some topics pose real challenges to our usual scientific methods even though they are fascinating and often puzzled over by nonscientists.[1] Cultural differences in taste preferences are one such interesting but underclarified topic. I do not undertake here the difficult task of presenting a new and complete analytic framework for this topic but hope instead to draw more attention to the important phenomenon of collective taste preferences, which seems to typify every food culture.[2]

We sometimes notice with our tongues and noses that a particular ethnic cuisine has a pattern of flavors repeated in many dishes. In time, we realize that this pattern is the favorite taste of that cuisine. It can nonetheless remain difficult for outsiders to understand why that taste is preferred, for what is considered a good flavor in one culinary culture may not be considered good universally. Yet cultural anthropologists—who, while still relatively young, must live in a foreign culinary environment for an extended period—often reach the point when unfamiliar foreign tastes first become tolerable, then become tasty, and may finally be internalized as among their favorites. Others besides anthropologists with cross-cultural contacts can also come to appreciate foreign flavors. But this type of appreciation is usually only acquired through repeated experiences of the flavors in question.

Despite this human capacity for adaptability, many people experience severe culture shock when first encountering a new cuisine. Some even feel so bewildered by a totally bizarre flavor that they cease craving exotic tastes altogether and retreat to their old familiar diets. Others, even after years of living in a foreign society, may continue to search among unfamiliar foods in the hopes of finding substitutes—however inadequate—for the diets of the societies where they grew up. In the midst of a foreign culinary culture, they seek consolation in flavors similar to their remembered favorites. Their refusal to give up the tastes of their childhoods, even in difficult situations, unveils the obstinate nature of flavor preferences. Such preferences often give people what appear to be permanent reference points in the judgment of all flavors.

Whether we adapt to foreign tastes or not, there is apparently a deeply embedded boundary, both psychological and physiological, that divides the experiences of our tongues and noses into two categories: our own culture's tastes and foreign tastes. This boundary does not come to the conscious surface when we are relaxed in our own dietary cultures. Rather, it is sensed to varying degrees when we encounter unfamiliar flavors. The experience of foreign tastes draws our attention not only to the boundary but also to our own culture's taste pattern, of which we are normally unaware.

Why is it that the familiar taste of our own culinary culture seems right, proper, or even just neutral, while foreign tastes seem exotic, wrong, or sometimes even repulsive? It is too easy to answer that taste is a matter of habit and that habits cannot be explained. I wish instead to consider the cultural patterning of tastes among people who share approximately the same culinary arts and knowledge. I call this pattern the culture's standard taste; it provides a sense of taste appropriateness, serving as a baseline for their judgments of flavors over the entire course of life. Admittedly, a single society can have more than one pattern of standard taste, depending on the breadth and complexity of its culinary history. Moreover, individuals can become comfortable with several different patterns, based on what foods they were regularly exposed to during childhood, that is, what foods educated their senses. People raised in a multicultural environment certainly seem more likely to acquire versatility in their culinary preferences.

What is a standard taste, then? It could easily be misunderstood as a typical dish or a well-known menu considered representative of a particular ethnic cuisine. Such dishes and menus can be stereotypes that are emphasized and sometimes shaped by outsiders' imaginations; they do not necessarily represent the typical taste of the culinary culture in question. One such example is the stereotyped image of Japanese food. World-famous raw fish in the form of sushi and sashimi have given the impression, clearly wrong, that the Japanese have long been raw fish eaters.[3] The habit of eating fish completely raw spread throughout Japan only in relatively recent times after sanitary conditions had improved through the development of transportation measures and cold storage systems.[4] In fact, the habit of eating raw fish in Japan has its oldest origin in a dish called *nare-zushi* in which the fish is not actually raw. Instead, the fish is fermented with salt and steamed rice. For understanding the Japanese enthusiasm for seafood, the long history of fermented fish flavors is a better guide than today's fashionable taste of raw fish.[5]

As in this example, stereotypes tend to emphasize superficial features of a cuisine by overfocusing on ingredients, seasonings, or cooking techniques that are unknown or uncommon elsewhere. By contrast, the standard taste that I have in mind here is not necessarily accorded much attention. It is related more closely to the underlying processes of cooking than to the visible and stylistic externals of the finished form. It is a particular type of flavor achieved by the combination of specific ingredients and associated cooking processes.

Throughout human history, in each society the initial availability of local foods prompted development of suitable processing and cooking methods. The linking of ingredients and specialized techniques is a cultural creation that often takes a long time—the accumulated effort of generations—to achieve. In some cases, however, standard tastes have shorter histories. A standard taste can form and become pervasive in a cuisine through the inspiration provided by a nonnative food at first considered exotic. In Korean cuisine, for example, red chili—an indispensable ingredient for the basic flavor both of *kimchi* and hot red pepper paste (*koch'ujang*)—was first introduced at the end of the sixteenth century (Kang 2000, 241–43; Lee 1999, 28; Shu et al. 1985, 103–113; and Yoon 2005, 418–20), a relatively recent point in the history of Korean cooking. The Korean case demonstrates that standard tastes can change, to some extent, through acceptance of foreign ingredients and flavors.[6] Whether it took a long time or not for a standard taste to be established is not really the point. Rather, what makes a taste standard is its wide acceptance as an indispensable flavor for many dishes. It is thus accepted by people who share a culture and incorporate the standard taste as a basic aspect of their culinary arts.

Standard tastes are deeply associated with particular ingredients and specialized preparation techniques. Nevertheless, our understanding of standard tastes should not be reduced to mere inventories of ingredients and procedures. What is most important about a standard taste is its flavoring effect whereby the ingredients and techniques reliably produce a certain range of expected tastes collectively preferred by tongues trained in a particular culinary culture. The preferred flavor always has an acceptable range for variation, although where the margins should lie is forever a cause of arguments. Because the standard taste is actually a range of acceptable flavors, new ingredients can sometimes fit into existing cooking processes or can substitute for other ingredients. Sometimes a new ingredient can even come regularly or permanently to replace a former ingredient (see the essay by Osborn in this volume). Such a change in a basic ingredient can lead to a new direction for or the refinement of a standard taste. This occurred with Japanese food when fermented soy-based sauces gradually replaced fermented fish-based sauces. New ingredients and substitutes can thus trigger changes in standard tastes.

Often enough, the standardized favorite flavors of an ethnic cuisine are made from combinations of an amino acid with other ingredients that add special aromas or gustatory sensations (see, for example, the essay by Cwiertka and Moriya on Korean soyfoods in this volume).[7] These basic flavors serve as the foundation for the overall taste of many dishes, imparting common characteristics that we instinctively associate with that cuisine.

Standard Taste: The Japanese Case

In contemporary Japanese cuisine, the standard taste has two major elements: (1) a kind of fish stock, dashi, that is an infusion of kelp and dried fish, and (2) fermented soybean products, either soy sauce or miso, which is a paste. In many Japanese recipes, these two elements play an important role in producing or subtly sustaining the typical overall flavor.

The traditional soup, *misoshiru*, is an everyday dish made mostly of these two elements. Other popular dishes such as *nimono* (stews) and other simmered or braised meats and vegetables must contain these two elements as basic flavorings, lest the cook fail to produce the expected tastes. But major dishes are not the only ones with this flavor pattern. Even side dishes and condiments—such as dip for a first course of sashimi or sauces for tempura (deep-fried foods)—also must include dashi and soy sauce, although usually inconspicuously.

The reason that dashi and fermented soy evolved into the standard taste of Japanese cuisine is suggested by Naomichi Ishige's famous theory of *umami-bunkaken*, or the "*umami* cultural area" (Ishige and Ruddle 1990, 333–59).[8] *Umami* means a taste of protein derived from the amino acid glutamate, whose flavor is sometimes enhanced by certain nucleotides. These chemicals naturally occur in various foods including fish, kelp, shellfish, meat, fermented products, and mushrooms.

The peoples of East and Southeast Asia have long been keen on such *umami* elements in their diets. In ancient times they developed *umami* seasonings, such as fish sauces in Southeast Asia and fermented soy products in China. Fish sauces, soy-based sauces, or both have become indispensable parts of all East and Southeast Asian cuisines, thereby giving rise to the *umami* cultural area. This predilection for *umami* is why both seafood stock and soybean extracts became basic components of Japanese standard taste.

According to Ishige (Ishige and Ruddle 1990), the *umami* cultural area can be divided into two subregions based on the salted and fermented *umami* sauces the people prefer. People in the East Asian region—with China at its center—prefer sauces made from fermented grains and beans. People in Southeast Asia, by contrast, prefer sauces made from fermented fish. This dichotomy should be understood as a marker of relative preferences, of course, indicating general differences between two large culture areas; there is no rigid boundary demarcating peoples in this very vibrantly interacting region.

Japan belongs to the first subregion today, since soy sauce is used constantly all over the country, whereas fish sauce is unfamiliar to most contemporary Japanese. However, locally made, fermented fish sauces such as *shotsuru, ishiri-shoyu,* and *ikanago-shoyu*[9] are still in use in some places in Japan. The long-standing existence of such local fish sauces offers proof that the Japanese share an ancient culinary history with the peoples of Southeast Asia in spite of the many Chinese influences on Japan's overall culture. The presence of dashi in everyday Japanese cuisine apparently represents a continuation of that Southeast Asian tradition.

Origins of the Components

The two major ingredients in dashi have an extensive history in Japan. *Kombu,*[10] or kelp, was first mentioned in the *Shokunihongi,*[11] a forty-volume history about eighth-century Japan that was completed in AD 797. According to this work, in AD 715 during the Nara Era—and even earlier—*kombu* was a precious tribute from the Ezo ethnic group in northern Japan to the court of the central government. In the Heian era (794 to the later twelfth century AD), *kombu* was sent to temples for the vegetarian diets of Buddhist monks. After the mid-Kamakura Era (in the thirteenth century), trade between Hokkaido, the Ezo-dominated area, and the mainland increased. It became easier to transport *kombu* from Hokkaido through the Sea of Japan to a port in the Wakasa region and then on to the city of Kyoto. Beginning in the early Edo era (1603–1868), well-developed sea trade brought *kombu* to Osaka, from which it spread even to Kyushu and the southernmost Japanese islands in what is now Okinawa Prefecture.

The use of *kombu* for dashi is said to have begun during the Genroku period (1688–1704). By the mid-Edo era in the Keihanshin district (the Kyoto-Osaka-Kobe area), cooking with *kombu*-infused dashi was popular even among ordinary people. *Kombu* has since become an indispensable ingredient for dashi in the wider area of western Japan's Kansai region.

The other main ingredient in dashi is dried fish, particularly the highly appreciated *katsuo-bushi,* or skipjack (striped bonito), that has been steamed, smoked, sometimes fermented, and then dried. *Katsuo* (skipjack)[12] was eaten as early as the first century BC in the Yayoi Era. It was perhaps initially consumed raw, although according to the *Teijohzakki*[13] from the late Edo era (1843), even in very ancient times it was used only in a dried form. In any case, by the Nara era (eighth century AD) it was referred to in official writings on wooden tablets as *katauo* (meaning "solid dried fish"), apparently a proto form of *katsuo-bushi.* In that era, boiling water infused with *katauo* was used to make a seasoning extract.

The name *katsuo-bushi* first appeared in the Muromachi era (approximately 1333 to 1573), although a similar use of dried skipjack was recorded during the Kamakura era (late twelfth century to 1333). A method of fermenting *katsuo-bushi* with mold developed extensively during the Edo period (1603–1868). In the Tokyo-centered Kanto region, the flavor of *katsuo-bushi* broth is highly valued and much preferred over that of *kombu.* This pattern contrasts sharply with the Kansai-region preference for *kombu* or a combination of *kombu* and *katsuo* flavors.

As Ehara (1997, 53) indicates, it is strange that cheaper dried fish for dashi, which must have been used in the past and are still daily consumed today throughout Japan, hardly appear in the historical writings. This omission may indicate that miscellaneous dried fish were too common to be mentioned in official documents or literature. In spite of their low status, such miscellaneous dried fish have been important for various kinds of dashi, especially for traditional noodle soups that require strong, thick broths.

By contrast with the origins of fish- and kelp-based broths, the other component of Japanese standard taste, fermented soy, has its origin in

Chinese culinary culture. Soy sauce and miso paste arose from an early seasoning called *hishio* in Japanese and *jiang* in Chinese.[14] This condiment was not divided into the liquid form (Japanese shoyu) and paste (Japanese miso) as it is today.

Hishio in Japanese originally refers to salt-fermented foods such as grains, fish, meat, or vegetables. Japanese historians posit that salting food was not originally a means of preserving the foods but rather a way to preserve precious sea salt by preventing it from absorbing moisture from the air. It is argued that unchecked deliquescence unpleasantly altered salt in taste and quality. The best way to keep the quality of salt stable was to preserve it in food (Higuchi 1987[1959], 76–77; Hirashima 1973, 68).

The various types of *hishio* gradually evolved into three categories of food: salted soy and grain varieties, which later developed into seasonings such as shoyu and miso, salted fish and meats (*shiokara* in Japanese), and pickled vegetables (*tsukemono* in Japanese).

There are two major explanations for how *hishio* was introduced to Japan. One is that Koreans who settled in the Owari, Mino, and Ohmi regions (central and western Japan) during the Asuka era (sixth century to AD 710) taught the Japanese the manufacturing process. At that time it was called *Koma-bishio* (Korean *jiang*) in Japanese, and it was soy-based. The other view is that *hishio* developed from *Tang ji*—Chinese dried fermented soybeans—brought by Ganjin, a Buddhist monk who came from China in AD 753. It appears that the story of older origins has merit (although both stories may be true), since according to the Taihoritsuryo, a law code from AD 701, some form of *hishio* was already being made in certain localities.

In those days *hishio* was so precious that the government provided it as a salary for high-ranking officials. In the Heian era, *tera-nattoh* (dried fermented soybeans made in Buddhist temples and developed from the original Chinese recipe) was used as a seasoning, and *hishio* was provided to the royalty and nobility. *Hishio* must have separated naturally into the paste (miso) and liquid (shoyu) during its storage, and people must have used both.

Thus, from the archaic mixture called *jiang*, *miso* first developed. During the Heian era (794 to the later twelfth century AD), as rice farming expanded in Japan, rice was added to the soybeans in the original continental recipe as another important ingredient. The use of rice in miso began the significant adaptation of continental *jiang* to Japanese preferences. Such localization increased as miso became widely accepted in Japan.

During the Kamakura era (later twelfth century to AD 1333), miso became popular among the people living in Zen Buddhist temples, and miso recipes such as *misoni,* simmered vegetables seasoned with miso, developed. In the later Kamakura era, as Japanese soybean production increased, miso became affordable even to ordinary people.

One famous explanation about the origins of soyfoods in Japan maintains that a Japanese Zen Buddhist monk, Kakushin, went to study in Hangzhou, China, during the Kamakura era and brought the recipe for *Kinzanji-miso* to his hometown, presently known as Yuasa-Cho of Wakayama Prefecture in Japan. The miso was named after the temple with which he was affiliated during his training in China. It is a kind of *name-miso*—literally, "lick miso"—that is served plain as an accompaniment to rice or alcoholic drinks. This usage contrasts with the typical utilization of the common, contemporary type of miso as an ingredient in cooking.

It is said that due to the difference of ingredients and climate in Japan, the locally produced *Kinzanji-miso* became unexpectedly soft and watery, yielding a clear liquid in the bottom of the cask. This liquid was later developed into *tamari-shoyu,* the dark, thick precursor of today's forms of soy sauce. Manufacturers in the town of Yuasa produced and distributed it in the sixteenth century.[15] Yuasa is thus deemed the place where the first type of shoyu (soy sauce) was invented.

Misoshiru (miso soup), one of the well-known principal items of the Japanese diet, was developed during the Muromachi era (approximately AD 1333–1573), after earthenware mortars and wooden pestles came to be widely used to break down coarse-grained miso. More recipes developed during the Edo era (1603–1868), when miso manufacturing spread to many areas of the country. By the end of the Edo era, sophisticated processing skills and devices had tremendously improved miso's flavor.

Although miso and shoyu both developed from antecedent *hishio,* the use of shoyu was limited to people in the upper layers of society as a luxury seasoning until the Edo period, whereas miso became popular among ordinary people as early as the Muromachi era (approximately AD 1333–1573). One reason that miso became more common is that once the standard method and recipe had been established, it was easier for ordinary people to produce at home than was shoyu. Shoyu making was more costly in small-scale production, since only a limited amount of liquid could be obtained from the ingredients, whereas with miso there were no residual wastes. The expression *temae-miso* (literally "taking pride in one's homemade miso"), which figuratively means "singing one's own praises," apparently arose during this period, when homemade miso became common in the Japanese countryside.

Although shoyu became widespread at a later time than miso, once it did become popular it developed into many varieties. *Usukuchi-shoyu,* a light-colored soy sauce, was first produced in 1587 in the place presently known as Tatsuno City of Hyogo Prefecture. It is one of the typically localized versions of soy sauce. To this day it is preferred in western Japan, where not only the taste but also the appearance of food is highly valued, as it does not impart any dark color to foods.

Shoyu especially developed throughout the Edo era. Soy sauce delivered from the town of Yuasa to Tokyo around 1640 was called *kudari-shoyu* and was considered superior to other types. It was further developed in the Tokyo region, where fresh seafood was abundant, in order to adjust its taste to complement the various types of fish locally caught and enjoyed. These developments created *koikuchi-shoyu,* the special dark soy sauce of Japan. Noda and Choshi of Chiba Prefecture developed as production centers of *koikuchi-shoyu* in the Kanto region (east Japan). This invention gave fermented soy a particularly Japanese flavor. During the eighteenth and nineteenth centuries, not only the locals but also Europeans gave high marks to its sophistication (Tanaka 1999, 12).

Whether homemade or bought from specialized manufacturers, both miso and shoyu have come to be widely accepted as seasonings, especially since the later Edo period (the early nineteenth century). During that time various dishes that are still cooked today were developed and popularized. Many of today's traditional dishes have their roots in this fairly recent period, when not only shoyu but also more sophisticated and developed dashi ingredients became accessible to ordinary people. Thus, the basic combination of the Japanese standard taste, shoyu and dashi, must have emerged during this period, when all the ingredients and materials became not only available but also affordable to the vast majority of the Japanese people.

The Persistent Nature of the Standard Taste

From the time when *jiang* was introduced to the periods when *katsuo-bushi* (specially prepared dried skipjack) and later kelp began to be used for dashi broth, some thousand years passed. These were the ingredients that would come together into a harmonious standard taste. But it was later still, toward the end of the Edo era (early nineteenth century), that all the major elements—miso, shoyu, *kombu,* and *katsuo-bushi*—finally became affordable enough for ordinary people that they could invent new recipes and include these flavors in their daily diets. Once these flavors were easily available, it took less than a hundred years for them to thoroughly permeate Japanese cuisine.

As noted earlier, the length of time needed for a standard taste to become well established is variable. But once a standard taste has become pervasive in a cuisine, it tends to persist, whether it has a very long history of development or a fairly recent origin. Although a standard taste is sometimes under assault from a different set of flavors, it still manages to endure. This is not to say, however, that it cannot gradually be replaced by some other standard taste emergent in a people's foodways.

It is likely that the standard tastes of many diets around the world will be stubbornly resilient, even though they are now being challenged by sweeping waves of globalization. The Japanese diet is a case in point.

Recently in Japan, traditional home cooking—dubbed "mothers' taste"—is becoming a trend again. Such cooking is becoming popular because the cuisine incorporates copious vegetables and seafood and employs less fatty cooking methods than the dominant Westernized diet, which is heavy on fat, meat, and sweets. People now perceive the old ways as healthier and nutritionally more balanced. Home cooking is thus a kind of culinary critique of the modern diet, which is associated with many lifestyle diseases such as obesity, diabetes, and arteriosclerosis. The Japanese had little experience of such diseases in the past.

The trend is also spurred by the praises of mass media, which portray home cooking as an authentic tradition from the country's past. The return to mothers' taste is thus reminiscent of the slow-food movement initiated in Italy. It appears that anti–fast-food movements are now developing in many parts of the world to varying degrees, although it is not always clear whether they have been influenced by Italy's slow-food movement or whether they embody spontaneous resistance within each culture to the ongoing drastic changes challenging their traditional diets.

In any case, Japan's back-to-authentic-eating trend celebrates the *obanzai* ("everyday fare") of the traditional vegetable-laden Kyoto diet in particular and, more generally, the *osohzai* ("daily food") of all good old-fashioned Japanese foodways.[16] Such time-honored Japanese cuisine is being reviewed and reevaluated by mass media. Moreover, recent tourists visiting Kyoto have been attracted to restaurants touting special full-course *obanzai* menus and to stores in the city's Nishiki market that feature so-called traditional health-oriented, natural foods such as tofu, *yuba* (bean curd sheets), and sweets made from soymilk. Even fresh vegetables, each with a regional brand name, are much in demand among the tourists for their image of locally based tradition and authenticity. Yet another reason that *obanzai* and *osohzai* menus are now being reappreciated, aside from their appeal to the health-conscious and those seeking authenticity, is that for slow foods, their cooking is relatively simple and does not take a long time, which also suits the busy people of today.

Yet in the midst of this trend, fast food continues to develop more and more forms and is provided through ever-expanding channels. Convenience stores are one such channel, where fast food is making rapid progress in meeting increasing consumer demands; it seems that they wish to buy some new ready-to-eat food at all times. The competition among convenience stores has grown so fierce that they have even been forced to offer quality food in spite of customers' usual demand for instant products. In this paradoxical situation, convenience stores have come to offer some high-quality foods with higher prices. One of their higher-grade lines features the authentic tastes of good old-fashioned household menus for lunch boxes. Thus, the back-to-tradition trend is reflected in fast-food products as well as in slow foods.

The Japanese craving for *osohzai* tastes even today, despite the market availability of almost any foreign food, demonstrates the persisting nature of the standard taste. It indicates that the basic flavor pairing of shoyu and dashi is still so deeply imprinted on the Japanese that it remains a reference point to which people can return at any time, even after many years of exploring exotic flavors. In fact, the standard taste is often reproduced or perceived even in foreign dishes. Striving to please Japanese diners, some cooks add shoyu to other countries' recipes. When trying their hands at foreign cuisines, many Japanese cooks also unconsciously gravitate toward flavors similar to Japanese food. Whatever is most similar to the Japanese standard taste is what gets prepared; thus, many ethnic dishes come to taste somewhat like Japanese cuisine. For example, so-called Indian curry often has a flavor of shoyu.

It is even claimed that a very popular Japanese cigarette has a flavor similar to shoyu. These examples show how the standard taste can ground people's taste judgments. Often it is used to judge the flavors of a foreign cuisine, although that other cuisine arises from a different standard taste and is supposed to be cooked and to taste accordingly rather than to fit with the pattern of the local foods. We thus see how the standard taste tends to affect people's senses once it has been fully internalized.

Ongoing and Prospective Changes

Although Japan's standard taste is still sustained both in the slow- and fast-food markets, changes in the components are inevitably taking place. In the latter half of the twentieth century, ready-made instant stock largely replaced homemade dashi. Instant stock has a stronger taste than the delicate flavor of the original and natural infusion. The taste of chemically concentrated glutamate is sensed more quickly and lasts longer on the tongue than the natural levels of glutamate in home-cooked dashi. Accustomed now to the taste of synthetic seasonings, the people no longer have the patience to slowly savor the natural taste on their tongues. Instead they seek the instantly sensible flavor of artificial stock.

By contrast, the tastes of shoyu, miso, and other fermented soy products are becoming lighter nowadays. This is because salt fermentation, long used worldwide as a means of food preservation, is becoming outdated. Cold storage techniques and transportation systems are so developed that people no longer depend on fermentation to safeguard their food against spoilage. Hence, salt fermentation is becoming a totally dispensable luxury, done only to delight the tongue.

This change of major preservation method initiated a change in taste preferences. Now that strong fermentation is unnecessary, a light hint of fermented flavor and aroma are commonly sought after, and people are less and less likely to prefer a rich salty taste anymore. In addition, recent concerns about health appear to have prompted somewhat less use of salt in developed countries, although many processed foods such as soups and chips are still high in salt. In any case, the health concern has probably further led to a reduction of salt in fermented foods.[17]

Japan's standard taste has thus been modified to consist of the easily sensible taste of dashi stock and the lightly fermented taste of shoyu. Yet this modified standard still adheres to the basic framework of dashi and shoyu. It has simply been adjusted to the needs and tastes of today's people with what are actually relatively modest changes to the traditional recipes.

The use of ready-made stock is apparently an irreversible trend worldwide, and so the artificial taste of chemical seasoning will likely prevail in most cuisines. If other fundamental changes were to occur in the future, I suppose they could consist of alterations in the tastes of fermented foods. It is unclear whether we are heading for a loss of fermented tastes in our varied food cultures or whether instead we are taking those flavors back in waves of food nostalgia. Gauging the extent to which Italy's slow-food movement is inspiring people in other dietary cultures will be an important aspect of any attempt to predict world food trends. Yet no matter how the fashion for slow food or other similar movements resists the globalization of local diets, the globalizing waves cannot really be kept away. Foreign products and cuisines enter local food markets and industries in this era when communication and transportation networks connect even the most remote areas of the world. Resistance will be a matter of balance between globalization and the preservation of local foodways. People committed to local culinary cultures must ask themselves to what extent they should accept globalizing trends. If they wish to keep their old ways at least partially intact, they must acknowledge that their daily choices on food matters powerfully shape the futures of their dietary cultures.

Notes

1. I would like to express my deepest gratitude here to the editors: Professor Sidney W. Mintz, for offering me the opportunity to engage in food research; Professor Chee-Beng Tan, who first initiated me to the topic of soyfoods through his chaired session in Chengdu; and especially Dr. Christine M. Du Bois, who lavishly extended her help and support not only in editing the text but also in clarifying ideas and concepts through patiently repeated discussions. Although I owe it mostly to her devoted efforts that I could complete my work, any errors or mistakes, if found in the text, should not be ascribed to anyone but myself.

2. It seems oxymoronic that studies of food cultures infrequently deal with taste. Questions such as "What tastes good to this society?" or "How can we predict the difference between something that tastes good and something that tastes bad?" are insufficiently raised by academics. Instead, academics often concentrate on other details about foodstuffs or on the social phenomena with which foods are either directly or indirectly related. I have been wondering why taste is not a focus of food studies even though it is such an important part of human cultures. In this light, here I suggest a viewpoint that may be useful for understanding taste in particular societies.

3. Historians generally agree that eating raw fish in the form of *sashimi* began during the Muromachi era (approximately 1333 to 1573) (see Watanabe 1964, 145; Okuyama 2001, 181). *Sashimi* became a formal course in the category of *namamono,* or uncooked food, just when soy sauce, an indispensable accompaniment for *sashimi,* was developing. However, at that time the category of uncooked food was not completely separated from those of *namasu* (vinegared food) and *aemono* (generally, food marinated in sauces including vinegar or some sour ingredient). Hence, few seafood dishes were served completely raw, since the vinegar partly cooked them. Raw seafood dishes thus evolved from fish cooked with vinegar. As

for the history of sushi, the original form, developed during the Nara era (710–784), was fermented fish or animal meat with salted and steamed rice. This archaic sushi was called *nare-zushi.* Initially, the rice was not eaten. Today's sushi developed from this ancient precursor (Watanabe 1964, 61, 216–24; see also Hibino 1992; Hibino 1997; and Ishige and Ruddle 1990).

4. Watanabe (1964, 289–90) indicates that beginning in 1899, a big ice manufacturing company in Tokyo supplied fifty tons of ice every day. This supply made possible the transportation of fresh raw fish to areas where only salted or dried fish had been eaten. This development fits with the observation that ordinary Japanese who lived far from the sea could not enjoy fresh raw fish until the latter half of the Meiji era (1868–1912), although raw fish recipes had already appeared in print and had been known to the whole nation.

5. *Nare-zushi,* or fish fermented with rice and salt, is still eaten in some parts of Japan as a special local delicacy reminiscent of old-time foodways. Although its flavor was once very common in Japanese cuisine, it is itself no longer widespread.

6. According to Kang (2000, 37), after chilis were accepted Korean cuisine shifted to a preference for "seasoned flavors," by contrast with the former taste for "light flavors." This is a good example of how newly acquired ingredients can be incorporated into existing cooking processes and create a new harmony of flavors, a harmony that eventually becomes a central part of the cuisine.

7. Despite its importance, glutamate is not always recognized as a component of a culture's standard taste. Such may be the case with the glutamate in the broths and sauces of traditional French cuisine.

8. For detailed explanations of *umami,* see also Kohno (1997) and Tanaka (1999, 22–24).

9. For further information about local shoyu varieties, see Aspect Inc. (1999, 87) and Okuyama (2001).

10. The history of *kombu* in this essay is based on the descriptions in Matsushita (1991) and Okada (2003).

11. This work is one of six formal documents of national history (the *Rikkokushi*) compiled during both the Nara (710–784) and Heian (794 to the later twelfth century AD) eras. This document reports that Suganokimikomahiru, the leader of the Ezo ethnic group, explained to the court in 715 that his family had presented them with *kombu* for generations (Miyashita 1994, 212).

12. This history of *katsuo-bushi* is reconstructed from descriptions in Ehara (1997), Matsushita (1991), and Okada (2003).

13. This is a collection of miscellaneous records and studies on the origins and changes of customs of the Samurai class. Ise Sadatake wrote it in 1843 for the convenience of his descendants.

14. The development of *hishio,* miso, and shoyu outlined in this essay is based on Hirashima (1973, 68–69), Imai and Matsumoto (1996, 116–20), Kanzaki (1987,

105–14), Maeda (1994, 270–73), Okada (2003, 224–26, 435–36), Okuyama (2001, 383–85), Tanaka (1999, 11–21, 391–94), and Yoshikawa and Ohori (2002, 62–64, 74–80).

15. According to Shurtleff and Aoyagi (2007), tamari was first sold in Yuasa in AD 1290. Naomichi Ishige (2000), by contrast, places the first commercialization in the sixteenth century. The difference in dates reflects the degree of commercialization discussed.

16. *Osohzai* has almost the same meaning as *obanzai*. The latter, a word from the Kyoto regional dialect, was reinterpreted and spread in the media by Shige Ohmura, a Japanese home cuisine specialist. She was a public intellectual engaged in preserving traditional Kyoto folk foodways.

17. Preference for a lightly salted taste is common in developed countries, while in developing Asian societies, such as the Philippines where I do fieldwork, a richly salty taste is still frequently preferred, especially among the poor. This is true despite the government's and doctors' recommendations that people consume less salt. The traditional preference for highly salty flavors may stem from the reliance of the poor on an otherwise rather bland rice diet. This example and others suggest that changes in preferences for salty foods, including fermented ones, may have much to do with modernization and rising standards of living.

References

Aspect Inc., eds. 1999. *Shihou no Chomiryo 1: Shoyu* [*Shoyu: Japanese "Shoyu" Sauce Book, Catalog, and Cooking Guide*]. Tokyo: Aspect, Inc.

Ehara, Satoru. 1997. "Shokuseikatsu Gendaishi no Ichishiten: Katsuobushi wo Chushin ni Shite" ["A Perspective on Modern Dietary History from the Viewpoint Centered on '*Katsuobushi*.'"] In Noboru Haga and Hiroko Ishikawa, eds., *Nihon no Shokubunka* [*Japanese Dietary History*], Vol. 4, 43–64. Tokyo: Yuhikaku.

Hibino, Terutoshi. 1992. "Sushi." In Matsunosuke Nishiyama et al., eds., *Tabemono Nihonshi Souran* [*Historical Survey of Foods in Japan*], 108–9. Tokyo: Shinjinbutsu Ohrai Sha.

———. 1997. *Sushi no Kao: Jidai ga Motometa Aji no Kakumei* [*The Appearance of Sushi: Taste Revolutions Sought through the Ages*]. Tokyo: Taikosha.

Higuchi, Kiyoyuki. 1987[1959]. *Nihon Shokumotsu Shi: Shoku Seikatsu no Rekishi* [*Japanese Food History: Transitions in Dietary Life*], rev. ed. Tokyo: Shibata Shoten.

Hirashima, Hiromasa. 1973. *Mono to Ningen no Bunkashi, Shio* [*Salt in the Cultural History of Things and Humans*], Vol. 7. Tokyo: Hosei University Press.

Imai, Seiichi, and Isao Matsumoto. 1996. "Shoyu Miso Johzou to Nyuusan Hakkou no Yakuwari" ["The Role of Lactic Acid Bacteria in the Processing of Shoyu and Miso"]. In Michio Ozaki, ed., *Nyuusan Hakkou no Bunkafu* [*Cultural Historiography of Lactic Acid Fermentation*], 116–45. Tokyo: Chuo Hoki.

Ishige, Naomichi. 2000. "Japan." In Kenneth F. Kiple and Kriemhild Coneè Ornelas, eds., *The Cambridge World History of Food*, 1175–83. Cambridge: Cambridge University Press.

Ishige, Naomichi, and Dae-Seong Jung. 1995. *Shokubunka Nyuumon* [*Introduction to Dietary Culture*]. Tokyo: Kohdansha.

Ishige, Naomichi and Kenneth Ruddle. 1990. *Gyosho to Narezushi no Kenkyu: Monsun Ajia no Shokujibunka* [*Study of Fish Sauce and Nare-zushi: Dietary Cultures of Monsoon Asia*]. Tokyo: Iwanami Shoten.

Kang, In-Hee. 2000. *Kankoku Shokuseikatsushi: Genshi Kara Gendai Made* [*Korean Dietary History: From Ancient Times to the Present*]. Translated into Japanese by Soon-E Hyun from the original Korean edition of 1978, later revised and republished in Korean in 1990. Tokyo: Fujiwara Shoten.

Kanzaki, Noritake. 1987. *Nihonjin wa Nani wo Tabete Kitaka?* [*What Have the Japanese Been Eating?*] Tokyo: Ohtsuki Shoten.

Kohno, Tomomi. 1997. *Aji no Bunkashi* [*A Cultural History of Taste*]. Tokyo: Sekai Shoin.

Lee, Seong-Woo. 1999. *Kankoku Ryori Bunkashi* [*History of Korean Culinary Culture*]. Translated into Japanese by Dae-Seong Jung and Naoko Sasaki from the original Korean edition published in 1985. Tokyo: Heibonsha.

Maeda, Toshiie. 1994. "Shoyu" and "Miso." In Matsunosuke Nishiyama et al., eds., *Tabemono Nihonshi Sohran* [*Comprehensive Dictionary of Foods in Japanese History*], 270–73. Tokyo: Shinjinbutsu Ohrai Sha.

Matsushita, Sachiko. 1991. *Iwai no Shokubunka* [*Dietary Culture of Festive Occasions*]. Tokyo: Tokyo Bijutsu.

Miyashita, Akira. 1994. "Kombu." In Matsunosuke Nishiyama et al., eds., *Tabemono Nihonshi Sohran* [*Comprehensive Dictionary of Foods in Japanese History*], 212. Tokyo: Shinjinbutsu Ohrai Sha.

Nishiyama, Matsunosuke, et al., eds. 1994. *Tabemono Nihonshi Sohran* [*Comprehensive Dictionary of Foods in Japanese History*]. Tokyo: Shinjinbutsu Ohrai Sha.

Okada, Tetsu. 2003. *Tabemono Kigen Jiten* [*Dictionary of Food Origins*]. Tokyo: Tokyodo.

Okuyama, Masuroh. 2001. *Mikaku Jiten: Nihon Ryori* [*Dictionary of Taste: Japanese Cuisine*]. Tokyo: Tokyodo.

Shu, Tassei, Dae-Seong Jung, and Sasuke Nakao. 1985. *Ajia no Shokubunka* [*Asian Food Culture*]. Osaka, Japan: Osaka Shoseki.

Shurtleff, William, and Akiko Aoyagi. 2007. "History of Soy Sauce, Shoyu, and Tamari." http://www.soyinfocenter.com/HSS/soy_sauce3.php.

Tanaka, Norio. 1999. *Shoyu Kara Sekai wo Miru: Noda wo Chushin to Shita Higashi Katsushika Chihou no Taigai Kankei Gaikohshi to Shoyu* [*Looking at the World through Shoyu: Shoyu and Foreign Trade History of the Noda and Higashi Katsushika Region*]. Nagareyama, Japan: Ron Shoboh.

Watanabe, Minoru. 1964. *Nihon Shoku Seikatsushi* [*History of Japanese Dietary Life*]. Tokyo: Yoshikawa Kohbunkan.

Yoon, Seo-Seok. 2005. *Kankoku Shokuseikatsu Bunka no Rekishi* [*History of Korean Dietary Culture*]. Translated into Japanese by Michio Sasaki from the original Korean edition, *Woorinara Sikseanghwal Munhwae Yoksa,* published by Shin Kwang through Shin Won Agency Co. in Korea in 1999. Tokyo: Akashi Shoten.

Yoshikawa, Seiji, and Yasuyoshi Ohori. 2002. *Nihon: Shoku no Rekishi Chizu* [*Historical Map of Food: Japan*]. Tokyo: NHK Press.

8

Fermented Soyfoods in South Korea

The Industrialization of Tradition

KATARZYNA J. CWIERTKA AND AKIKO MORIYA

"Koreans can hardly be Korean if they don't eat *toenjang*" (fermented bean paste)
Kim Il Sung in Cumings (1997, 396)

"The true taste that *only* Koreans are able to appreciate can come from no other food but *chang*"
Han and Han (1995, 26, emphasis added)

Introduction

Half a century ago, hunger was a common feature of life for the majority of South Koreans.[1] Three and a half decades (1910–45) of economic exploitation under Japanese colonial rule were followed by the devastation of the Korean War (1950–53). The 1948 division into two Korean states, the Democratic People's Republic of Korea in the north (industrialized and rich in mineral resources) and the Republic of Korea in the south (abundant in fertile rice paddies) paralyzed economic growth, condemning each half to the reestablishment of the economic components cut out of a functioning national economy. Throughout the 1950s, South Korea remained heavily dependent upon foreign aid, and even in the early 1960s the country was ranked among the world's poorest nations along with Burma, Congo, India, and Kenya (Nelson 2000, 6, 10).

The rapid economic development of the last three decades increased the per capita income from US$150 in 1960 to $10,548 in 1996 and enabled the country to become the eleventh-largest economy in the world (Pemberton 2002, 76). Urbanization proceeded at a spectacular tempo. While in

1960 city dwellers comprised 28.3 percent of Korea's[2] population, a quarter of a century later they had expanded to 65.4 percent.[3] More than half of them resided in the metropolitan cities of Seoul and Pusan. This has meant much more than just a geographic relocation. Of the country's forty-one million people, more than twenty-seven million lived and worked in social and economic settings that were far removed from those of their parents and grandparents. Their new places of residence made it practically impossible for such migrants to engage in the home production and processing of staples (Brandt 1971, 49–51; Hart 2001, 27, 42–43).

As the economy grew, the country's diet underwent changes. By 1990, average levels of expenditure on foodstuffs as a percentage of the household budget (the so-called Engels Coefficient) dropped to 32 percent (Nelson 2000, 73). Adjustments usually accompanying economic affluence, such as declines in the consumption of cereals and increases in the shares of meat, fish, vegetables, and fruit in the diet, advanced rapidly. Annual per capita rice consumption, for example, dropped from 132.4 kilograms (kg) in 1980 to 102.4 kg in 1997. Barley—formerly a food of considerable importance because, although less liked than rice, it was strongly promoted by the government to discourage grain imports—has now been abandoned by most people; consumption has declined from 36.8 kg per person in 1965 to 1.5 kg in 1996 (Pemberton 2002, 77). Per capita consumption of foodstuffs of animal origin such as beef, pork, chicken, eggs, milk, and dairy products had risen from 5.5 kg in 1965 to 93.7 kg in 1996. The consumption of industrially processed foods such as biscuits and commercially prepared meals increased significantly, and the percentage of an average household's food budget dedicated to eating out rose from 5.8 percent in 1982 to 22.5 percent a decade later (Nelson 2002, 74). By the 1990s, abundance and variety became the key attributes of the South Korean food scene. Laura Nelson sketched the new circumstances as follows:

> Street vendors built high pyramids of apples, oranges, and pears. Vending machines sold a range of South Korean and imported soft drinks. The shelves of neighborhood shops were filled with snack foods: chips, cookies, crackers, ramen, and chocolates, and supermarkets offered aisles packed with cereals, staples, snack foods as well as fresh vegetables, fresh fish and fresh meat. Prepared meals were offered at sidewalk stalls, quick Korean-cuisine food spots, fast-food joints, and high-class restaurants. South Korea had also become relatively open to imported foods of all kinds (Nelson 2000, 74–75).

Insufficient food supply has definitely disappeared as a social problem in South Korea, and the majority of the population today can even afford to indulge in foreign culinary trends. During the 1980s and 1990s, the Korean fast-food industry experienced tremendous growth. As of 2001, the major players on the market included Lotteria (752 outlets), BBQ (1400 outlets), McDonald's (321 outlets), KFC (236 outlets), Popeye's (185 outlets), and Burger King (113 outlets) (Jung and Kim 2003, 13). The coffee giant Starbucks is the most recent addition to the range of multinational chain stores in Korea. In 2007, the company operated 153 outlets in Seoul and 74 in the rest of the country.[4]

However, foreign food remains largely within a snack and dining-out category, only sporadically featuring in home cooking. With the exception of convenience foods such as pizza, Chinese-Japanese noodle soup (*ramyŏn*), and occasionally cooked pasta or Japanese-style curry,[5] foreign dishes rarely find their way into Korean kitchens.[6] The "rice-soup-*kimch'i* pickles[7]-side dishes" pattern remains the guiding principle of the majority of Korean meals, and even at the end of the twentieth century young brides continue to make an effort to learn to cook like the groom's mother (Potrzeba Lett 1998, 144). It should be pointed out, however, that certain foreign foods have by now firmly established themselves as components of a Korean-style meal. For example, variations of coleslaw often appear as a side dish alongside traditional stews and greens, and various kinds of sausage are not infrequently featured on the table, either as simply pan-fried, as *chŏn* (dipped in flour and egg, then pan-fried), or as ingredients in Korean stews.

Crowds of (overwhelmingly young) customers at McDonald's and the ice-cream parlor Baskin Robbins by no means indicate that Koreans are eager to abandon their native diet. To be sure, there is a certain ambivalence toward achieving a globalized lifestyle while losing Korean identity in the process (Nelson 2000, 25), and a preference for foreign food is interpreted by some Koreans as a sign of conspicuous consumption and vanity (Bak[8] 1997, 150). However, as foreign products and institutions become ubiquitous, people tend to see them increasingly as features of their daily lives and even begin to perceive them as "native" rather than "foreign."[9] A Starbucks outlet is not always a reminder of the encroachment of multinationals; it can also be regarded simply as a convenient meeting or resting place (figure 5).

Familiarity with foreign food trends appears to have made Koreans more conscious of their own culinary heritage. Even if the consumption of fresh

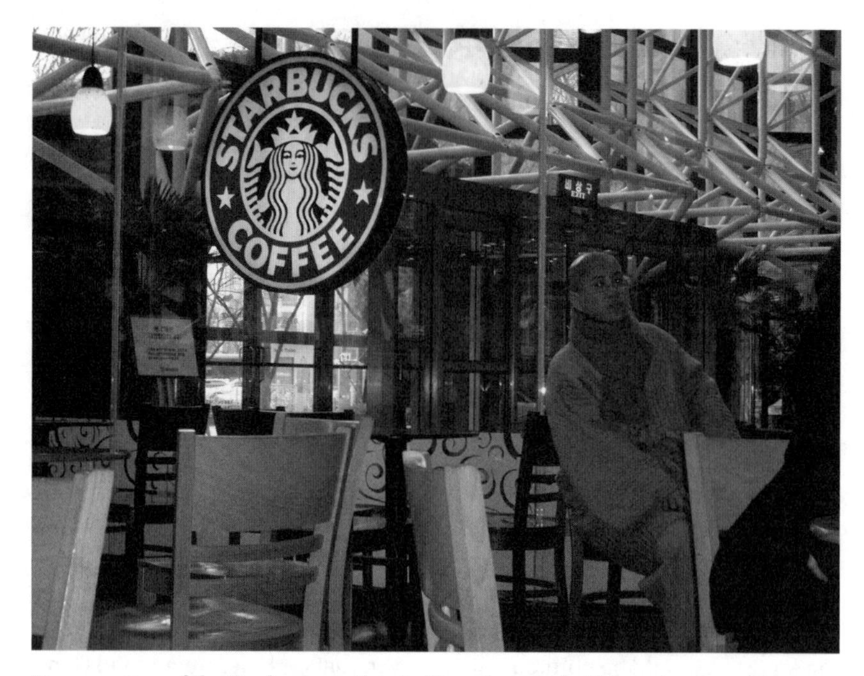

Figure 5. One of the Starbucks outlets in Korea's capital. Although not regular customers, nuns and monks are not an unusual sight at the Korean Starbucks. (Photo by K. J. Cwiertka, January 2005)

vegetables and meat as well as fruit, snacks, and instant foods increases and if the *kimch'i* pickles, rice, and soyfoods that had in the past dominated every meal appear in ever-declining quantities on Korean tables today (Korean Nutrition Society 1989, 90, 162–63), these items continue to play a central role in the Korean diet. To eat Korean food becomes increasingly a matter of conscious decision rather than the taken-for-granted act of the past. Taste, price, convenience, fashion, health consciousness, and cultural attitudes are the major motives that—in differing degree and varying order—influence the food choices of contemporary Koreans.

Soybeans constitute a fundamental component of the Korean diet. They appear on the table in a wide range of forms. Whole soybeans are boiled with other beans, rice, and other cereals (*k'ongbap*) or are mashed into a creamy soup that is usually served in the summer with noodles and julienned cucumber (*k'ongguksu*). Soybean sprouts are utilized as an ingredient in a variety of soups, stews, and stir-fries. A mainstay of daily menus is *k'ongnamul much'im*, blanched soybean sprouts seasoned with green onions, garlic, salt (or sometimes soy sauce), sesame oil, and crushed sesame seeds. Several kinds of soybean curd of different firmness are used in Korean cooking depending on whether it is to be fried, braised, or simmered. Fresh curd cut into squares and arranged with pieces of *kimch'i* pickles serves as a popular snack with alcoholic beverages (*tubu kimch'i*). When mixed with minced meat, bean curd can also be employed as a filling for dumplings (*mandu*) that are then fried or steamed. Roasted soybeans and roasted soybean flour are indispensable ingredients in many traditional desserts (*kwaja, ttŏk*).

During the last two decades, soymilk has joined the roster of popular soybean products in Korea. Despite a humble beginning in the 1960s as a substitute for cow's milk for children with lactose intolerance, it has by now become a daily beverage. It is drunk during meals as well as between them.

These soyfoods are by all means vital components of the Korean diet. However, in terms of significance they fall behind the crown jewels of Korean cuisine—fermented soyfoods (*chang*)—because *chang* is what determines the taste of most dishes.

The Soul of Korean Cuisine

Fermented soyfoods, which are often referred to by their generic name "*chang*," have played a central role in Korean cooking throughout its history. The soybean fermentation process is generally considered to be of Chinese origin (Huang 2000, 346–74), but Korean scholars claim that their ancestors are the founders of the *chang* culture of East Asia (i.e., Yi 1984, 15–16, 145–48; Kwon 1995, 19; Yi 1999, 21–32; Lee 2001, 70–71). Sorting out this dispute lies outside the scope of this essay. It appears, however, that the issue is much larger than the origin of fermented soyfoods alone. The technology of making *chang* from soybeans is documented by Korean researchers to have originated and developed in the kingdom of Koguryŏ, the most northerly of the three kingdoms into which the Korean peninsula was divided between the fourth and seventh centuries, and the kingdom of Parhae, a Manchurian kingdom established in 698 by the heirs and successors of the kings of Koguryŏ (Pratt and Rutt 1999, 226, 340–41). The Chinese government claims both Koguryŏ and Parhae as part of the history of China, and this interpretation has recently aroused tension in the region.[10]

It needs to be mentioned that Huang's volume *Fermentations and Food Science,* the most impressive historical work on the subject, does not address the fermented soyfoods of Korea, although it treats the Japanese case quite extensively. The reference to fermented soyfoods in Korea in the main text of the volume reads as follows: "But the spread of fermented soyfoods did not stop at Japan. We see similar products in Korea (*jang, doen jang*), Vietnam, Thailand, Indonesia (*taucho, kechap*) and Malaysia (*taucheo*). They all owe their origin to the ancient ferment, *chhü* (or *koji* in Japanese), which was developed initially to support the brewing of alcoholic drinks from grains as shown in Chapter (c)" (Huang 2000, 378). Huang's research can be usefully extended to the Korean peninsula, where fermented soyfoods have played a dietary role that is hard to overestimate. These foods can certainly be labeled the soul of Korean cuisine.

The culture of fermented condiments made of soybeans began to take shape in Korea during the Three Kingdoms period (57 BC–AD 668). A few centuries later, two major fermented soybean products—the liquid *kanjang* (soy sauce) and the solid *toenjang* (soybean paste)—developed (Han'guk Munhwachae Poho Chaedan 2001, 16–17). The third and most distinctive condiment in the Korean soybean trinity—hot red pepper paste (*koch'ujang*)—came into being much later after the introduction of red peppers into Korea at the end of the sixteenth century. The first references to this new variation of soybean paste in historical documents dates back to the second half of the seventeenth century (Lee 2001, 79).

For the last three hundred years, these three types of *chang* have constituted the very foundation of Korean taste, along with garlic, green onions, and hot red peppers (Han and Han 1995, 23–32). Hi Soo Shin Hepinstall[11] (2001, 24) writes that "there are three essential Korean sauces: soy sauce (kanjang), fermented soybean paste (toenjang), and hot red pepper paste (koch'ujang). They are primarily responsible for the character and unique flavor of Korean food. Traditionally, the sauces were made once a year and stored in a dozen or more large and small earthenware crocks placed on the backyard *changdokdae* (sauce-crock pad), a standard feature of every Korean home."

With the exception of sweets, *kimch'i* pickles, and rice,[12] it is difficult to find a Korean dish that does not contain one or another kind of *chang* or that is not customarily served with a dipping sauce based on some *chang* (Han and Han 1995, 25). Soy sauce, soybean paste, and hot red pepper paste are standard flavorings in soups (*kuk, t'ang*), stews (*tchigae*), and braised dishes (*chorim*). Meat is usually marinated in soy sauce or red pepper paste before it is sautéed or grilled, and dressings for greens often include soy sauce or soybean paste. Different varieties of *chang*, often mixed with vinegar or sesame oil, also appear on the table as dipping sauces. Due to the use of soy sauce (often in small quantities) in a wide range of dishes, in terms of quantity this is the most important type of *chang* in Korean cooking. However, all three play an equally important role in providing Korean cuisine with its distinctive taste.

The long-lasting centrality of *chang* in Korean cuisine is reflected in numerous sayings and proverbs. The dependence on *chang* for the flavor of most dishes, for example, is proclaimed in the expression "the taste of food is the taste of *chang*." The high value placed on *chang* is mirrored in a saying among exasperated women about how difficult and demanding husbands can sometimes be: "even twelve pots of *koch'ujang* can't please a husband." Another proverb declares that "the politics of a region are best understood by tasting its liquor, and the conditions in a household are best understood by tasting its *chang*," indicating the importance of *chang* in the management of the Korean household (Han and Han 1995, 23, 50).

The manufacture and storage of *chang* constituted a key concern of women, who were solely responsible for the production and cooking of food (Hart 2001, 102). The two major events that marked the passage of time in the Korean household were the pickling of *kimch'i* in late autumn and a range of activities related to the production of soybean pastes and sauces (Han and Han 1995, 24). In comparison with pickling *kimch'i*, the production of *chang* was a much more complicated chore, because it consisted of several tasks that had to be performed repeatedly at different times of the year.

First of all, the fermentation starter *meju*—dried lumps of fermented soybean mash—had to be manufactured. This took place in early winter after the *kimch'i* pickling had been completed. The mash was made of soybeans soaked in water and then boiled and shaped into lumps (bricks, discs, cones, or balls) that were next dried in the sun for several days and left for up to two weeks in a warm place to ferment. During this procedure the mold *Aspergillus oryzae* grew on the surface, and bacteria of *Bacillus* species multiplied inside each lump (Lee 2001, 71). Afterward, *meju* chunks had to be left to dry in the sun yet again for several weeks.[13] Great care was required when performing these chores; incorrect handling could mean being left without the most important ingredient for manufacturing *chang*.

In early spring, *meju* had to be immersed in brine in the ratio 2:4:1.2 (*meju*, water, salt) so that the salt concentration of the mash oscillated around 20 percent. Charcoal and red chili pepper were added to the mixture; the former was supposed to remove impurities, and the latter was used to sterilize the ingredients. The pulp was then placed in a large crock where amino acids and sugars formed by the breakdown of the soybeans were exuded, becoming part of the brine, and salt-tolerant yeasts had a chance to grow. After a few months, the mixture acquired a dark brown color and meaty flavor. At this stage, *toenjang* and *kanjang* were not yet separated from each other. The liquid was drained from the pulp and then boiled and left to mature for forty to sixty days, and this turned into the traditional Korean soy sauce that could keep for several years. The mash that remained after the liquid had been drained was mixed with salt, packed tightly in a jar, and then left to ferment in the sun for another month. The result was the classic Korean soybean paste (National Academy of the Korean Language 2002, 65–68).

The third major type of Korean *chang*, red chili pepper paste, is a product of a separate process unrelated to the one described above, but fermented *meju* is its vital ingredient. Porridge is first made of rice, wheat, or barley flour. It is then mixed with malt powder. Powdered *meju* and red pepper powder are added to this mixture, and the paste is placed in a crock and left in a sunny place for about a month. During fermentation, the meaty flavor from hydrolyzed proteins and the sweet taste of hydrolyzed starches mix with the pungent tang of chili pepper, resulting in a distinctive taste (Lee 2001, 78; National Academy of the Korean Language 2002, 69–70).

The enduring centrality of *chang* manufacture and storage in each Korean household is reflected in proverbs, expressions, and superstitions that relate to these chores. For example, it was considered a bad omen for a household if the taste of *chang* differed from the condiments prepared in previous years. Women, who were exclusively responsible for the manufacture of fermented soyfoods, took utmost care to replicate precisely the procedures that had previously resulted in successful products. Days were carefully selected to begin the undertakings, and menstruating women and women who had recently given birth were kept away from the scene, as were strangers.

As the proverb "when a good daughter-in-law enters the house, the taste of *chang* improves" indicates, *chang*-making skills were considered crucial to women's status. Many old sayings also warned women about various dangers related to the making and storing of *chang*. For example, finding vermin in the crocks was said to forecast disaster in the family (Han and Han 1995, 49–51, 56).

The manufacture of soy sauce, soybean paste, and red pepper paste were strictly a home affair for centuries. Preparation methods and taste varied considerably, not only by region but also because each family had its own recipes handed down from generation to generation (Shin Hepinstall 2001, xvi). Because the taste of Korean dishes largely depends on the taste of *chang*, the cooking in each household acquired its distinctive flavor through the use of its homemade sauces. Consuming the same *chang* created a bond among the members of the family.[14]

This was still the case a few decades ago. Today, however, more than 80 percent of Korean households consume factory-made soy sauce (Nongsu Ch'uksan Sinmun 2003, 348). The reliance on factory-made *koch'ujang* and *toenjang* is much lower, but it is rising fast. For example, between 1998 and 2002 the yearly production of *koch'ujang* increased from 86.515 tons to 138.653 tons, and production of *toenjang* increased from 114.347 tons to 161.634 tons.[15]

The gradual shift from homemade to factory-made *chang* continues to have a powerful effect on the Korean diet in two respects. On the one hand, the taste of Korean home cooking has gradually become uniform, losing the distinctiveness provided by differences in taste among the *chang* products manufactured in different households. This is particularly true for soy sauce, which, as noted above, has been more frequently replaced by the commercial product than any other condiment.

On the other hand, the changes that the *chang* market underwent during recent years inspired the diversification of production and product development. Although in the past wealthy cooks possessed the resources to use different varieties of *kanjang, toenjang,* and *koch'ujang* depending on the dishes they prepared,[16] peasant households, which constituted the overwhelming majority of the Korean population, resorted to the basic three. In this respect, with the soybean-processing industry achieving an increasing degree of sophistication, we can speak of democratization and of increasing variety in taste as Korean homemakers begin to diversify their use of sauces.

The Industrialization of *Chang* Manufacture

The very first soy sauce factory on Korean soil was the Yamamoto Soy Sauce Brewery (Yamamoto shōyu jōzōjō), which began to operate in the port of Pusan, at the southeastern tip of the peninsula, in 1885 or 1886 (Yi 1999, 88).[17] Like similar factories that mushroomed in the ensuing decades, this factory was aimed at the Japanese settlers who began to pour into Korea impelled by the desire for economic improvement. By 1910, the Japanese residents of Korea constituted the largest overseas community of Japanese in the world (Duus 1995, 289).

After decades of intervention in the country's affairs, starting with the forced opening of Korean ports in 1876, Japan seized and occupied Korea in 1910. It remained in Japanese hands until 1945. Unlike Western colonial powers who had relied heavily on native administrators, Japan imported from the homeland a large number of its own people—competent and loyal personnel for the high and lower ranks of the colonial establishment and for the offices of Japanese corporations in the colony. By 1939, the Japanese population in Korea had reached 650,000, or 3 percent of the entire population of the peninsula.[18] Most Japanese resided in urban areas and settled in about two dozen large towns and cities (Duus 1995, 324).

Restaurants, inns, teashops, and brothels were the first enterprises to provide services for Japanese residents in the Korean treaty ports, soon to be followed by sake brewers and soy sauce manufacturers (Duus 1984, 158). Japanese city dwellers, as the majority of Japanese residents in Korea were, relied heavily on commercial producers for their two major fermented soyfoods: soy sauce (shōyu) and soybean paste (miso) (Hirano 1971, 30–45). This was particularly true for soy sauce, which had been almost entirely commercialized in premodern Japan. From the late sixteenth century onward a new Chinese method for soy sauce manufacture began to spread in Japan, replacing the Korean method described earlier. The new technology was complicated and labor-intensive and was therefore suited only for large-scale manufacture (Ishige 2001, 114–15). Hosking described it concisely as follows:

> [G]rains of whole wheat are parched and cracked and soybeans are steamed. These are then mixed with spores of the mold *Aspergillus oryzae* and incubated for three days, making the kōji. This kōji is added to a brine solution, the result, now called *moromi,* being put into huge cedar casks holding up to two thousand gallons and left to mature for at least two summers. When ready, the *moromi* is pressed in cotton sacks under heavy weight, a process that extracts crude soy oil as well as soy sauce. The oil rises to the surface and is removed. The soy sauce is pasteurized and bottled. The best quality takes two years to make (Hosking 1996, 220).

It was this method rather than the Korean one that was used in soy sauce factories operating in Korea from the late nineteenth century onward. These enterprises were primarily owned and managed by Japanese entrepreneurs,[19] and their products were chiefly aimed at Japanese communities in Korea. We may surmise that urban Koreans might also have become consumers of the Japanese-style soy sauce, but it is difficult to assess to what extent.

According to 1940 statistics, 69 Japanese soy processing factories were in operation throughout Korea, employing in all 843 people (Yi 1999, 98). This translated into an average of twelve workers per factory, but factory size varied. Most were small, employing five to fifty workers, but Shimaya Jōzō Co., Ltd., in Seoul and Fujichū Shōyu Co., Ltd., in Taejŏn, for example, counted more than one hundred employees each, Koreans among them (Chōsen kōgyō kyōkai 1940, 252).

After Korea's liberation, when the Japanese hurried home leaving their business ventures behind, former employees took over the factories, setting the stage for the transformation of *chang* manufacture in post-1945 Korea (Yi 1999, 91, 114–15). Several of these pioneering establishments, such as Sempio Foods[20] in Seoul, Jinmi Foods in Taejŏn, and Monggo Foods in Masan, still operate successfully today (Yi 1999, 131). The pioneers concentrated on soy sauce manufacture, as this was the focus of their predecessors. Soy sauce played a far more profound role in urban Japanese cooking than soybean paste had (Ishige 2001, 115).

As the Japanese who left Korea were the primary consumers of factory-made soy sauce, however, the business was at first far from successful. The outbreak of the Korean War (1950–53) marked the turning point for the soy sauce industry in Korea. The orders for the troops provided work for thirty-five factories, and several more profited from a large share of the population's having been driven from one part of the country to another by the war (Yi 1999, 115–16). At the time of the cease-fire, Sempio was on its way to becoming a national brand, advertising its soy sauce as "Happy News for Homemakers" (Kim et al. 1996, 11). By 1958, more than a hundred commercial manufacturers of *chang* were in operation throughout South Korea.

It needs to be clarified at this point that from the 1930s onward in Japan, some manufacturers began to use a new and efficient chemical method of soy sauce manufacture, which soon spread to the colonies (Yi 1999, 215–16). The method relied on artificially breaking down the protein obtained from defatted soybeans, thereby producing amino acids.[21] It normally takes one to three days to produce chemical soy sauce (in English often called HVP soy sauce, which stands for "hydrolyzed vegetable protein"), as opposed to the several months needed to brew the classic product. Its taste, however, is inferior to the fermented product and requires additives in order to achieve a flavor, color, and taste that approach the original. In practice, many manufactures mixed fermented and chemical sauces in order to achieve some balance between product quality and production efficiency.

The shortage of resources that followed the outbreak of the Sino-Japanese War (1937–45) had a direct effect on soy sauce manufacture. In 1941 the Japanese government ordered soy sauce factories to concentrate their production on the chemical method (Kakugi Kettei 1941). Consequently, the Japanese factories that were taken over by Korean entrepreneurs after 1945 already relied heavily on acid-decomposed soy sauce.

Following the explosive rise of soy sauce manufacturers in the 1950s, the 1960s gave the Korean fermented soyfood industry administrative and legal backbone. The Korean Cooperative of Fermented Soyfoods Industry (Taehan Changnyu Kongŏp Hyŏptong Chohap) was established in 1962, and the first official standards for the manufacture of fermented soyfoods were issued five years later (Yi 1999, 116). Interestingly, the Japanese method of brewing as well as the chemical method were both defined as standard, and before the regulations were modified in 1993, it was legally impossible to produce soy sauce for retail sale by the traditional Korean brewing method. Weighing these facts, the anthropologist Chu Young-ha would write that Korean food-processing technology had not yet managed to free itself from the Japanese colonial grip (Chu 2000, 110).

Throughout the 1970s and 1980s, the Korean *chang* industry experienced continuous growth (Nongsu Ch'uksan Sinmun 2003, 342–43). Urbanization was not the only incentive for the increasing popularity of factory-made fermented soyfoods. The so-called new village movement (*saemaŭl undong*)—launched in 1971 by President Park Chung Hee (1917–79) and aimed at revitalizing the countryside and modernizing its conservative outlook and practices—encouraged Koreans to replace the primitive produce of home brewing with modern factory-made products (Pratt and Rutt 1999, 395–96; Yi 1999, 125–26).

Despite the growth of the industry, in the early 1970s the overwhelming majority of the population still consumed homemade *chang*. The main reason behind the reluctance to abandon homemade soyfoods—along with the high price and unsatisfactory taste of the commercial products—was the lack of trust in their quality. This suspicion was nourished by the fact that the overwhelming majority of soy sauce on the Korean market was either pure chemical soy sauce or, at best, a mixture of the classic Japanese soy sauce and its chemical version, referred to as mixed soy sauce (*honhap kanjang*). In 2002, *honhap kanjang* constituted 69.1 percent of all soy sauce retailed in South Korea. Fermented Japanese-style soy sauce accounted for 27.5 percent, and the so-called *chosŏn kanjang*—a product manufactured on the basis of the traditional Korean methods—comprised a mere 3.4 percent of sales (Nongsu Ch'uksan Sinmun 2003, 349).[22]

Increasing media exposure of the alleged harmful effects of chemical soy sauce on human health created a negative image for the industry in general, affecting soybean paste and hot red pepper paste sales as well. The issue became an object of public debate for the first time in 1968, and two major storms of criticism relating to the soy sauce industry followed in 1985 and 1996 (Yi 1999, 217–42). With the standard of living rising along with the health consciousness of the population, consumers became increasingly concerned with the quality and safety of the food they purchased. Public pressure resulted in reforms in the industry, which were reflected in several bankruptcies and takeovers. The number of corporations producing soy sauce declined sharply, from 140 in 1970 to 81 in 2003.[23]

A preference toward a return to traditional products is clearly reflected in statistics. Between 1993 and 1997, sales of mixed soy sauce dropped from 75.6 to 69 percent, while those of fermented soy sauce increased from 3.3 to 10.5 percent (Yi 1999, 159). Manufacturers predict that the latter will come to dominate the South Korean market in the near future.

The prospects for commercialization of soybean paste and hot red pepper paste remain promising as the quality of the products keeps improving, which fosters consumer trust. The market is by no means saturated. As of 2002, only 49.1 percent of South Korean households used industrially produced *koch'ujang*, and merely 28.3 percent relied on commercially made *toenjang* (figure 6).[24] As the generations of homemakers who still take up the time- and labor-consuming chore of making *chang* gradually pass on, the industry can count on a continuous rise in sales.

Conclusion: *Chang* and Korean Identity

In his 1977 article on housing in Korea, Boudewijn Walraven proclaimed that Koreans would have difficulty living in urban apartments because these were completely inappropriate for the storage and manufacture of fermented foods.

> Where is one to leave kimch'i crocks in an apartment? Where to place the huge containers with hot red pepper paste, soy sauce and soybean paste? A traditional Korean house has a special place in the backyard, where 5 to 8 of such containers stand. An apartment is far too small for making kimch'i:

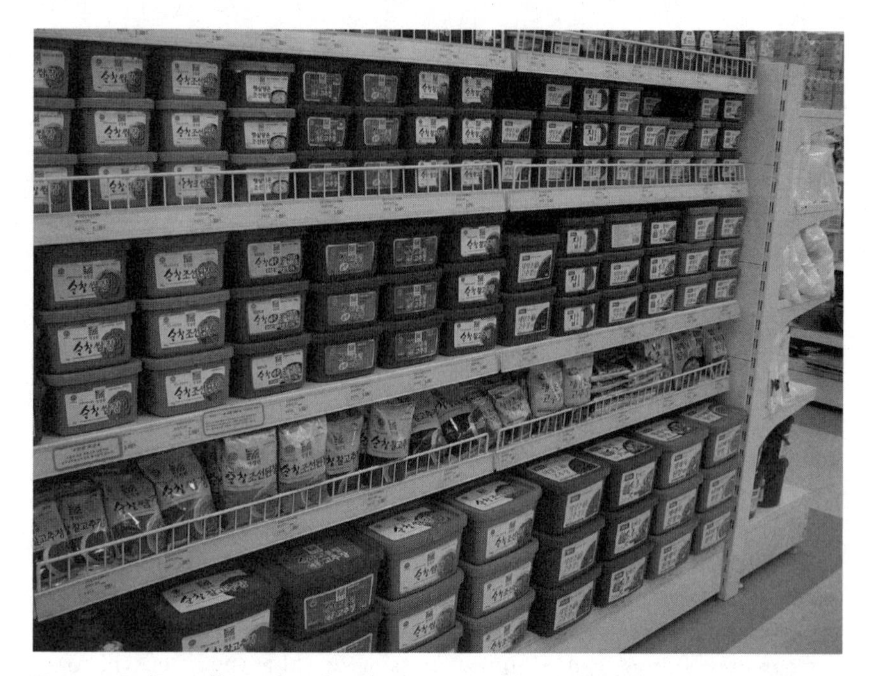

Figure 6. Industrially produced soybean paste and hot red pepper paste gradually replace the homemade product. Note the different sizes of containers. (Photo by K. J. Cwiertka, November 2003)

> there is simply too little space to spread the ingredients and let them dry in the sun. Moreover, how is one to ensure without the ondol[25] the constant temperatures that are so important in making soy sauce and soybean paste? One can buy them on the market of course, but it is a common knowledge that these are poor substitutes. As long as Koreans will remain finicky in this respect, they will not be eager to reside in apartments, regardless of how many have been built in recent years (Walraven 1977, 54).

A quarter of a century after these words were published, large-scale apartment blocks (*ap'at'ŭ tanji*) are ubiquitous in Korea (Gelézeau 2001), and indeed, Koreans are increasingly relying on the factory-made surrogates for their daily *chang*. How did this change affect their attitudes toward the soul of their cuisine?

It appears that the more ordinary Koreans become detached from the production of *chang*, the more prominent the place it captures in Korean cultural imagery. Half a century ago, lumps of *meju* attached to the roof, and crocks with fermented soybeans constituted a fundamental element of the Korean landscape. Today, *meju* lumps are difficult to spot, and sauce crocks evoke feelings of nostalgia, as in Hi Soo Shin Hepinstall's recollection of her childhood:

> During most of my childhood, the food for our kitchen came from our own land—fresh vegetables from our backyard and rice and grain from our fields in the countryside. . . . In the center of the backyard, a few steps from the kitchen's back door and surrounded by flowerbeds and terraced vegetable gardens, was a raised stone platform (*changdokdae*) where we kept twenty or so large and small crocks for storing the three basic sauces: soy sauce, fermented soybean paste, and hot red pepper paste (Shin Hepinstall 2001, 4).

Vanishing lifestyles, including home *chang* manufacture, have been increasingly singled out in the last two decades as an important part of Korea's cultural heritage. Remainders of old Korea that managed to escape the modernizing effect of the *saemaŭl* movement are now placed under the protection of the government. For example, the local government of Sunch'ang, a town in North Chŏlla Province celebrated for its superb hot red pepper paste that at one time was offered as a tribute to the king, actively participates in preserving the manufacturing tradition through its Koch'ujang Village project (Kim 2002). The inhabitants of Hahoe Village near Andong, the most well-known government-sanctioned traditional village, are expected to carry on their daily chores, including the making of *chang*, as if time had stood still (figure 7).[26]

It is hard to believe that only three decades ago, sauce-crock pads were considered symbols of backwardness by the authorities, and getting rid of them was praised as an important step toward Korean advancement (Yi 1999, 125–26). The changing attitude toward *chang* making during the last half century—from a taken-for-granted, mundane chore to an object of reproach and finally to the icon of Korean cultural heritage—reflects the transformation of Korean society.

It seems that economic affluence and a growing familiarity with foreign culinary trends over the last two decades have fostered an emerging pride in Korean culinary heritage and have inspired the use of Korean cuisine as a cultural and national symbol. As Raymond Grew (1999, 11) has pointedly observed, it is awareness of others and greater freedom of choice that cause the issues of identity to arise, and it is consciousness of change that stimulates the inventive uses of tradition.

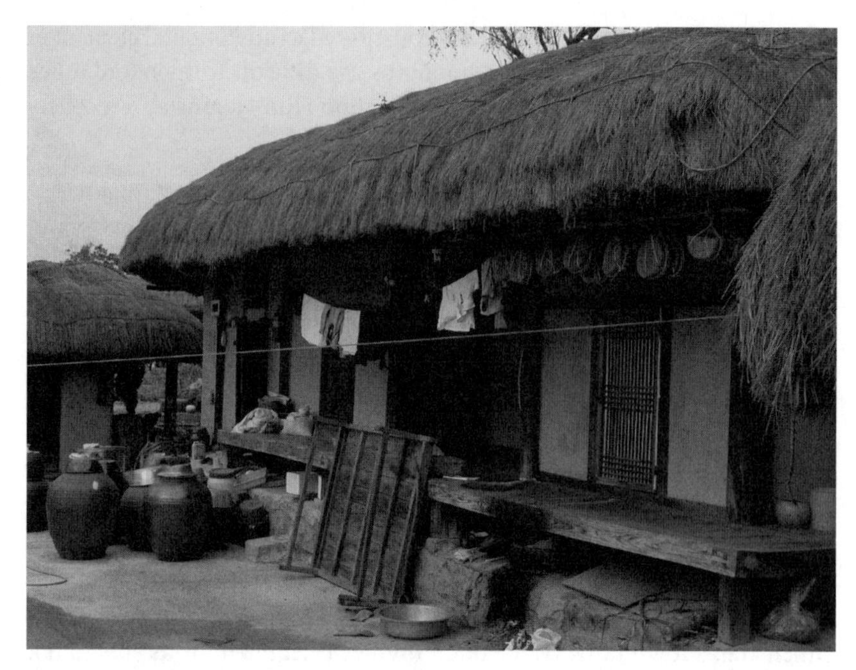

Figure 7. A snapshot from the Hahoe Folk Village, near Andong. Note the *meju* attached to the roof and sauce crocks. (Photo by K. J. Cwiertka, October 2003)

In contemporary Korea, cuisine constitutes one of the most powerful flags of identity, a medium through which national identity operates at the level of the ordinary man and woman on the street.[27] Michael Billig's concept of banal nationalism in the sense of an ubiquitous, mundane reminder of nationhood, is of particular relevance here (Palmer 1998, 181–82). In the Korean case, the role of food as a medium that evokes the feeling of unity is particularly pronounced because of its pungent taste (deriving from hot red peppers) and strong smell (deriving from garlic, spring onions, and fermented soyfoods), signals that have in the past discouraged non-Koreans from appreciating Korean cuisine.[28]

To be sure, the South Korean government is actively promoting Korean cuisine abroad,[29] and most Koreans appear to find satisfaction in the growing popularity of their foods in Japan, the United States, and Europe. At the same time, however, they seem to find comfort in the conviction that only Koreans are fully able to appreciate the distinctive and complex flavor of native Korean cooking. And they are increasingly aware that they owe it to *chang*.

Notes

1. We are grateful to the editors of this volume for their comments and suggestions. We would also like to thank Professor Isao Kumakura for introducing us to each other. He thought that we might form a good research team, and as always, he was right. This research has been funded by the Netherlands Organization of Scientific Research to which we are also grateful.

2. Throughout this essay, the word "Korea" or "Korean" will refer to the entire Korean peninsula in relation to pre-1948 developments and to the Republic of Korea (South Korea) when discussing events that took place following the division of the peninsula.

3. As of 2001, 82 percent of Koreans lived in urban areas (Jung and Kim 2003, 1).

4. Starbucks Company, www.istarbucks.co.kr/store/store_map01.asp.

5. Japanese curry is a British-Indian dish, and *ramyŏn* is a Chinese noodle soup, both modified by the Japanese in the early twentieth century (Ohnuma 2002; Ishige 2001, 157). It should be pointed out, however, that Koreans perceive curry as well as *ramyŏn* as native rather than foreign dishes.

6. A 1988 study indicated that the majority of Korean homemakers made regular use of instant foods, but almost two-thirds of them generally adhered to traditional cooking. The younger the age, the more housewives were inclined to have nontraditional meals. However, this did not mean that they cooked non-Korean meals but rather that they frequently served breakfasts of milk and bread and relied more on instant foods (Hart 2001, 104–7). Of course, much has changed since the time of this study. Today, young homemakers often cook pasta and Western-style green salads with chicken or tuna, while toast and sandwiches regularly appear at breakfasts and lunches. However, the repertoire is limited.

7. The most internationally known Korean food, it is a kind of fermented vegetable, which is pickled with salt and then fermented with lactic acid. The addition of hot red pepper powder, green onions, garlic, and ginger gives it a red color and pungent taste. For more information, see Chu (1995) and Walraven (2002, 97–101).

8. When transcribing Korean words and names, we followed the McCune-Reischauer romanization system except when the English transcription was already established (i.e., Hollym) or if authors used their own transcription when publishing in English (i.e., Bak 1997; Lee 2001). When transcribing Japanese words, we have used the Hepburn romanization system.

9. Examples of this phenomenon are too plentiful to mention here. See Walvin (1997).

10. The issue has received extensive media coverage. See, for example, Yu (2004).

11. Shin Hepinstall is the author of a highly acclaimed Korean cookbook in English.

12. Although it is not a regular practice, local *kimch'i* recipes that include soy sauce do exist (Han 1999, 50). Rice is customarily cooked without the addition of *chang*, but one of the most popular Korean dishes, *pibimbap* ("mixed rice"), consists of a bowl of rice topped with fresh and cooked vegetables and *koch'ujang* that are supposed to be mixed together before eating.

13. See also Osgood (1951, 86).

14. This is also why relatives who still go to the trouble to make *chang* at home often distribute the product among family members living in urban areas. By doing so, they retain the bond within the family. These observations are based on fieldwork conducted by Akiko Moriya among elderly Koreans.

15. Internal publication of the Korean Cooperative of Fermented Soyfoods Industry, consulted on the premises of the cooperative in June 2004.

16. For example, four basic types of Korean soy sauce can be distinguished: (1) *ch'ŏng kanjang*, light soy sauce that has been stored for less than two years, usually used for soups; (2) *chung kanjang*, soy sauce stored for three to four years, used in soups and greens; (3) *chin kanjang*, dark soy sauce, slightly sweet, stored more than five years, used in simmered and steamed dishes; (4) *chin kanjang* (written with a different ideogram than no. 3), the best soy sauce of dark color and sweet taste, stored for ten years or more (Yi 2003, 48).

17. It seems most probable that Yi made a mistake when calculating the date for the Western calendar as 1886. The *Register of Korean Factories* mentions the eighteenth year of the Meiji era as the year in which this brewery was established, which translates into 1885 (Chōsen kōgyō kyōkai 1940, 253).

18. This colonists-to-colonized ratio is remarkable when compared to .2 percent in French Indochina, .7 percent in British Malaya, and .4 percent in the Netherlands East Indies (Delissen 2000, 126–27).

19. Company registers indicate that soy sauce factories owned and/or managed by Koreans began to emerge from the late 1920s onward. More research is necessary, however, in order to assess the role of Korean entrepreneurs in the industry before 1945.

20. The correct transcription should be "Saemp'yo," but here we follow the transcriptions commonly used by the companies themselves.

21. This product is known in Japanese as *aminosankai shōyu* and in Korean as *sanbunhae kanjang* or *aminosan kanjang*.

22. This source does not mention pure chemical soy sauce. According to Yi (1999, 159), in 1997 this product constituted 20.5 percent of soy sauce manufacture.

23. Internal publication of the Korean Cooperative of Fermented Soyfoods Industry, consulted on the premises of the cooperative in June 2004.

24. For comparison, the figure for *kanjang* is 83.1 percent (Nongsu Ch'uksan Sinmun 2003, 348).

25. This is the typical Korean system of heating a house with flues passing under the floor: the fire for the morning meal heats the room for the day, and the fire for the evening meal heats the room for the night (Pratt and Rutt 1999, 326).

26. The picture shows a very poor and rather messy house. In a more affluent household, the crocks would be kept on a raised platform as Shin Hepinstall describes.

27. This is clearly reflected in the centrality of the topic in the English-language research on Korean foodways. See, for example, Bak (1997), Han (1994), Pemberton (2002), Reinschmidt (2001), and Walraven (2002).

28. See, for example, Han (1994), and chapter 4 in Yuh (2002).

29. English-language journals that introduce Korea to the world, such as *Koreana* and *Korea Now,* regularly feature articles on Korean cuisine, and its salutary qualities are frequently emphasized (Korean Overseas Culture and Information Service 1998, 27–42; Walraven 2002, 100).

References

Bak, Sangmee. 1997. "McDonald's in Seoul: Food Choices, Identity, and Nationalism." In James L. Watson, ed., *Golden Arches East: McDonald's in East Asia,* 126–60. Stanford, CA: Stanford University Press.

Brandt, Vincent S. R. 1971. *A Korean Village: Between Farm and Sea.* Cambridge: Harvard University Press.

Chōsen Kōgyō Kyōkai. 1940. *Chōsen Kōjō Meibo* [*Register of Korean Factories*]. Keijō: Chōsen Kōgyō Kyōkai.

Chu, Young-ha. 1995. "Origin and Change in *Kimch'i* Culture." *Korea Journal* 35(2): 18–33.

———. 2000. *Ŭmsik Chŏnjaeng, Munhwa Chŏnjaeng* [*Food War, Culture War*]. Seoul: Sagyejŏl.

Cumings, Bruce. 1997. *Korea's Place in the Sun: A Modern History.* New York: Norton.

Delissen, Alain. 2000. "Denied and Besieged: The Japanese of Korea, 1876–1945." In Robert Bickers and Christian Henriot, eds., *New Frontiers: Imperialism's New Communities in East Asia, 1842–1953,* 125–45. Manchester, UK: Manchester University Press.

Duus, Peter. 1984. "Economic Dimensions of Meiji Imperialism: The Case of Korea, 1895–1910." In Ramon H. Myers and Mark R. Peattie, eds., *The Japanese Colonial Empire, 1895–1945,* 128–63. Princeton, NJ: Princeton University Press.

———. 1995. *The Abacus and the Sword: The Japanese Penetration of Korea, 1895–1910.* Berkeley: University of California Press.

Gelézeau, Valérie. 2003. *Séoul, Ville Géante, Cités Radieuses.* Paris: CNRS.

Grew, Raymond. 1999. "Food and Global History." In Raymond Grew, ed., *Food in Global History,* 1–29. Boulder, CO: Westview.

Han, Kyung-koo. 1994. "Some Foods Are Good to Think: Kimchi and the Epitomization of National Character." Paper presented at the Association for Asian Studies Meeting in Boston. Also published as "Ŏttŏn Ŭmsig-ŭn Saenggak Hagi-e Chot'a: Kimch'i-wa Han'guk Minjoksŏng ŭi Chŏngsu." *Han'guk Munhwa Illyuhak* 26: 51–68.

Han, Pong-nyŏ. 1999. *Uri-ga Chŏngmal Araya hal uri Kimch'i Paek Kaji* [*The Hundred Kinds of Kimch'i We Really Should Know*]. Seoul: Hyŏnamsa.

Han, Pong-nyŏ, and Pok-chin Han. 1995. *Chongga Chip Siŏmŏni Chang Tamgŭnŭn pŏp* [*Chang Recipes from the Mother-in-Law in the Head Family's House*]. Seoul: Tungji.

Han'guk Munhwachae Poho Chaedan. 2001. *Han'guk Ŭmsik Taegwan,* Che 4, *Kwŏn: Palhyo, Chŏjang, Kagong Sikp'um* [*Survey of Korean Cuisine,* Vol. 4, *Fermented, Preserved, and Processed Foods*]. Seoul: Hollym.

Hart, Dennis. 2001. *From Tradition to Consumption: Construction of a Capitalist Culture in South Korea.* Seoul: Jimoondang.

Hirano, Masaaki. 1971. "Shōyu no Rekishi: Sono Yurai to Hattatsu" ["The History of Soy Sauce: Its Origins and Development"]. In Heiji Tamura and Masaaki Hirano, eds., *Shōyu no Hon,* 2–44. Tokyo: Shibata Shoten.

Hosking, Richard. 1996. *A Dictionary of Japanese Food: Ingredients and Culture.* Tokyo: Charles E. Tuttle.

Huang, Hsing Tsung. 2000. *Science and Civilisation in China,* Vol. 6, *Biology and Biological Technology,* Pt. 5, *Fermentations and Food Science.* Cambridge: Cambridge University Press.

Ishige, Naomichi. 2001. *The History and Culture of Japanese Food.* London: Kegan Paul.

Jung, Jaechul, and Hun-hee Kim. 2003. "American Fast Food Industry in Korea." Research paper 903M16. London, Ontario, Canada: Ivey School of Business, University of Western Ontario.

Kakugi Kettei. 1941. "Kyūsoku Shokuryō Taisaku ni kan Suru ken" ["Concerning Quick Processed Foods As Countermeasures to Food Scarcity"]. Cabinet decision issued on September 26, 1941. http://www.ndl.go.jp/horei_jp/kakugi/bib/bib00350.htm.

Kim, Min-hee. 2002. "A Mother's Cooking Has No Rivals." *Korea Now* 31(10): 24–25.

Kim, Ŭng-dŏk, et al., eds. 1996. *Hanguk Kwanggo 100 Nyŏn, ha* [*100 Years of Korean Advertising,* Vol. 2]. Seoul: Hanguk Kwankko Yŏnguwŏn.

Korean Nutrition Society. 1989. *Korean Nutrition Resource Data.* Seoul: Shinkwang Publishing.

Korean Overseas Culture and Information Service. 1998. "Kimchi and Pulgogi: Two Healthy Korean Foods." In *A Guide to Korean Cultural Heritage,* 26–43. Seoul: Korean Overseas Culture and Information Service.

Kwon, Tai-Wan. 1995. "The Role of Soybeans in the Korean Rice Diet." *Korean and Korean American Studies Bulletin* 6(1): 19–22.

Lee, Cherl-Ho. 2001. *Fermentation Technology in Korea.* Seoul: Korea University Press.

National Academy of the Korean Language. 2002. *An Illustrated Guide to Korean Culture: 233 Traditional Key Words.* Seoul: Hakgojae.

Nelson, Laura C. 2000. *Measured Excess: Status, Gender, and Consumer Nationalism in South Korea.* New York: Columbia University Press.

Nongsu Ch'uksan Sinmun. 2003. *Hanguk Sikp'um Yŏngam* [*Yearbook of Korean Foods*]. Seoul: Nongsu Ch'uksan Sinmun.
Ohnuma, Keiko. 2002. "Curry Rice: Gaijin Gold. How the British Version of an Indian Dish Turned Japanese." In Alan Davidson and Helen Saberi, eds., *The Wider Shores of Gastronomy: Twenty Years of the Best Food Writing from the Journal Petit Propos Culinaires*, 160–67. Berkeley: Ten Speed.
Osgood, Cornelius. 1951. *The Koreans and Their Culture*. New York: Ronald Press.
Palmer, Catherine. 1998. "From Theory to Practice: Experiencing the Nation in Everyday Life." *Journal of Material Culture* 3(2): 175–99.
Pemberton, Robert. 2002. "Wild-Gathered Food As Countercurrents to Dietary Globalisation in South Korea." In Katarzyna Cwiertka with Boudewijn Walraven, eds., *Asian Food: The Global and the Local*, 76–94. Honolulu: University of Hawaii Press.
Potrzeba Lett, Denise. 1998. *In Pursuit of Status: The Making of South Korea's "New Middle Class."* Cambridge: Harvard University Asia Center.
Pratt, Keith, and Richard Rutt. 1999. *Korea: A Historical and Cultural Dictionary*. Richmond, UK: Curzon.
Reinschmidt, Michael. 2001. "The Korean Rice Burger: Hybridization and Stabilization of Rice As a Cultural Icon." Paper presented at the Annual Meeting of the American Anthropological Association, Washington, DC.
Shin Hepinstall, Hi Soo. 2001. *Growing Up in the Korean Kitchen: A Cookbook*. Berkeley: Ten Speed.
Walraven, Boudewijn C. A. 1977. "Wonen in Korea" ["Living in Korea"]. *Verre Naasten Naderbij* 11(2): 45–56.
———. 2002. "Bardot Soup and Confucians' Meat: Food and Korean Identity in Global Context." In Katarzyna Cwiertka with Boudewijn Walraven, eds., *Asian Food: The Global and the Local*, 95–115. Honolulu: University of Hawaii Press.
Walvin, James. 1997. *Fruits of Empire: Exotic Produce and British Taste, 1660–1800*. Houndmills and London: Macmillan.
Yi, Ch'un-ja, et al. 2003. *Chang*. Seoul: Taewŏnsa.
Yi, Han-ch'ang. 1999. *Chang: Yŏksa-wa Munhwa-wa Kongŏp* [*Chang: History, Culture, and Industry*]. Seoul: Sinkwang Ch'ulp'ansa.
Yi, Song-u. 1984. *Han'guk Sikpum Munhwasa* [*Cultural History of Korean Foods*]. Seoul: Kyomunsa.
Yu, Shiyu. 2004. "Sino-Korean Relations: Lessons in Antiquity." http://www.atimes.com/atimes/China/FA06Ad01.html.
Yuh, Ji-Yeon. 2002. *Beyond the Shadow of Camptown: Korean Military Brides in America*. New York: New York University Press.

9

Tofu in Vietnamese Life

CAN VAN NGUYEN

Translated by Duong Thanh Nguyen

The Origins of Tofu in Vietnam

ORAL HISTORY AND DIRECT DOCUMENTARY EVIDENCE

Tofu is a popular food in daily Vietnamese life.[1] In rural and urban areas, in the mountains and deltas, it would be hard to find anyone who eats rice but never eats tofu. Most Vietnamese consider tofu a traditional, cheap, and well-liked dish.

To discover the origins of tofu in Vietnam, we investigated trade villages specializing in its production. Elderly informants told us that it is a hereditary trade, handed down from generation to generation for a long time. They know that the ancestors who brought this trade were Chinese, but as far as the villagers can tell, when and how this skill came to Vietnam is unknown and unrecorded.

Their perception of historical gaps is a reality, for after years of war many kinds of old scripts and documents have been lost. For instance, the *Dai Viet Su Ky Toan Thu* (*Complete Set of Dai Viet History*) is the most reliable historical book on Vietnam.[2] According to its introductory chapter, it was written by Le Van Huu (AD 1230–1322) and completed in 1272 with a total of thirty volumes (*Complete Set of Dai Viet History*, 1983). But in fact, no original is available today, and some scholars doubt that there were thirty volumes. The version we read today was edited and printed in 1697 by the next epoch of historians after Le Van Huu. This problem illustrates the difficulty of finding reliable documents regarding the origin of a popular food such as tofu.

We have found only two early books that mention soybeans and tofu. The first is the *Van Dai Loai Ngu* by Le Quy Don (AD 1723–1783). In his discussion of grains, he mentions *dai dau*, or soybean (Le Quy Don 1962 [18th C.]). The second book where we found mention of soy is the *Nu Cong Thang Lam* by Le Huu Trac (AD 1720–1791). Concerning soybeans, he stated that *dau nanh* (another name for soy) is sweet and warm and is good for recovery after an injury, for the beauty of women, for bone marrow, for vitality, and as an antidote for ingested toxins. He pointed out nourishing agents in tofu, known today as amino acids and vitamins. He also introduced two ways to process soy and eight vegetarian dishes made with tofu (Le Huu Trac 1971 [18th C.]).

Le Quy Don and Le Huu Trac are two famous Vietnamese polymaths of the eighteenth century. We can deduce that tofu must have existed and become popular in Vietnam no later than the eighteenth century since these scholars carefully studied it and discussed it in their books. Both men were born at the beginning of eighteenth century; hence, tofu was quite possibly present in Vietnam in the seventeenth century.

However, according to some scholars, tofu entered Vietnam even earlier, in the tenth to eleventh century. Their reasoning merits consideration.

EVIDENCE FOR THE EARLIER DIFFUSION OF TOFU

Scholars list four reasons why the diffusion of tofu plausibly occurred far earlier than the time of Le Quy Don and Le Huu Trac. All four reasons are forms of circumstantial evidence.

Mass migrations between China and Vietnam. Relations between China and Vietnam have existed for more than two thousand years. Not only did Chinese imperial envoys impart cultural information to small groups of Vietnamese leaders, but the migration of thousands of people due to wars[3] also spread cultural knowledge. The Vietnamese might have learned about making tofu from the Chinese.

Migrations of Chinese and Vietnamese Buddhists. The book *Thien Uyen Tap Anh* of the Vietnam Buddhist Congregation, considered to be from the period of the Tran dynasty (thirteenth to fourteenth century AD), shows specific links between China and Vietnam. It states that "the Buddhist master Vo Ngon Thong (?–AD 826) came from Quang Dong (Guangdong), China. . . . In December 820 he came to Kien So temple (now in Gia Lam district, Hanoi) to meditate and founded the 'Vo Ngon Thong' sect in Vietnam" (Vietnam Buddhist Church 1990).

In other paragraphs, the book also states that "the Buddhist master Bien Tai came from Quang Chau (Guangzhou), China to meditate at Pho Ninh temple, Tu Liem, Hanoi in the period of the Emperor Ly Thanh Tong of the Ly dynasty" (1054–1071) and "the Venerable Tinh Khong (AD 1091–1170) from Phuc Chau (Fuzhou), China, traveled south to Khai Quoc temple, Vietnam when he was 30 years old" (Vietnam Buddhist Church 1990).

Moreover, not only did Chinese monks travel to Vietnam, but also Vietnamese monks who belonged to the Thien Vo Ngo Thong or Ti Ni Da Luu Chi sects went to China to meditate. In this period, some Vietnamese monks may have learned to make and use tofu, or Chinese monks may have brought it with them to Vietnam and popularized it in Vietnamese temples.

Exchanges between the imperial governments of China and Vietnam. There was also frequent interaction between the imperial governments of China and Vietnam. The *Complete Set of Dai Viet History* (1983) mentions that in the spring of AD 1007, the Vietnamese emperor sent two envoys to the Song dynasty in China to deliver rhinoceros as a tribute and to ask for *The Great Tang* prayer book. In the spring of 1009 they returned successfully with the book. Moreover, in September 1020 another envoy went to China, again requesting and receiving the same prayer book. This demonstrates that in the Ly dynasty, Vietnamese emperors were interested in Buddhism and in popular Chinese sects. We can deduce that Vietnamese representatives might have eaten tofu at imperial parties in China and that they also might have asked for training in how to make it.

One of Le Quy Don's books, the *Kien Van Tieu Luc* (1997 [18th C.]), recounts a relevant story of a Vietnamese emperor's illness. In the time of the Tran dynasty (thirteenth–fourteenth centuries) or perhaps the Ly dynasty (eleventh and twelfth centuries AD)—Le Quy Don mentions two possible periods—the land was often flooded. One year, the emperor had a soreness in his eyes that none of the royal doctors could cure. The emperor had a dream that he would be fine and that the flooding would stop if he threw one person into the river as a sacrifice the very next day.

So the next day, soldiers caught an oil-vending couple, as they were the first to appear by the river. The emperor ordered the soldiers not to force them into the river but rather to tell them the problem and only to throw them into the river if they volunteered. After listening to the persuasions of imperial officials, the couple agreed to jump into the river to cure the eyes of the emperor and save the people from the flood. Before they died, they were asked what kind of food they would like to have in posthumous offerings to them. The answer from the husband was "steamed sticky rice and chicken"; his answer for dessert was "bean soup."

Although tofu is not mentioned in this allusion to bean soup, we can surmise that what was meant was tofu soup. Possibly at that time, tofu had existed in Vietnam for only a short time, so it was seen as a special, good, and valuable food. Only the emperor, the high officials, and the monks of famous pagodas could have this luxury in their daily meals. To a poor, ordinary person such as the oil vendor, tofu was a food of high rank, indeed of the same rank as the steamed sticky rice and chicken. It would be something he could only taste posthumously during a special event such as the anniversary of his death. This would be why he asked for bean soup for dessert. There would be no reason for him to choose an ordinary soup.

Vietnamese folk songs and sayings. These suggest an ancient origin for tofu in Vietnam. We may examine, for example, the lines to a song recommending that "If you want to enjoy tofu with traditional Chinese soy sauce, sharpen your knife and scissors, shave your head, and become a monk."

This little song suggests that tofu first appeared in Vietnam in the temples. In the beginning, it was an appetizing and exotic food. Hence, many people wanted to taste it, and there was no other way to do so than to go to a temple. The folk song also suggests that Buddhism was popular at the time and that many people did, in fact, become monks. There are, of course, many reasons to become a monk, but the people sometimes explained the popularity of the monk's life by saying that those who chose it simply wanted "to enjoy tofu with Chinese soy sauce."

For the above reasons, we may assume that tofu perhaps came from China to Vietnam via the monks. As previously noted, Chinese monks went to Vietnam, and Vietnamese monks apparently went to China to study in turn. Alternatively, perhaps the introduction came about through the trips of imperial envoys seeking Buddhist knowledge. The envoys probably brought seeds from China to Vietnam to plant in temple gardens for soybeans that were then used to make tofu. Later, tofu was popularized. These origins help explain why all tofu trade villages[4] claim Chinese individuals as the ancestors of their trade. Tofu appeared in Vietnam thanks to the cultural exchange between China and Vietnam, especially the process of propagating Buddhism. The introduction possibly happened in the tenth to eleventh centuries, in the Ly-Tran dynasties in Vietnam and the Song dynasty in China. It was the peak period of Buddhism in Vietnam, and there was a regular exchange with Chinese Buddhism.

Furthermore, other pundits have argued that in the Tang dynasty in China, in the seventh to tenth centuries AD, there was already a comprehensive exchange between the two countries. For instance, when the Chinese Emperor Duong Minh Hoang reigned, he ordered the fast transport of litchi from Vietnam to his palace, fast in order to keep the litchi fresh so that Duong Quy Phi (the royal second-rank wife) could enjoy the taste. Such exchanges suggest that it is even possible that tofu entered Vietnam before the Ly-Tran dynasties.

Nevertheless, these are only theories, as it is impossible discern the precise history of tofu in Vietnam.

The Role of Tofu in Vietnamese Life

As we have outlined above, tofu entered Vietnam through the development and exchange of Buddhism. For this reason, since ancient times ordinary Vietnamese have been eating vegetarian dishes every day, including tofu, in accord with their beliefs that vegetarian food is clean and promotes tranquility.

At first, imperial rules required vegetarian foods on the altar when emperors prayed to heaven. A great many trays of sticky rice and vegetarian foods as well as many, many dishes in each tray were clearly recorded in the book *Lich Trieu Hien Chuong Loai Chi*, written by Phan Huy Chu (1961). It was because tofu was already a vegetarian food in the temples that it appeared early in sacred royal meals. Later, tofu became prevalent in Vietnamese daily life as a religiously appropriate food for certain days on the calendar (Soc and Vong).[5]

Practitioners of Vietnamese traditional medicine also discovered health-promoting qualities of tofu. As noted earlier, according to Le Huu Trac tofu is both an appetizing food with many nutritious components and also a medicine. This is perhaps why tofu soon became popular in Vietnam: it satisfied important nutritional needs. This role becomes apparent when we consider that since ancient times the Vietnamese have had a diet high in starch. For human beings engaged in hard physical labor, the first requirement is to feel full after a meal. For this reason, starchy foods are quite common and very important.

Yet Vietnamese life was hard, and rice and sweet potato at no time met all the people's needs. They were frequently threatened with starvation. Particularly in mountainous areas and in the bare-hilled midlands, the land is often parched and not very fertile. Rice and sweet potato are difficult to grow. Fortunately, soybeans partly met the people's needs in those areas. During the period before the harvest of other crops, boiled soybeans supplied protein and calories, enabling human survival. Ripe soybeans could be stored a long time for later use or else used immediately if necessary.

A member of the *Fabaceae* family, soy is easy to cultivate, prevents erosion, and fixes nitrogen in its roots, thereby enhancing soil fertility. For this reason soy was planted in crop rotations. When maize was later introduced to Vietnam, maize and soy were grown together in intercropping systems.

Moreover, soy has proved easy for Vietnamese to store and preserve. After the harvest, ripe soybeans are bound in sheaves on the vine, hung in the kitchen or around the house, and taken down to make tofu when needed. Since during the Vietnamese rainy season the constant rain and cold wind make it hard for people to go to market, Vietnamese farming families find it quite convenient during that period to use stored soybeans for tofu.

These many useful agronomic and storage qualities of soy encouraged its rapid adoption, especially in mountainous and midland areas. Its popularity in Vietnamese villages and urban trading areas is evident even in the naming of streets. For example, in Hanoi most of the thirty-six oldest streets were named for the goods sold there. A street near the Red River, which has a wharf for the exchange of goods between Hanoi and other areas, is called Hang Dau (the street where they sell soybeans). Formerly this street was a center for the sale of beans and soybean products such as tofu and soybean sprouts.

Tofu in Vietnamese Cuisine

Because tofu is a delicious food that can be processed in many ways, it quickly became popular in Vietnam. In some areas, after the period of the Ly and Tran dynasties there appeared a religious practice called meditate at home. This practice attracted those who could not become monks yet wished to recite Buddhist scriptures and pray. Although such individuals were not consistent vegetarians, they did abstain from meat on specific days of particular weeks. These home meditators learned many different ways to process tofu. Sometimes their tofu cuisine corresponded to specific religious regulations—for instance, on the second day of the third week of each month, tofu cooked with brine and dried tangerine is required as the second dish for breakfast, and stewed tofu is required as the second dish for dinner. On the fifth day of the fourth week in a vegetarian month, the dinner should have a dish made with tofu, fermented tofu, and taro. First, mix fermented tofu with regular tofu, then boil this mixture with taro in fresh coconut milk.

The monks, farming families, and home meditators developed simple ways to make the tofu itself. There are two important steps in the process: grinding the soybeans with water to make a proteinaceous solution, and heating and curdling the solution into a custard.

For the first step, even before the Common Era the Vietnamese knew how to grind beans with simple stone tools to separate the hulls from the cotyledons (inner beans). Later, when they began making tofu, they used this method of grinding.

Still later, the Vietnamese discovered how to use round-shaped stone mortars. They would remove the soybeans' hulls, put the beans into water, and then grind the mixture to make the solution. The quantity of water in this step was flexible, so it was quite easy for people to do from a technical point of view, although it was hard physical work. (Nowadays, most city markets include tofu producers. These producers use electric grinders to prepare the protein solution. The process is quite fast, and the solution is smooth.)

It is not clear how the second step—heating and curdling—was accomplished in the distant past. In the *Nu Cong Thang Lam* (1971 [18th C.]), however, Le Huu Trac discussed two methods of curdling:

> Method #1: Filter residues out of the solution, boil it, and then pour in a salt solution [made from a coagulating salt such as magnesium chloride] or gypsum powder to make the soy solids rise to the surface. Gather the curd, squeeze the water out, cover the curd with canvas, and put it into a frame.
>
> Method #2: Filter out residues, pour water in, and boil. After boiling, add a little prepared sour water and boil again. Use a chopstick to stir lightly until the soy solids rise to the surface. Cover with smooth canvas and put into a frame (figure 8).

According to our survey, the second way is more popular in contemporary Vietnam because the material for preparing the sour water is readily available: fruits such as lemon, dracontomelum, or star fruit; sour leaves such as those from the *veo* or tamarind plants; or the products of starch fermentation, such as vinegar or other ferments. Elderly informants who

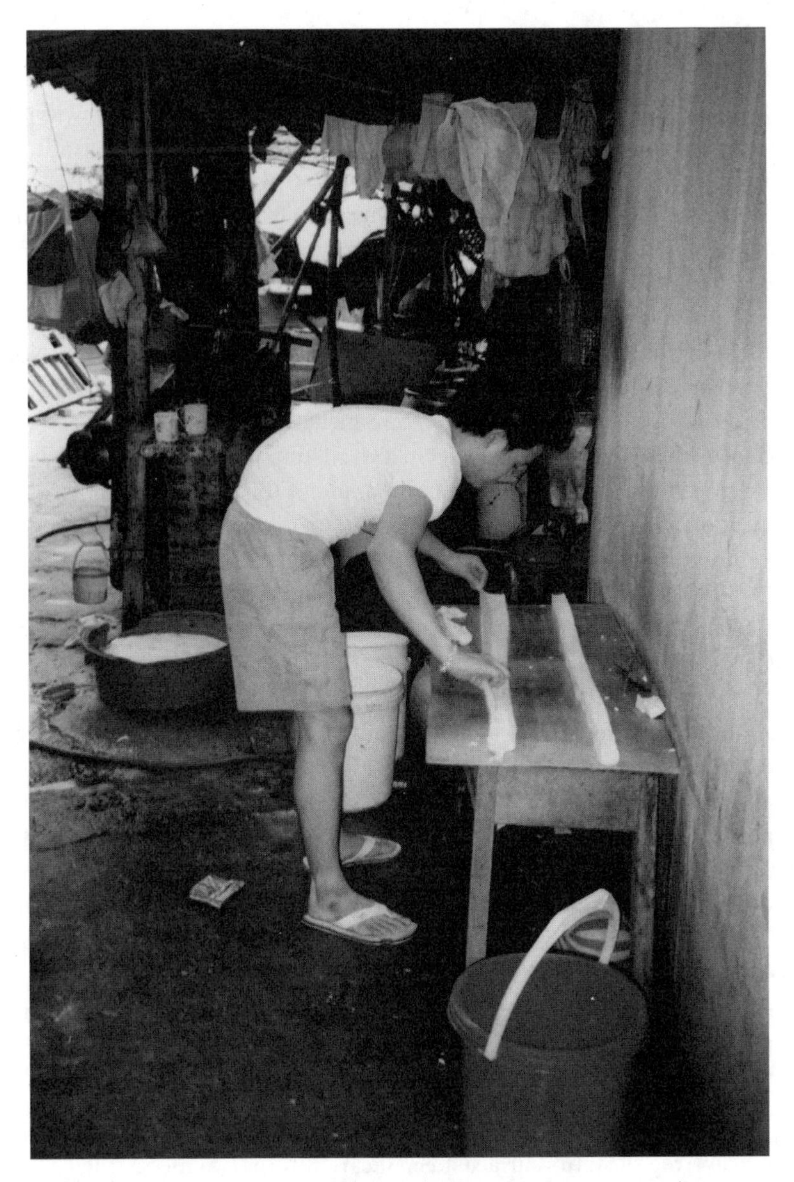

Figure 8. Tofu making in Hanoi, Vietnam. (Photo by C. B. Tan, 2003)

used to make tofu noted that just how sour the water is affects the alkalinity of the solution, thereby determining the size of the solid. Proper pH is key to preparing a smooth, soft, and perfumed tofu. Sour materials also give the tofu special flavors. Each trade village—and even each tofu-producing family—has its own recipe for making the sour water.

In contemporary daily life, the Vietnamese use tofu in multiple forms. Many of these can be sorted into four categories: vegetarian dishes, nonvegetarian dishes, vegetarian soup, and nonvegetarian soup.

Examples of the vegetarian dishes are boiled tofu, tofu cooked with soybean-made meat substitutes, and tofu cooked with mushrooms. Nonvegetarian dishes include tofu stewed with egg, tofu stuffed with shrimp and meat, tofu simmered with tortoise meat, tofu cooked with dry pork, and tofu cooked with rice vermicelli and shrimp paste.

Vegetarian soup dishes are usually made of tofu with various types of plant root, stalk, seed, or fruit, such as potato, tomato, taro, squash, Indian taro, lotus seeds, lotus tubers, carambola (star fruit), or bamboo shoot. When the soup is cooked with many of these ingredients, it is simply called mixed vegetable soup. Nonvegetarian soups can be made by boiling tofu with plant roots and meat, such as fish or barbecued spareribs.

In addition, grilled tofu sells in the marketplaces, especially in the mountainous areas of Vietnam. The tofu is grilled to a golden color, sold, and then used in many different dishes. They include snail with green banana, tortoise with green banana, and catfish or eel simmered with banana. When cooked with grilled tofu, these dishes have more flavor and extra fat and sweetness. For many people, grilled tofu has become an integral component of simmered dishes. For similar reasons, most soups with plant roots or fruits incorporate tofu, and grilled tofu sliced into small pieces goes into vegetable salads and noodle soups.

In Le Huu Trac's *Nu Cong Thang Lam* (1971 [18th C.]) we find tofu dishes popular in ancient Vietnam:

1. *Tofu soaked in soy sauce:* Use five parts tofu and one part salt. Put a layer of tofu in a dish and sprinkle a layer of salt on it, completely covering the tofu's surface. Keep it carefully for two nights, then steam, and then soak in soy sauce for use over the next several days.
2. *Vegetarian shredded soy "meat":* Boil water and rice with the wild "Vang" plant until the rice turns red. Strain the rice out of the water. Roast the rice and then pound it into small pieces (called "thinh").

Steam tofu, slice it into small pieces, and allow to sit for 5 to 6 days until a white mold grows on it that has the appearance of cat's hair. Roast salt, mix it with the "thinh," and then add four parts tofu to every one part of the "thinh"-salt mixture. Pour some good wine over it, cover, and allow it to sit for two or three months to enhance the taste through fermentation.

3. "*Vegetarian chao*": Boil tofu for ten minutes until it is well done, strain and dry it, and grill it to a golden color and fine flavor. Cool and slice into small pieces. Roast sesame seeds with salt, grind some galingale root, and mix these three ingredients together. Taste and adjust seasoning if desired. Mix the tofu with the seasoning mix. Loosely wrap with leaves of the *lot* plant or lettuce, and eat.

As for contemporary life, *The Dictionary of Vietnamese Foods* (Nguyen Loan 1996) provides recipes for modern gourmet tofu dishes:

1. *Tofu fry with lemon grass:* Mix lemon grass, saffron, and chili together and mince them to make a condiment. Make diagonal surface cuts in tofu to enhance its absorption of this condiment. Marinate for an hour. Deep-fat fry the tofu in vegetable oil until golden. Eat with shrimp sauce.
2. *Tofu roll with corn:* Pound corn to a pulp, and mix with scallion, pepper, salt, and *nang* root (cassava). Layer the corn mixture onto thinly sliced tofu and roll the tofu up tightly. Clean mushrooms, soak them in salty water for at least a half hour, and cut an onion into tiny cubes. Heat coconut milk, add soy sauce, salt, sugar, and pepper. Once this stock is boiling, add the tofu to let it absorb the flavor of the soup. Then add the mushrooms, onion, and some *nang* powder that has been mixed with cashew oil. Bring to a boil. Serve as a soup.
3. *Sweet and sour breaded tofu:* Cut tofu into thick slices. Set aside. Clean straw mushrooms, soak them in salty water for at least a half hour, and slice into thread-like pieces. Mix the mushrooms with corn batter. Mince scallion and cut mung bean vermicelli noodles into short pieces; mix them well and season with pepper and salt. Mix all of the above ingredients into a paste and spread them on the surface of the tofu. Deep-fat fry the seasoned, coated tofu to a golden color. Mix fresh coconut milk with *nang* starch (tapioca), fish sauce, salt, sugar, and lime juice, and then boil. Finally, put

sliced onion into the liquid, completing the sweet and sour flavor. Pour this liquid onto the tofu before eating.

4. *Steamed tofu and meat:* Crush tofu until it is smooth, decant the water, and mix with soy sauce, liquid lard, monosodium glutamate, and sliced green onion. Mince lean meat and season with fish sauce, salt, and pepper. Put the tofu paste into a steamer basin with the meat paste on top of it. Steam the layers. Cut in aesthetic diagonals before serving. Can be served with coriander.

In contrast to the elaborate recipes above, today the most popular tofu dishes cooked in Vietnamese families include:

1. *Boiled tofu (dau phu luoc):* Boil tofu for about ten minutes. Drain. Before serving, cut tofu into smaller cubes. This boiled tofu can be eaten with different Vietnamese sauces, among which the best-liked are shrimp paste (cham mam tom), small shrimp sauce (cham mam chua), fish sauce with lime juice (cham mam chanh), and soy sauce (dau tuong).
2. *Tofu cooked with tomatoes (dau phu sot ca chua):* Pan fry thin, square pieces of tofu to golden on both sides. Set aside. Add more oil to the pan, heat, stir-fry some pieces of ginger until they release a nice aroma, and then add sliced tomatoes. Lower the heat and add water to simmer the tomato until partly liquefied. Add tofu and seasoning (salt, sugar, fish sauce). Return to high heat and boil for a few seconds.

In addition, vegetarian and nonvegetarian tofu soups, as previously discussed, are quite popular. Moreover, people use gypsum to make tofu for a sweet custard (*tao pho*). This custard is a flavorful and nutritious dessert, good for children and the elderly (see the discussion of bean curd custard in Tan's essay in this volume).

Other Soybean Uses

Soymilk is made approximately like tofu, except that the curdling of the liquid is omitted, and sugar is added. Before carbonated beverages became widespread, during the hot summers when the need to drink is high, soymilk was the favorite Vietnamese drink. Today each family can still produce soymilk for themselves. The beans must be soaked in water until they are soft, and then they are ground with water in a special processor. After filtering, this liquid is brought to a boil. Then the soy milk is ready for drinking.

The Vietnamese also use soybeans to make various sauces that are indispensable to their traditional cuisine. These sauces have been considered so valuable that during the Le dynasty (seventeenth–eighteenth centuries AD), regulations required the payment of jars of soy sauce (*cham dau tuong*) to officials in border areas, such as those between Vietnam and China, between Vietnam and today's Laos, and between Vietnam and the ancient kingdoms of Chan Lap and Chiem Thanh (both in what is now the southern part of Vietnam). Individuals taking literature examinations to obtain bureaucratic positions within the imperial governments were required to make similar payments to the proctors.

Today, as vegetarian food is gaining in popularity, tofu is also processed to form mock-meat dishes, such as vegetarian fish, vegetarian barbecued spareribs, vegetarian chicken, and vegetarian pork-pie. These dishes are sometimes used when people pray to the ancestors.

For all these reasons, many Vietnamese regard tofu not as foreign but rather as long-standing, traditional, and indispensable in daily life.

Notes

1. This article benefited from the assistance of Chee-Beng Tan, Chan Yuk Wah, and Christine Du Bois.

2. Dai Viet is the former name of Vietnam.

3. There were many wars between China and Vietnam throughout their ancient history. For example, during the late Song dynasty of the thirteenth century, an army of the Chinese general, Trieu Tung, escaped to Vietnam and later joined the famous Vietnamese general Tran Hung Dao to fight against the Yuan dynasty's invasion.

4. In April and May 2004, I visited four tofu-producing villages and conducted interviews with families producing tofu. These included Mo Village, Mai Dong Village, and Chem Village in Hanoi and Thuan Thanh Village in Bac Ninh Province.

5. This is the old Chinese nomenclature for two particular days in a calendar month. Soc is the first day of the month, and Vong is the fifteenth day.

References

Complete Set of Dai Viet History. 1983. Hanoi: Social Science Publishing House.

Le Huu Trac. 1971 [18th C.]. *Nu Cong Thang Lam*. Hanoi: Women's Publishing House.

Le Quy Don. 1962. [18th C.]. *Van Dai Loai Ngu.* Hanoi: Culture Publishing House.

———. 1997. [18th C.]. *Kien Van Tieu Luc.* Hanoi: Social Science Publishing House.

Nguyen Loan. 1996. *Dictionary of Vietnamese Foods.* Hanoi: Culture and Information Publishing House.

Phan Huy Chu. 1961. *Lich Trieu Hien Chuong Loai Chi,* Vol. 2. Hanoi: History Publishing House.

Vietnam Buddhist Church. 1990. *Thien Uyen Tap Anh.* Hanoi: Literature Publishing House.

10

Soyfoods in Indonesia

MYRA SIDHARTA

Introduction

When the United States invaded Iraq in March 2003, anti-American demonstrators demanded an end to diplomatic relations with the United States.[1] Probably none of them was aware that the United States had been Indonesia's main supplier of soybeans for many years. Hence, a diplomatic rupture could have cut off supplies of a staple food that has kept Indonesians alive and in good health for centuries. The stability of that trade relationship and the familiarity of U.S. beans led Indonesian soyfood manufacturers to prefer U.S. beans to those of other countries.

Soybeans have been used as food for many centuries in Indonesia, although it is not possible to fix a firm date for their introduction. British explorers and colonialists indicated that soy was present in Sumatra in the seventeenth century (Dampier 1729, 2:28; Bradley 1732, 2:150).[2] Later Sir Stamford Raffles, who was lieutenant governor in the Archipelago from 1812 to 1816, mentioned the *kédélé* (soybean) as one of the important legumes grown in Java (Raffles 1982, 117).[3] He also noted that the Chinese there prepared soy sauce from *kédélé*.

The Chinese, who first came to the archipelago as traders seeking spices and exotic merchandise (such as shark fins, pearls, Bird of Paradise feathers, etc.), probably also brought soybeans and the techniques of bean curd manufacture. In due time they decided to settle. In all likelihood, they looked for the means to produce their own foodstuffs. It is known that they planted their own legumes and greatly influenced local cuisine.

The *Serat Centini,* a classic Javanese text, mentions the use of *tempe* (*tempeh*) and calls it a nutritious food. Unlike tofu (bean curd), for which the beans are ground and first made into soymilk, tempe is made of whole beans that, after cleaning and dehulling, are pressed and fermented and then sold as cakes in various forms.

Today soybean products are among the most popular foods in Indonesia and are enjoyed by the rich as well as the poor of all ethnic origins. These products include not only tofu but also two traditional soyfoods not often found in other countries, *oncom* and *tempe,* that are manufactured in the villages of Indonesia.

The Promotion of Soybeans

Soybean cultivation lags far behind demand in Indonesia, in part because soy meal is needed as poultry feed. During the period 1991–96, seven hundred thousand tons of soy were imported yearly from the United States. In 1996 alone, their value came to US$517.636 million (Adisarwato and Windiarto 1999).

This dependence on imports has led the government to explore ways to improve soybean cultivation, meanwhile seeking optimum soil conditions to make this possible. There are now several plantations operating in the hilly areas of Java and Sumatra and additional research on the island of Papua, but soybean production is still inadequate.

This is not the first time that pushing up soybean production has been thought necessary. Under Dutch colonial rule and in view of the population explosion especially on the island of Java, several attempts to expand production were made. Unfortunately, however, after the disastrously expensive Java War, in 1830 the Dutch introduced the *cultuurstelsel,* or cultivation and consignment system. This system introduced tobacco, tea, and coffee plantations on a large scale and led to both deforestation and wildlife extinction. Its objective was to force up the commercial production of agricultural export commodities in order to replenish the Dutch colonial treasury, but it resulted in many abuses and was halted in 1870. Among the problems it caused was the reduction of time that peasants had to plant crops needed for daily consumption, such as rice and soybeans. Yet the need for new protein sources that would be inexpensive and easy to process became acute because people were poor and had to work hard for their daily nourishment.

In that era, Dutch experts were well aware of the nutritional value of the soybean. For a medical conference in Paris in 1889, a certain Dr. B. Stokvis commissioned the Kohler Bakery in Amsterdam to bake bread and biscuits from soybean flour and presented them as low-carbohydrate products, recommended for patients suffering from diabetes (Greshof 1890a, 347–56). The Dutch experts also recommended that soybeans be planted as a second crop in the rice fields in Indonesia, next to corn and sweet potatoes.

Yet the Dutch in Indonesia were never really attracted to soybean products and for the most part stuck to their own food, for which the ingredients had to be imported. There was thus an abundance of cheese and butter for their daily needs. According to nineteenth-century botanist G. Greshof, the people of West Java preferred to eat soybeans fried or roasted, which was why the Dutch were never attracted to the food, since whole soybeans can be difficult to digest. The people of Central and East Java had tempe, however, which was their main staple (Greshof 1890b, 435).

It was the Eurasians who were more adventurous in their food choices and commonly ate the same food as the native Indonesians. Eurasians were almost always the offspring of a European father and an Indonesian mother who did traditional Indonesian cooking for the family. After Indonesian independence, when the Dutch were moving back to Holland, many Eurasians of Dutch descent as well as Indonesian Chinese left Indonesia to settle elsewhere. They brought Indonesian food with them, including tempe and tofu. Indeed, some people moving to the Netherlands in that period were advised to learn to make tofu and tempe for extra income.

Finding the Netherlands too small and the climate too cold and unpredictable, many of these same people emigrated anew for other more spacious countries with better climates such as the United States (particularly California), Canada (Vancouver), and South America, to which they also brought *tempe.*

The Story of Tofu in Indonesia

Since the essays in this volume by Tan and Nguyen discuss the making of tofu, here we confine ourselves to its Indonesian history. We have no documented information as to the origin of tofu in the Archipelago and must rely on oral tradition among the people of Kediri, a city in East Java. Kediri's people claim that tofu came to their city first, brought by the troops of Kublai Khan in 1292.

As confirmed by historical records, the story begins when Kublai Khan demanded tribute from the Javanese king Kertanegara of Singosari, but the king refused to comply with Kublai Khan's request. Kublai Khan's special envoy, sent to Java in AD 1289, was humiliated by Kertanegara, and his face was disfigured by order of the Javanese court. Kublai Khan sent an army of twenty thousand soldiers to punish the king. Meanwhile, however, Jayakatawang, king of the eastern Javanese realm of Kediri, had conquered Singosari and killed Kertanegara.

Raden Wijaya, Kertanegara's son-in-law, vowed revenge. Luckily for him, the Mongol expedition landed in Surabaya. Raden Wijaya was able to direct the ships through the Brantas River to Kediri, lead the army into victorious battle, and establish the illustrious Majapahit Kingdom, which maintained its rule into the fifteenth century (Fruin Mees 1920).

The place where the Mongol ships anchored in Kediri is now called Jung Biru (Blue Junks), but of course the junks are nowhere to be seen. Kublai Khan's ships had cooking galleys; it seems reasonable to assume that some were equipped for making tofu. Today many tofu shops can be found in Kediri, where they offer tofu in a great variety, from soft custardlike cakes to the more solid *takua.*

The city of Kediri has identified itself with tofu. On the occasion of its 1,123rd anniversary, in the year 2000, a giant tofu measuring 80 × 80 × 60 cm and weighing 300 kg was made to mark the occasion. A replica can be found in the Indonesian Museum of Records in Semarang; the original was donated to several orphanages (City of Kediri 2000; Asita 2000). Today, tofu shops have become tourist destinations; tourists are brought to these shops to enjoy tofu for breakfast or as a teatime snack. For the snacks, the tofu is thinly sliced, flavored, and baked. In appearance it is similar to potato chips, particularly the Pringles brand popular in North America. Many tourists leave the shops carrying bags of the tofu snacks along with other specialties of the city and its environs.

Another city famous throughout the Archipelago for its tofu is Sumedang, a town in the hills of West Java, some two hundred kilometers south of Jakarta. Although lacking so sensational a history as Kediri, Sumedang was founded about a century ago by a Chinese known by the name of Ong Kino who sold his tofu there and became renowned for the way he deep-fried it (as *tahu pong*). Nowadays visitors to Sumedang are greeted by hundreds of signboards advertising *tahu pong* at various restaurants and shops. Vendors carrying plastic bags filled with the merchandise retail their wares in the streets far beyond the city's borders.

Tahu pong is tofu cut into cubes measuring about four centimeters on each side and deep-fried until crispy outside but still soft inside. It is offered in restaurants with a thin chili sauce. In Jakarta, roadside hawkers in traditional markets and bustling streets offer the same food, freshly fried, because they have brought their cooking utensils along, including a liquid gas container for their cooking fuel. The tofu is sprinkled only with a little salt and some fresh green *cabe rawit* (small, hot green chili). *Tempe* is offered in the same way, with hawkers busily meeting the demands of buyers. One hawker, selling in front of the gate of Jakarta's *Pasar Baru,* a street lined with fashionable boutiques and shops, talked proudly to me of the many celebrities who are his customers.

Indonesia's *Oncom*

The dregs of the early steps in tofu processing (known as soy pulp or by the Japanese word *okara*) are sold to the local cattle industry for use as animal feed, as well as to villagers, who process the sediment further to make *oncom. Oncom* is a fermented soybean (or peanut) product that is locally consumed but has a limited range of uses. It has a brilliant orange color from *Neurospora* mold (Shurtleff and Aoyagi 2007a) and is pressed into a thin block. Known all over Java, it is only consumed by those individuals who appreciate its distinctive taste. To many its flavor seems stale, but fortunately it takes on the flavors of spices when cooked. It is either fried as a snack or used instead of meat in several dishes. Most popular is the *pepes oncom,* for which the *oncom* is mixed with spices and then wrapped in banana leaves and grilled.

Tempe: What Is It, and How Is It Made?

Tempe is a molded cake produced by the fermentation of dehulled, soaked, and cooked soybeans. To make *tempe,* first the beans are sorted, cleaned, and then cooked in water for about half an hour. After that, they are left to stand for one night, in order to allow an acid to form that prevents contamination from certain unwanted bacteria. The next day the beans are dehulled by putting them through a special device. Traditionally the beans were trampled to remove the hulls, but this is now considered unhygienic and is no longer practiced. After the hull has been removed, the beans are reheated until they are fully cooked, then strained, and finally cooled.

Meanwhile, a traditional fermentation starter has been prepared by allowing the mold *Rhizopus oligosporus* to grow on *waru* (*Hibiscus*) leaves.

To speed up the process of mold formation, a starter may also be taken from a previous batch of *tempe*. The mold is then mixed into the beans; afterward the mixture is wrapped either in banana leaves or perforated plastic bags. We have also seen it spread out on a shallow wooden basin and covered with a perforated plastic sheet. After thirty-six hours, the *tempe* is ready to be consumed. A white film can be seen on the surface of the beans (Budi Santoso 1993, 24–31). It is this *Rhizopus* mold that holds the beans together and makes the *tempe* easy to slice. Each 100 grams of *tempe* contains 10.9 grams of protein, the equivalent of the protein in 1.6 cups of milk, 1.9 eggs, or 3.1 ounces of local steak. It is also a good source of vitamins B1 (thiamin), B2 (riboflavin), B3 (niacin), B6, iron, and folic acid. *Tempe* made by traditional methods also contains vitamin B12, which is very important for strict vegetarians. Moreover, *tempe* is cholesterol-free and contains no salt.

The waste from the manufacture of *tempe* is a liquid containing the hulls of the beans and some unprocessed cotyledon that was sloughed off during dehulling. To make good use of this waste, some *tempe* makers keep cattle; one of those with whom I spoke has eight cows he feeds with the waste. In this manner, he keeps his environment clean and derives additional income from selling cow's milk.

Tempe can be used in many recipes and is also used as a meat substitute by vegetarians. However, it is most commonly rubbed with crushed onion and salt and then fried and eaten. Near Malang, where one village had about twenty *tempe* manufacturers, I observed *tempe* sliced thinly, coated with flour mixed with spices and then deep-fried to make a crispy snack.

To understand the popularity of *tempe* in Java, we need to understand Javanese eating habits. Eating a full meal with one's entire family happens only occasionally, as during a celebration. By contrast, on every ordinary morning after cooking, the housewife puts the dishes on the table, and the members of the family eat whenever they like. Yet because snacks are offered by door-to-door salespeople throughout the day, a proper meal is sometimes only eaten in the evening. To help prevent the food from getting stale, the housewife uses plenty of spices and herbs, especially tamarind. *Tempe* fits well with these habits, as it stays fresh for a day or two without refrigeration, while meat and fish would spoil during the same length of time. In addition, among farmers meals are prepared in order to be brought to the fields. Without equipment to warm the food, people eat the meal cold; *tempe*, which is tasty at any temperature, becomes especially useful in these circumstances.

The Story of *Tempe*

The ancient history of *tempe* is unknown, but it apparently first developed in Indonesia. This product is found mainly on the island of Java or in regions to which the Javanese have migrated. According to historian Hieronymus Budi Santoso, *tempe* is mentioned in the Serat Centini, a Javanese classic of the late eighteenth century AD (Budi Santoso 1993, 13).[4] There, *tempe* is recommended as nutritious, good-tasting food. Some scholars theorize that soy *tempe* derived "from an application to soybeans of an earlier fermentation used on coconuts, perhaps the now famous coconut presscake tempeh (*tempeh bongkrek*)" (Shurtleff and Aoyagi 2007b, 1).

Since the 1970s, the Department of Education has disseminated booklets in an attempt to spread *tempe* manufacture throughout the Archipelago. These booklets, printed in Bahasa Indonesia side by side with the local dialect, are simple to follow, especially by using the illustrations (Anonymous 1989). However, this educational effort has not been successful. Better results have been obtained by sending makers of tofu and *tempe* to islands such as Timor, Central Sulawesi, and Papua (West New Guinea) where the extra protein was most needed. A report in the *Kompas* daily newspaper for September 2, 2002, tells us that the people of Papua Province now have tofu and *tempe* on their daily menus whenever there is not enough fish available. Five manufacturers who migrated from Central Java to New Guinea in 1977 are all doing very well. At present there are twenty-five manufacturers throughout Papua, each processing 50 kg of soybeans into tofu or *tempe* daily. But their efforts to teach the Papuans to make tofu and *tempe* have not been a success because the Papuans shun messy work with water (Kewa Ama 2002).

The popularity of soyfoods on Java makes this island first in processing soybeans into food products (specifically, *tempe*) as compared to the other islands of the Archipelago. According to the census of 2000, there are 83.8 million Javanese living in Indonesia, constituting 41.71 percent of the total population (Suryadinata, Arifin, and Ananta 2003, 31). The Javanese are not the only Indonesians who eat *tempe*. If we include other ethnic groups as well, half of the total population of 205 million are probably *tempe* eaters.

To this day, *tempe* making is a village home industry. Indeed, in many Javanese villages people almost seem to live by making *tempe* alone. In Sanan, a village on the outskirts of the city of Malang, as many as 358 *tempe* makers can be found. Together they produce an average of twenty thousand kilograms of *tempe* daily, some sold in the market and others by vendors who go door-to-door in the city and deliver to their clients. A large part of the product is sliced into thin pieces and then deep-fried and sold as snacks, for which the village has become famous.

Tempelan is a village in Central Java with a long history of *tempe* making, but there are also villages with a shorter history that are just as proud of their specialties. The village of Tegalparang in South Jakarta has twenty *tempe* makers, and some of them boast of having restaurants as their customers. Sometimes people order large quantities to take with them when they go abroad. This is why there are current experiments with preserving *tempe* and why we now have vacuum-packed and frozen *tempe*.

For the domestic market, *tempe* is usually sold in the form of cakes wrapped in banana leaves or plastic sheets. Also seen lately is *tempe* in the form of tubes whereby long, thin plastic bags are filled with the soy cake. Some specialties are individually wrapped in banana leaves, in various shapes. The *tempe* from Malang, for instance, is wrapped as small triangles; others may be in tubes, squares, or rectangles.

Other Soyfoods

Soy sauce used to be made at home, using recipes faithfully handed down from generation to generation, even as they varied from region to region (on soy sauce, see the essays by Cwiertka and Moriya and by Ozeki in this volume). The regional differences remain. In Central Java, where people like to eat sweet food, the soy sauce is thick and tastes sweet. Black soybeans are preferred to make this sauce, since they have a special flavor and add to the blackness of the sauce. The sweetness comes from brown palm sugar, which also contributes to the special aroma of the sauce. Spices are added to make the sauce tasty and can become the mark of the identity of a particular brand or region. Some makers add cloves or cinnamon, but in the Chinese areas, Chinese spices such as *pekak* (star anise), *pekchi* (cinnamon flower), and *ang hua* (red flowers) are used. In the coastal city of Indramayu in West Java, some fish oil is added to make the sauce taste like seafood.

Highly salted soy sauce is also made and is used by the Chinese. Also here we find different tastes as marks of the makers. In Jakarta, the most sought-after type is the *Jembatan* (bridge) brand, which is made in the Chinatown area. We also find Japanese soy sauces on store shelves, for they too are popular, as is the so-called *kecap Inggris* (English soy sauce), which is a locally manufactured kind of Worcestershire sauce. For cooking, at times different kinds of soy sauces are mixed.

Taoco, or fermented soybeans, constitute a condiment still made at home, which varies from region to region. The best-quality products come from Cianjur, a town in the hills of West Java, and from Medan, a town in Sumatra, where the population is mostly Chinese. *Taoco* is a soybean paste similar to miso. It is made the same way as miso by adding grain to the beans and fermenting with a mold. There is also a semifluid variant of this product, as the beans are not mashed but instead are left whole or halved within liquid. Because of the liquid, the product is sold in bottles.

As mentioned earlier, historically the West Javanese liked to eat soybeans fried or grilled. This is still noticeable when they use fried soybeans to garnish certain dishes. In such cases, the fried beans are mixed with fried shredded coconut and seasoned to taste. Another version is the ground fried soybean, which adds flavor to the dish. Soybean flour, in other words, is also used as seasoning. Cooked whole soybeans are also eaten, but unlike the Japanese and Koreans who like the young beans fresh from their pods or served outside their pods as snacks, Indonesians cook soybeans either in soups or as a dessert sprinkled with ground coconut and sugar.

Soybean custard, or *kembang tahu* (literally, bean curd flower), is eaten as a snack or a dessert with a light, sweet ginger sauce. It is usually sold by vendors who go door-to-door or station themselves in the marketplace awaiting customers. According to one vendor, the manufacturer of *kembang tahu* brings the containers to a meeting place where vendors wait to buy their stock and then disperse to bring the custard to buyers. At receptions and big parties, custard is commonly offered by the caterers and enjoys an increasing popularity with party guests.

Nata de soya is an edible cellulose product deposited by bacteria growing in tofu whey (the liquid left over from tofu manufacture after the desired solids have been curdled out). The *nata de soya* is a kind of jelly, to be consumed as dessert. This product has been promoted to minimize the waste product of tofu, which endangered the environment by encouraging growth of unwanted molds. A similar product, *nata de coco,* is very popular in Indonesia, but *nata de soya* is not as easily available. A large part is exported, mainly to Japan. Experts are also exploring possible industrial applications for this product in the high-tech nonfood industries (Basrah Enie 1998). Because of its strength, it appears quite suitable for manufacturing membranes for sound systems. Further uses are possible as well in adhesives, cosmetics, packaging, and the making of plywood.

Soygurt production is still in the experimental stage but seems promising because soymilk is very popular and is a developing home industry.

Yogurt from cow's milk is very popular, and food experts expect soygurt to become equally so.

Soybean oil from locally cultivated beans is produced by a single factory for use as salad and cooking oil. However, this oil is usually mixed with other oils that also have high proportions of polyunsaturated fatty acids.

Because of increasingly modern ways of life, which impel people toward sophisticated menus, soy flour has good prospects for the future in recipes such as cakes, cream, pasta, etc. In small quantities, the soy flour enhances the texture and moisture retention of such products.

Soy Products As Source of Protein

Data from Indonesia's Central Statistics Bureau indicate that consumption of nonaquatic meat in Indonesia is low compared to that of other countries. In 2003, meat consumption was 7.10 kg per capita, as compared to 39 kg in China and 25.97 kg in Japan. Other Southeast Asian countries such as Malaysia, the Philippines, and Thailand show figures of around 25 kg.[5]

Not all the provinces in Indonesia show the same eating habits, however. Some provinces, especially those close to the sea, prefer fish to meat. In addition, there is a relatively high intake of protein through legumes in two provinces on the island of Java, the cradle of *tempe,* compared to, for example, the low-protein intake through legumes on the island of Sulawesi, where the main protein source is fish.

Statistics for 1996, 1999, and 2002 illustrate the importance of soy protein to Javanese diets. The economic crisis struck many countries in Southeast Asia in 1997 and 1998. Its effects were still felt in 1999, and full recovery came only in 2002. Statisticians and nutritionists in Indonesia consequently saw an overall drop in protein intake in 1999 and a recovery by 2002 to the 1996 levels. The intake of legumes rose, however, in Central and East Java, even as meat intake dropped. The primary legume that provided protein during the economic downturn was soy.

Conclusion

For *tempe* and tofu there are hundreds of recipes, and new uses and recipes are regularly added by women's magazines and magazines specializing in food. The old traditional recipes used by the Chinese are generally also used by native Indonesians, sometimes under different names. For example, stuffed tofu has become very popular among Indonesians, but rather than call it by its Chinese name of *yong taufu,* they call it by the Chinese word for a completely different dish, *siomay* (in China this word refers to dumplings of a kind not eaten in Indonesia). Sometimes tofu is used to replace meat or chicken, as in *tahu balado.* In the original dish, chicken or meat is fried, and a mixture of chili, garlic, onion, and lemon grass is poured over it. Tofu here transforms the dish into vegetarian and thus less expensive fare.

Culinary experts and housewives are constantly looking for new uses for soybean products. The increasing consumption of soyfoods is thus not due solely to the population explosion but is in part the result of the housewife's creativity.

President Sukarno, who led Indonesia from 1945 to 1966, repeatedly directed his people not to be a nation of *tempe.* By that he meant that they should not remain people who, like Indonesians during colonial times, had to live by eating cheap food such as *tempe.* Little did he know that not only would Indonesians continue to eat *tempe* but also that *tempe* would reach a higher level of lifestyle. *Tempe* is now enjoyed by celebrities and is also served in the Presidential Palace as part of the National Menu. Similarly, other soybean products are gaining in popularity as Indonesians experiment and innovate with this versatile bean.

Notes

1. I wish to thank the Ford Foundation Indonesia—particularly Ms. Suzanne Siskel—for sponsoring my trip to Chengdu to participate in the Eighth Symposium on Chinese Dietary Culture. Thanks also to Professor Chee-Beng Tan for encouraging me to research soyfoods in Indonesia. This essay benefited from the editorial guidance of Dr. Christine Du Bois and Professor Sidney Mintz.

2. I am grateful to Professor Andrew F. Smith, Theodore Hymowitz, and William Shurtleff for this information.

3. Raffles used the word *kédélé* instead of the present *kedelai.*

4. The *Serat Centini* is a classic, consisting of thirteen books written in the old Javanese script and language. The Javanese treat it as a kind of encyclopedia that explains Javanese culture, including religion, spiritualism, history, traditions, food, and everyday life. It is also consulted to ascertain which are auspicious days and what events are omens. It was probably written beginning in the late eighteenth century and presented to Sultan Pakubuwono V in 1815.

5. Note that all of the statistics in this paragraph refer to meat consumption, not to protein intake. In addition to protein, meat contains large amounts of water and also fat to varying degrees. Note also that data from the United Nations Food and Agriculture Organization show higher figures for all these countries.

They also show Malaysia's meat consumption outpacing that of Japan. Indonesia remains clearly at the bottom of the list for meat consumption, however. See the Food Balance Sheets at http://faostat.fao.org/site/502/default.aspx.

References

Adisarwato, T., and Rini Windiarto. 1999. *Meningkatkan Hasil Panen Kedelai* [*To Improve the Output of Soybeans*]. Yogyakarta: Swadaya.

Anonymous. 1989. *Membuat Tempe Dan Raginya* [*To Make Tempe and Its Mold*]. Timor Timur: Departemen Pendidikan dan Kebudayaan.

Asita, K. D. 2000. "Kota Kediri Berulang Tahun" ["The City of Kediri Celebrates Its Birthday"]. *Kompas* (daily newspaper), July 8, p. 11.

Basrah Enie, A. 1998. "A Study on the Development of a Nata de Soya Processing Industry from Tofu Whey." In Lilis Nuraida and Sedarnawati Yasni, eds., *Prosiding Seminar Pengembangan, Pengolahan Dan Penggunaan Kedelai Selain Tempe* [*Proceedings of the Seminar on Development—Processing and Use of Kedelai Other Than for Tempe*], 43–55. Bogor, Indonesia: Center for Food and Nutrition Studies and the American Soybean Association.

Bradley, Richard. 1732. *The Country Housewife and Lady's Director,* 6th ed., Pt. 2. Project Gutenberg EBook #7262.

Budi Santoso, Hieronymus. 1993. *Pembuatan Tempe Dan Tahu Kedelai.* [*Manufacturing Tempe and Tofu from Soybeans*]. Yogyakarta, Indonesia: Penerbit Kanisius.

City of Kediri, Indonesia. "1123 Tahun Kota Kediri" ["1123 Years of the City of Kediri"]. Brochure. July 1, 2000.

Dampier, William. 1729. *Voyages around the World: A Voyage to New Holland.* 2 vols. London: James Knapton.

Fruin Mees, W. 1920. *Geschiedenis van Java, dl 1, Hindoetijdperk* [*History of Java, Part I, the Hindu Era*]. Weltevreden (Jakarta), Indonesia: W. Kolff.

Greshof, G. 1890a. "De Soja Boon en Hare Betekenis als Voedingsmiddel in Nederlandsch Indië" ["The Soybean and Its Meaning As Food in the Netherlands-Indies"]. Pt. 1. *Tijdschrift voor Land, Tuinbouw en Boschcultuur* [*Journal of Agriculture, Horticulture and Forestry*]. Buitenzorg (Bogor), Indonesia: Departement voor Landbouw (Department of Agriculture). Jaargang [Volume] XV(3): 347–56.

———. 1890b. "De Soja Boon en Hare Betekenis als Voedingsmiddel in Nederlandsch Indië" ["The Soybean and Its Meaning As Food in the Netherlands-Indies"]. Pt. 2. *Tijdschrift voor Land, Tuinbouw en Boschcultuur* [*Journal of Agriculture, Horticulture and Forestry*]. Buitenzorg (Bogor), Indonesia: Departement voor Landbouw (Department of Agriculture) Jaargang [Volume] XV(4): 435.

Kewa Ama, Kornelis. 2002. "Sukses Memperkenalkan Tahu Tempe di Papua" ["Success with the Introduction of Tofu and Tempe in Papua"]. *Kompas* (daily newspaper), September 2, p. 27.

Nuraida, Lilis, and Sedarnawati Yasni, eds. 1998. *Prosiding Seminar Pengembangan, Pengolahan dan Penggunaan Kedelai Selain Tempe* [*Proceedings of the Seminar on Development—Processing and Use of Kedelai Other Than for Tempe*]. Bogor: Center for Food and Nutrition Studies and the American Soybean Association.

Raffles, Stamford. 1982 [1817]. *History of Java.* Petaling Jaya, Malaysia: Oxford University Press.

Shurtleff, William, and Akiko Aoyagi. 2007a. "History of Specialty Fermented Soyfoods." Lafayette, CA: Soyfoods Center. http://www.soyinfocenter.com/HSS/specialty_fermented.php.

———. 2007b. "History of Tempeh." Lafayette, CA: Soyfoods Center. http://www.soyinfocenter.com/HSS/specialty_fermented.php.

Suryadinata, Leo, Evi Nurvidya Arifin, and Aris Ananta. 2003. *Indonesia's Population, Ethnicity and Religion in a Changing Landscape.* Singapore: Institute of Southeast Asian Studies.

11

Social Context and Diet

Changing Soy Production and Consumption in the United States

CHRISTINE M. DU BOIS

Introduction

In the last century the world has witnessed the astonishing rise of U.S. soybean agriculture from negligible harvests to the production of 86.7 million metric tons in 2006–2007 (USDA 2008).[1] Soybeans have become the country's second most valuable crop[2] and most valuable agricultural export (Whitton 2004; USDA 2005; USDA 2006c). Agricultural analysts Smith and Circle aptly predicted that "it is not likely that such a tremendous increase in production will ever again be duplicated by soybeans or any other crop" in the United States (1972, 1). Consumption has been affected, too: soy protein and lecithin appear in small quantities in countless U.S. foods, and soy oil is prominent in the American diet. The tale of this expanding soy industry—or rather, industries (soy has played a role in the farming, grocery, beer, military, chemical, automotive, energy, paper, plywood, printing, and medical fields)—opens windows on many facets of American society. It is a story of enormous creativity, sedulous profit-seeking, shifting eating preferences, and controversy, all shaped by and in turn shaping global trends.

The history of soy in the United States is relevant not only to Americans but also to people in many other countries. This is because currently, the United States produces nearly a third of the world's soybeans (USDA 2008) and exports nearly half of its production, principally to Europe, Japan, Mexico, China, and Taiwan (Ash, Livezey, and Dohlman 2006, 13). The United States is the largest producer of soy today (USDA 2008).

The account below demonstrates the ecological and chemical constraints on how humans obtain and process foods as well as the long-term impacts that people with political and economic power make on dietary patterns (see Ross 1980, 1987). Yet in any given period a society's dietary patterns are not wholly dictated by these factors. While the tastes for certain foods and not others (and for certain combinations of foods and not others) are historically derived, they can at times be slower to respond to ecological changes or to changes in the political economy than some would wish. Culture is thus not merely a reflex of material and social constraints, although it is profoundly molded by them.

The case of soy repeatedly demonstrates this interplay between ecology, socioeconomic power, and culture. The middle of the twentieth century provides a good example. Having historically acquired a taste for bland cooking oils other than soy, Americans did not turn in droves to stronger-flavored soy oil during that period, although the soy industry and many in government desperately wanted them to. (Throughout this essay, the phrase "the soy industry" serves as shorthand for the many and varied farmers and companies dealing with soy production, processing, product formulation, marketing, and distribution.)[3] In this case, industry was forced to adapt to American tastes, not the other way around. The soy industry duly made changes in processing to lessen the oil's flavor, thus improving it from the viewpoint of most American consumers. At first the new, blander soy oil did not do well in exports south of the border, however, since Mexicans preferred stronger-tasting oil (Kahn 1991, 93–94). In a surprisingly few years, soy went on to become the most important oil in the American diet, just as the soy industry wished.

The Early Years

This complex interplay of forces affecting soy began with ex-sailor Samuel Bowen's plantings in Georgia in 1765; he used the crop to make soy noodles and sauce for export to Britain. The American Revolution apparently ended the business (Hymowitz and Harlan 1983) and was the first of several wars that would alter the course of U.S. soy history. Although soy seeds were reintroduced from Asia on a number of occasions throughout the 1800s, it was not until the end of the century that Americans would treat the plant as much more than a curiosity.

In 1887 Congress passed the Hatch Act, funding the development of state agricultural experiment stations. These stations, along with the interest that the U.S. Department of Agriculture (USDA) began taking in soy, promoted it as a farm crop. In 1898 the USDA started introducing new varieties of soy; in this they were aided by the enhanced Far Eastern trade ensuing in the aftermath of the Chinese-Japanese War of 1894–95 (USDA 1937; Mounts, Wolf, and Martinez 1987, 819). Over time, breeding programs with numerous varieties of soy enabled researchers to develop new strains with desired characteristics, such as better adaptation to U.S. soils and climates and higher oil content (USDA 1937, 1155, 1161; USDA 1975, 226). Eventually, USDA researchers William Morse and Howard Dorsett would go to East Asia, bringing back some forty-five hundred soy specimens. But that trip would occur during 1929–31 (Hymowitz 1984). Well before then, government efforts to study and promote soy set off a long chain of events leading to its current prominence in U.S. agriculture.

In the early twentieth century, soy in the United States was primarily a southern crop planted as forage for domestic animals and as a nitrogen-renewer for the soil; it was not generally planted for beans (USDA 1937, 1156–59). Soon after the Russo-Japanese War of 1904–5, however, the Japanese found themselves in control of surplus Manchurian soybeans grown to meet wartime needs. They exported many of these beans to Europe, where after the beans were crushed the oil was used for soap; the protein meal that remained was fed to dairy cattle (Bowdidge 1935, 6–8; Smith and Circle 1972, 4). This trade eventually spurred U.S. interest in likewise importing and crushing whole soybeans.

Interest in the whole beans grew during the World War I shortage of fats and oils, since the increasing quantity of processed soy oil imported from Manchuria was often of poor quality (Windish 1981, 12). Worries about the boll weevil infestation of U.S. cotton fields also stimulated attention to oils from sources other than cottonseeds (Mounts, Wolf, and Martinez 1987, 819; Wik 1972, 155; Anonymous 1916). In addition, during World War I protein-rich soy flour was used as a meat substitute (Mindell 1995, 16; Golbitz 1998, 5–6). In light of these varying events, some visionaries came to realize that the country could benefit from a robust domestic soy-processing industry and a domestic crop of beans to supply it.

In the meantime, the center of U.S. soy agriculture was shifting northward; by 1924 Illinois was the leading producer, a distinction it shares with Iowa today (USDA 2006a; Hymowitz 1987, 28). Rather rapidly thereafter, midwestern production far outstripped that of the South. The shift occurred not because southerners began growing less soy but rather because midwesterners became big soybean boosters (USDA n.d.).

They did so partly for agronomic reasons. First, corn farmers paid attention to advice from agricultural researchers on how to control the corn borer pest; in well-distributed bulletins from the University of Illinois, for example, "of the ten suggested controls, nine recommended [regular plantings of] soybeans" (Windish 1981, 66–67). Second, in 1920 scientists made a breakthrough in understanding soy's sensitivity to the length of the day, a phenomenon called photoperiodism. The new insight enabled breeders and farmers to select the best varieties for growth and timely maturation at the latitudes of the U.S. Midwest (Hymowitz 1990; USDA 1975, 226). Third, in 1934 cinch bugs decimated midwestern corn, oats, and wheat but left soybeans unscathed. Fortunately, "there was still time enough in the season to plant soybeans on those acres the cinch bug had annihilated" (Windish 1981, 67); that fall Illinois farmers harvested more than double the soybeans of the year before, 60 percent of the entire U.S. crop (USDA n.d.). Finally, soybeans "are less sensitive to drought than corn" (Powell 1971, 50). Soy was turning out to be an excellent alternate crop for farmers in the Corn Belt.

Plantings of midwestern soy were also prompted by the bold business gambles of seed and grain-processing entrepreneurs. The pivotal venture came with Illinois corn processor August Staley's 1921–22 announcement—through newspapers, farm magazines, pamphlets, letters, and service representatives who visited farming communities—that he would begin crushing soybeans in the fall of 1922. Staley guaranteed farmers that he would buy all they could grow (Shurtleff and Aoyagi 2007a, 5; Shurtleff and Aoyagi 2004a; Forrestal 1982, 56; Smith and Circle 1972, 4). In response, in the spring of 1922 Illinois farmers planted five times as many acres of soy as the year before (Windish 1981, 65–66). This development encouraged other businessmen to begin crushing.

The oil from these beans was mostly used in manufacturing, primarily in paints, soaps, and varnishes; the by-product protein meal was sold very cheaply as feed for domestic animals (Smith and Circle 1972, 5). As Smith and Circle explain, the early "growth of the soybean industry . . . was influenced more by the shortage of oil [for manufacturing] and its relatively high price than [by] the need for protein" (1972, 5).

More promotional efforts, including the colorful Soil and Soybean Special train carrying exhibits about soy and reaching some thirty-four thousand rural people during the spring of 1927 (Forrestal 1982, 65), also helped expand the soybean industry. Then in 1928 a coalition of farmers in New York sought soy meal for dairy cattle; in a multibusiness arrangement, Illinois farmers were guaranteed an acceptable minimum price for their soybeans—up to one million bushels—thus protecting farmers from a feared drop in prices due to potential oversupply (Smith and Circle 1972, 4; Windish 1981, 74, 200–201). Once again, acreage increased.

Other factors whipped up the startling soybean expansion. Crop improvement associations, working closely with university advisors, worked tirelessly to bring better seed to growers. They urged farmers to use only seed that was officially certified to be of desired varieties; uncertified seed, while perhaps cheaper or more convenient to purchase, was more likely to disappoint. The success of these organizations is illustrated by the case of a particular strain of the Manchu variety, winner of multiple farm show awards during 1924–26. By 1927 "nearly 76 percent of all known soybean growers in Illinois were using [this] strain[,] . . . a factor directly attributed to efforts of the Illinois Crop Improvement Association toward standardization" (Windish 1981, 128).

In addition to the concerted promotion of better seeds, improvements in agricultural machinery spurred soy farming. Soy became a popular crop around the same time that American farms became much more mechanized (Smith and Circle 1972, 3). Improvements in the quality and prices of tractors between 1910 and 1930 enabled farmers to tend their fields with far fewer draft animals (P. Johnson 1978, 73–109). This change freed up "between 55 and 80 million acres of cropland in the U.S." previously used as pasture (Powell 1971, 45). Obvious though it seems, it is not sufficiently discussed that by revolutionizing American agriculture, the internal combustion engine was a vital factor in opening the land to the mass production of soybeans.

Farm animals became by and large creatures raised for their meat or milk rather than for their horsepower, and they came to eat meat-enhancing foods such as soy meal rather than forage crops (which had included not only soy but also oats, other grasses, and the legumes clover and alfalfa) (Berlan 1991, 122). Within the space of twenty-five years beginning around 1920, there occurred an immense switch on American farms from foraging horses and mules to meal-eating hogs (Powell 1971, 46). The gradually increasing demand for soy meal stimulated soy plantings.

Soy agriculture also benefited significantly from the development of combine harvesters. First used to harvest soy in 1920 and found valuable in reducing losses caused by shattering of the pods (Liu 1997, 3), over the years adaptations of combines to make them suitable specifically for soy further reduced harvesting losses (Windish 1981, 55–56). Combines also reduced the need for farm labor; farmers were grateful for this change, since "the great tide of immigration which assured cheap labor was tapering off" (P. Johnson 1978, 73). The reduction of labor costs helped make domestically grown soybeans more competitive with beans grown in Asia (Smith and Circle 1972, 3).

But U.S. farmers needed extra aid to compete with inexpensive Asian soy. The U.S. Congress obliged with a series of controversial tariffs on soy imports from 1913 to 1936 (Windish 1981, 102–3). The most important of these was the Smoot-Hawley Tariff of 1930, pushed through Congress with the assistance of the American Soybean Association (ASA). Now protected, in the 1930s the young soybean industry flourished (Smith and Circle 1972, 4).

It flourished despite the Great Depression and indeed in part because of it. Farm revenues dropped so low during that period that Congress initiated programs to prop up crop prices. These programs paid farmers to plant less of certain crops in order to prevent crop supplies from outstripping demand, which would have caused prices to plunge. Crops under acreage restrictions included corn, wheat, and cotton. Since soy was deemed a soil-conserving crop, it was, by contrast, under no acreage restriction; "the plan was that soybeans were to be plowed under as green manure, but permission was regularly granted to harvest the crop" (Powell 1971, 49). Farmers increased anew their acreage of soy (Powell 1971; Smith and Circle 1972, 2, 5, 8–9).

The 1930s also saw notable advances in soy processing, utilization, financing, and research. In 1934 the Archer, Daniels, Midland Company (ADM) began deriving lecithin from crude soybean oil. Since that time, lecithin has been used (in small quantities) in a wide variety of food, industrial, and medical applications as an emulsifier, lubricant, animal-feed supplement, pigment dispersant, and softening agent (ADM n.d.a; n.d.b). In 1936 trading in soybean futures began at the Chicago Board of Trade (Windish 1981, 67), and the U.S. Regional Soybean Industrial Products Laboratory was established at the University of Illinois (Mounts, Wolf, and Martinez 1987, 820). Also in that year the first patent for a soy-based infant formula was granted, going to a doctor who had for years been supported by Seventh-day Adventists as a missionary in China (Johnson, Myers, and Burden 1992, 434). The following year, the Central Soya company erected a massive factory in Indiana for processing soy oil by German methods of solvent extraction, which provided a higher yield; by 1941 the company had advanced the process considerably, leading to improvements in the quality of the meal left behind after oil extraction (Shurtleff and Aoyagi 2004b).

The industrial possibilities for soy caught the attention of Henry Ford who, during the Great Depression, looked for ways to help American farmers by finding manufacturing uses for agricultural products. He was fascinated by the relationships between machine manufacture and the human genius for helping plants grow. Somewhat prophetically, he tried to reveal the potentialities for bringing these different phenomena closer together.[4]

During 1932–33 alone, scientists in his employ spent more than $1 million on soy research. This and later work invented or improved products such as soy plastics for automobile parts, soy shock absorber fluid, soy meat substitutes, soy coffee, and soy textiles. Many of these surprising items were displayed at the 1933–34 Chicago World's Fair in the Ford-sponsored Industrialized American Barn, an exhibit that spread soy's fame (Bryan 1990, 112–13; Wik 1972, 148–51; Nevins and Hill 1954, 491). Ford's use of soy in the manufacture of vehicles also stimulated soy farming in Michigan (Nevins and Hill 1954, 491).

But Ford was ahead of his time. During his life, most of the food and industrial applications for soy that so impassioned him did not really catch on. Research into soy industrial applications continues today, however. For example, recent high prices of petroleum have provoked greater interest in using soy oil for diesel. Likewise, research into uses of soy protein in foods acceptable to the American palate is increasingly important today.

The Emergence of a Superpower

The spring of 1941 was a turning point; in that year, for the first time more soy was planted for beans than for all other purposes combined (Hymowitz 1990). The following year the soy industry reached another milestone: under the impact of World War II, U.S. soybean production finally outstripped that of Manchuria (Shurtleff and Aoyagi 2007b, 1).

Despite the growth of the U.S. soy industry in the 1920s and 1930s, before World War II the United States had imported 40 percent of its fats and oils, primarily for use in foods (ASA n.d.; USDA 1945). But the war cut the United States off from its crucial Far Eastern suppliers. America's European allies were also deprived of their oil supplies and found themselves short of adequate protein (Powell 1971, 54; USDA 1945). In response to these deficits, the U.S. government urged "an all-out effort [to] increas[e] soybean production, astronomically" and guaranteed farmers relatively high prices for their beans (Windish 1981, 78; see also Powell 1971, 54). American farmers and processors gladly rose to the occasion, surmounting serious technical challenges along the way (USDA 1945; Walsh 1947, 26–27). Between 1940 and 1945, the number of acres harvested more than doubled (Golbitz 1999, 362).

Much of the increased production of beans came from switching land used for forage-variety soy to oil-bean varieties (Walsh 1947, 6). Indeed, by 1950 "90 percent of the crop was being harvested as beans" (Windish 1981, 97). This change and the spectacular growth of soy farming in the decades since the war (both in acreage and in average yield per acre) turned the United States into a global "soybean superpower" (Golbitz 1998, 5; Golbitz 1999, 362).

During World War II itself, soy was used in glue to hold U.S. torpedo boats together (Kahn 1991, 78); as a foam stabilizer in U.S. Navy fire extinguishers (soy protein has "marvelous fire-fighting properties") (USDA 1951, 605; see also Jenkins 1975, 33); in K rations, pork link sausage, and macaroni for the U.S. Army (Johnson, Myers, and Burden 1992, 430); and in the domestically consumed margarine that became a common substitute for increasingly scarce butter and lard (Powell 1971, 55; USDA 1975, 232–33; Walsh 1947). Although during the 1930s margarine consumption had already begun to rise and although an alliance of margarine producers and farmers had expanded the use of soy oil in margarine during that decade (Borth 1942, 211), the wartime exigencies of the 1940s were of major importance in creating an American market for soy oil as human food (USDA 1966, 123).

However, during that period ongoing problems with the flavor of soy oil forced manufacturers to limit its proportion in their margarine to no more than 30 percent (Mounts, Wolf, and Martinez 1987, 821; USDA 1993, 86). The flavor problem caused the soy industry so much worry that after the war Americans would abandon soy as other edible fats and oils became more available (USDA 1951, 575). Cooperative research among government, university, and industry laboratories came to the rescue, bringing ever-greater improvements to soy oil's flavor and shelf life (USDA 1951, 575–78; Mounts, Wolf, and Martinez 1987, 821; USDA 1993, 86–88). These improvements made possible a lasting shift from using soy oil in manufacturing to using it in human foods. The switch was critical to the soy industry's survival, since "cheap petroleum . . . after World War II" came largely to displace soy oil in manufacturing (Johnson, Myers, and Burden 1992, 442). Today, more than 95 percent of soy oil used in America is turned into human food (U.S. Census Bureau 2006, 6).

In the 1940s there was still a long way to go in promoting soy oil in the American diet, however. In addition to flavor issues, the postwar soy industry faced state and federal antimargarine laws (USDA 1975, 232; Windish 1981, 21; ASA n.d.). These laws, passed from the late 1800s forward at the behest of the dairy industry, placed taxes on margarine and in some states prohibited the use of yellow colorings that made margarine look more like butter. The soy and margarine industries succeeded in having these laws repealed, thus further promoting the use of soy oil as human food.

All the same, just after World War II Americans were not yet eating enough soy to prevent a problem of oversupply for the industry (ASA n.d.). During and just after the war, some of the surplus was used to make powdered soups such as Pea Soya, fed to starving refugees in Europe and Asia (Johnson, Myers, and Burden 1992, 430; Windish 1981, 15–16). Because of soy's role in nursing West Europeans back to health, some in the industry came to see the bean as an agent of freedom and democracy (Windish 1981, 25–27). Both patriotism and market interests goaded them to frustration with what they saw as an inadequate postwar demand for soy (see ASA n.d.). Now so successful at producing soybeans, they believed that American soy should be consumed in ever greater quantities, both at home and abroad.

Several factors soon relieved the economic pressure on them. For one, political changes and postwar economic problems prevented China from restoring its prewar soybean exports to Europe (Hapgood 1987, 80; Windish 1981, 27). U.S. soy producers eagerly filled the gap, assuming the new role of peacetime suppliers to Europe's recovering economies (Berlan, Bertrand, and Lebas 1999, 406). In addition, U.S. government farm policies during the Korean War raised the price per bushel of soybeans (Powell 1971, 57).

By that war's end, however, the soy industry once again faced a surplus (Powell 1971, 58). The 1954 enactment of Public Law 480 (also known as Food for Peace) helped to rectify this situation. The law, which authorized the exchange of excess agricultural commodities for foreign currency, had "an indirect, but effective, influence on the increase in soybean acreage through the disposal of surplus oil. . . . [I]t appears that the program has helped maintain favorable market prices for soybeans" (Powell 1971, 59). After 1954, under PL 480 exports of soybean oil rose approximately twenty-fivefold to around 1.3 billion pounds in 1961 (Powell 1971, 60). Moreover, beginning in 1966 soy oil and especially soy flour were blended with gelatinized cornmeal, dried milk, vitamins, and minerals to make corn-soya-milk (CSM), for years shipped to developing countries for malnourished people—especially preschoolers—also through the Food for Peace program (Wolf 1973, 3403; Johnson, Myers, and Burden 1992, 430). In recent years more than half a million metric tons of such soy products have been shipped overseas annually as part of U.S. feeding programs (U.S. Agency for International Development, personal communication, 2003).

In the meantime, three new food trends also aided the soy industry. Of only minor significance at first—but a harbinger of the future—was the increase in U.S. consumption of traditional Asian soyfoods. The Kikkoman Corporation noticed in the 1950s and 1960s that Americans began eating more often in Asian restaurants. U.S. military personnel who had served in World War II, in the postwar Japanese occupation, and in Korea had come back with a taste for Asian foods (Yates 1998, xiii). Kikkoman surmised that this change in the American palate could lead to increased use of soy sauce in home cooking. Hence, "the company first began prime time television advertising of its soy sauce in the United States during the 1956 presidential election returns. That was a full year before Americans saw TV ads for the Toyopet, the first car Toyota sold in the United States" (Yates 1998, xi).

By 1972, Kikkoman had decided to build a factory in Walworth, Wisconsin, the "first significant Japanese manufacturing facility ever built in the United States" and still "the largest soy sauce plant in the Western world" (Yates 1998, vii, xi). These moves both spurred and responded to the increasing U.S. consumption of soy sauce and other traditional soyfoods (Hesseltine 1983, 296; Yates 1998, xi).

The second, and to soy farmers far more important, food trend was the burgeoning postwar consumption of meat in industrialized nations. By 1973, "per capita consumption of chicken had increased by factors of 2, 4, and 15 in the United States, Europe, and Japan respectively" (Hapgood 1987, 80; see also Berlan 1991, 126). This extended meat binge coupled with advances in the conversion of soy meal into animal feed caused demand for soy to shoot upward. Meal evolved into the industry's number one revenue producer. It became number one not on a per-pound-of-finished-product basis (soy oil is worth more per pound than soy meal) but rather on a per-bushel-of-beans basis, since a bushel of beans yields more than four times more meal than oil (Ash, Livezey, and Dohlman 2006, 3–4).

Although soy meal had been used early in the twentieth century to feed cattle, its value in fattening swine and poultry was not established until later as scientists made advances in inactivating antinutritive factors in soy and in discovering the precise amounts of soy and other ingredients to mix in the feed for each type of animal (Smith and Circle 1972, 6–8). The late 1940s and early 1950s were critical years, when improved soy meals for poultry were introduced (Johnson, Myers, and Burden 1992, 429; Schaible 1970, 51). The eventual importance of poultry to the soy industry is illustrated by statistics from the 1990s, when chickens consumed significantly more soy protein than anyone else in America, some 40 percent of the yearly domestic supply. Swine were next at a bit under 30 percent (Johnson, Myers, and Burden 1992, 429; Golbitz 1998, 6; LMC 1999). In addition, pet food and fish farming provide valued markets for soy meal (Mounts, Wolf, and Martinez 1987, 823; PROMAR 2000; Hayes 1996). Despite growth of soyfood consumption in the United States, by 2005 humans still ate less than 3 percent of the domestic soy protein supply (Ash, Livezey, and Dohlman 2006, 3).

Raising animals for meat is an inefficient use of edible plants. In recent years, a pig has required more than three pounds of feed to produce a single pound of meat, and a chicken has required around two pounds (Anonymous 2006b; United Soybean Board, personal communication, 2003; see also Kahn 1991, 171). Thus, the great quantities of chicken and pork that Americans eat represent hefty prior sales of soy meal. Indeed, because Americans consume most of their soy indirectly through chicken and pork and because they eat so much of these meats, U.S. per capita use of soy is significantly higher than that of Japan. This is true even though Japanese consumption of chicken has risen dramatically (the levels previously had been quite low) and even though the Japanese are great consumers of tofu and other soy products, obtaining far more of their daily protein intake directly from soy than do Americans (Du Bois and Mintz 2003, 324–25; Hapgood 1987, 73; Johnson, Myers, and Burden 1992, 442). The fact is that as long as Americans eat plenty of meat—barring any serious new competitor in the feed market—U.S. farmers will continue to enjoy stable domestic demand for their soy meal.

The role of chicken in American cuisine requires an "enormous quantity of soybeans" (Powell 1971, 65) in another way as well. One important use of soy oil is as fat sold to fast-food restaurants for deep-fat frying. Already by the 1970s there were "40,000-plus carry-out fried chicken operations throughout the nation" (Powell 1971, 65); soy is the primary oil that these establishments have used. Thus, chickens not only consume much soy meal when alive but also utilize considerable soy oil when fried as a favorite American dish, well over 200 million pounds of soy oil yearly by the 1990s (Earley 1995; USDA 1999b).

Soy oil figures in a different way in the third important food trend that has helped the soy industry. As its flavor improved, soy oil in the United States began to be used much more often in liquid form as a home-cooking or salad oil (Mounts, Wolf, and Martinez 1987, 822; Golbitz 1999, 373). Since 1960, this latter market for soy oil has come very valuably to complement its niches in the semisolid and solid shortening and margarine markets (Mounts, Wolf, and Martinez 1987, 821–23). In the United States "soybean oil makes up about 80 percent of all the [liquid home-use] oils on the market. If the label says just 'vegetable oil,' there is a good chance that it is soy" (Messina, Messina, and Setchell 1994, 40; USDA 1999b). Consequently, today nearly half the soy oil consumed in the United States is used as liquid cooking or salad oil (U.S. Census Bureau 2006).

From a financial perspective, these many changes in the American diet helped turn soy into the "Cinderella crop" of the 1960s and early 1970s (Kahn 1991, 284; Smith and Circle 1972, 3). Its production and reputation had soared, and there were definitely profits to be made.

New Uses for Soy Protein

In addition to these food trends, other changes in the U.S. diet also affected the soy industry, although less steadily. One such change has been the gradually increasing human consumption of soy protein in a variety of new products. Americans' willingness to eat soy protein has gone hand in hand with the industry's development of techniques for extracting, concentrating, and texturizing soy. Most importantly, the industry has also made advances in rendering soy palatable to Americans by reducing or eliminating beany, grassy, and chalky flavors (Johnson, Myers, and Burden 1992; Rackis, Sessa, and Honig 1979).

Nudging Americans toward soy protein consumption was the USDA's 1971 decision allowing government reimbursement for use of vegetable proteins in the National School Lunch Program (Johnson, Myers, and Burden 1992, 438–39; Berlan, Bertrand, and Lebas 1999, 413). During the first year alone of such use, American schools served "23 million pounds of hydrated textured vegetable protein" mixed into meats; most of this vegetable protein came from soy (Johnson, Myers, and Burden 1992, 440).

Meat prices were soaring at the time (Ross 1980, 207), and just at the point when children were eating soy in school, their mothers were discovering its economizing virtues at the supermarket. Hoping to encourage shoppers to continue buying beef, grocers blended ground beef with soy-based extenders in a 3:1 meat-to-soy ratio, thereby helping to reduce the price of a package of meat by as much as 40 percent (Johnson, Myers, and Burden 1992, 440). Such blends eventually captured 25 percent of the ground meat market, but when beef prices dropped in 1973 the popularity of the blends faded. Consumers revealed their true attitude: that the blends were mere "substitutes" for real, pure meat, something that one would only buy out of financial necessity (Rackis, Sessa, and Honig 1979, 264; Johnson, Myers, and Burden 1992, 440). Afterward, "many food processors felt the need to reassure consumers that their products contained no 'fillers' or 'cereal additives'" (Golbitz 1998, 7).

The U.S. military was less finicky and more interested in financial savings: beginning in 1980, ground beef purchased by the Department of Defense "was extended 20 percent with textured soy protein" (USDA 1993, 129; see also Johnson, Myers, and Burden 1992, 440; Mindell 1995, 19). By the mid-1990s, "about a hundred million pounds of soy protein [were] served to [U.S.] armed forces each year" (Messina, Messina, and Setchell 1994, 40).

Meanwhile, new social movements were afoot that combined a sometimes mystical appreciation of the bean with hard-nosed appraisals of soy's potential in global diets. The countercultural movement among youths of the 1960s and early 1970s had made Asian philosophies, medical practices, belief systems, and foods—including soyfoods—more known in the United States. Also in the 1970s, "popular books such as Frances Moore Lappé's *Diet for a Small Planet,* and William Shurtleff and Akiko Aoyagi's *The Book of Tofu,* promoted vegetarian, soy-based diets" (Mindell 1995, 17; see also Messina, Messina, and Setchell 1994, 22–23). Thus, seen in light of its ancient role in Asian medicines (Mindell 1995, 15–16; Messina, Messina, and Setchell 1994, 36; Pitchford 1993), soy appeared to be an exceptionally healthful, psycho-spiritually invigorating and cleansing food. Seen in light of its protein efficiency, it also appeared to be a potential solution to world hunger. Among countercultural youths and the New Age movement that followed, soy was often understood in both lights simultaneously as a food that was morally correct and pure both for the individual and for humankind.

Consumption of soy protein—not only in traditional Asian forms, such as tofu, but also as analogs imitating U.S. meat and dairy products—began to rise. U.S. analogs were not new, having first been merchandised in the 1920s by Dr. John Harvey Kellogg, the breakfast cereal pioneer, and further developed by Seventh-day Adventists as part of their vegetarian lifestyle (Golbitz 1998, 6; Messina, Messina, and Setchell 1994, 37). But the New

Age eating that has become increasingly popular since the late 1970s has elevated the U.S. marketing and development of analogs—indeed of soyfoods of all kinds—to a new plane. The importance of New Age culinary choices has been joined by the impacts of a rising population of soy-eating Asian immigrants and the growing interest in soy on the part of medical researchers and the health journalists who report on their work.

Soymilk, imported into the United States from Asia in the early 1980s, has thus evolved into a $745 million overwhelmingly domestic industry. Soyfoods have become commonplace; by 2006, three-quarters of soy products purchased in the United States were sold in mainstream supermarkets. Such growth meant that between 1992 and 2004, U.S. soyfood sales grew from $300 million to $3.9 billion (Soyfoods Association of North America 2006).

In addition, medical reports about soy have boosted its status as a human food. In late 1999 the U.S. Food and Drug Administration (FDA) decreed that as long as manufacturers meet certain conditions, they can make claims on food labels linking consumption of soy protein to a potential reduction in the risk of heart disease. The claim is based on decades of nutritional research (Messina, Messina, and Setchell 1994, 100, 244). Some research has also suggested that eating plant hormones in soy, called isoflavones, can alleviate uncomfortable symptoms of menopause and could help prevent osteoporosis and certain cancers (Golbitz 1998, 13–14). Hence, although there is controversy among medical researchers about the safety of consuming soy isoflavones in foods or supplements—especially when added to foods in large quantities and when fed to certain subgroups in the population (Sigler 2000)—isoflavones are being incorporated in foods marketed for their purported health benefits (Burros 2000). Responding to this trend, in 1998 ADM opened the world's first factory dedicated to the large-scale production of isoflavones.

In January 2006, however, the prestigious American Heart Association cast scientific doubt on many of soy's touted health benefits (Sacks et al. 2006). The effects of the association's skepticism on the popular soyfoods market remain to be seen. For now, health-oriented functional foods, or nutraceuticals, are a booming market in the United States (Sabatini 2000). In the 1990s, soyfoods in particular were the "hottest growth area in the North American food industry, with sales growing at an annual rate of more than 30%" (Golbitz 1999, 16). Although sales growth is now down in the more normal single digits (Wright 2005), food manufacturers continue to explore ways to include soy protein or soy isoflavones in their recipes.[5]

Another trend encouraging human consumption of soy protein is vegetarianism among American youths. According to a 2005 Harris Interactive poll, approximately 3 percent of children ages eight to eighteen abstain completely from meat, poultry, fish, and seafood (Stahler 2005). Because soy is a good source of protein, vegetarians and semivegetarians consume it often, considerably more than do U.S. meat eaters. This trend is good news for natural-foods companies and soyfoods processors although perhaps bad news for soy farmers and bean processors, since American chickens destined for the dinner table eat so very much soy.

The movement toward vegetarianism—an outgrowth of increasing environmentalism among American youths (Fishman 2000)—is still small enough that the U.S. market for soy meal as animal feed remains huge. This situation could change, however, as demand for meat in ever more prosperous China could cause world meat prices to rise. Higher meat prices in the United States coupled with an increasing population and decreasing arable land could induce Americans to eat less meat and more pulses such as soy (cf. Pimentel et al. 1999).

Corporations would certainly find new ways to profit from this scenario, and certain companies would have a head start. Among them are those engaged in research on how conventional breeding can produce soy varieties particularly suited to soyfood production. For example, the small Schillinger Seed Company in Iowa has developed a variety that is especially suited to extrusion technology. Extrusion of soy protein makes its texture more meatlike; hence, this new variety of soy works well in meat analogs.

Shifts in U.S. Consumption of Fats

Another social change promoting soy came about in the mid-1980s as the nutritional research and lobbying group the Center for Science in the Public Interest began raising government and public awareness of the health risks posed by coconut, palm, and palm kernel oils. Then in 1987 heart attack survivor Phil Sokolof, a wealthy metal fabricator, began paying for full-page newspaper ads decrying manufacturers' use of tropical oils in prepared foods (see Kahn 1991, 229–30). His ads greatly increased public awareness of the dangers of such oils. Within two years the resulting outcry had pressured most manufacturers to stop using them.

Growing public concern about these saturated fats spurred companies to switch from tropical oils—and animal fats—to soy oil, which is much less saturated. For example, in 1990 Burger King announced that thereafter much of its menu (in particular french fries) would be cooked in "a blend of 20 percent peanut oil and 80 percent soybean oil" (Kahn 1991, 220) rather than in beef tallow as before. Other fast-food companies soon followed suit. The switch was a boon to the soy industry. Eventually, the switch would also provide some benefit to the environment: today, innovative companies are developing pleasant-smelling, less-polluting, and increasingly cost-effective diesel fuel based on soy oil, often soy oil left over from commercial deep-fat frying.[6] According to the National Biodiesel Board, "Hundreds of major [transportation] fleets use biodiesel, including all branches of the U.S. military, Yellowstone National Park, NASA, several state departments of transportation, major public utility fleets such as Florida Power & Light, cities such as Seattle, and more than 100 school districts" (National Biodiesel Board 2005). This usage of soy oil, while still very small compared to the amount of petroleum expended yearly for diesel, nevertheless is a positive move in the direction of altering America's energy consumption patterns.

The use of soy oil in processed American foods has turned out to be a curse, however. Medical researchers have found that, ironically, the partially hydrogenated soy oil that U.S. food industries and restaurants have widely employed in the past decade is even less healthy for the human heart than the saturated oils it replaced. Partially hydrogenated soy oil has been processed with hydrogen, which increases the time that it stays fresh on a supermarket shelf or in a deep-fat fryer. Unfortunately, partial hydrogenation also converts healthy fats into trans fats.[7] These fats have been found to be so artery-clogging that beginning in 2006 the FDA has required all packaged foods to list the amounts of trans fat they contain. In addition, the Board of Health of New York City voted in September of 2006 to ban trans fats in all of the city's 20,000 restaurants, a decision that could begin a nationwide trend (Lueck 2006).

Agricultural technology companies have responded to these events by developing new varieties of soy that require less hydrogenation. These varieties have relatively long shelf lives with significantly reduced trans fat. Monsanto announced the marketing of such a soybean, Vistive, in 2004, and in 2005 Kellogg announced that it would begin using oil from these beans in certain foods. Dupont's Pioneer High-Bred International teamed with Bunge, Ltd., to produce Nutrium™ Low Lin Soybean Oil, with properties similar to Vistive oil; Kellogg is likely to turn to this source of beans as well (see Barrionuevo 2005).[8]

Soy and Controversy

The overall effect of these many post–World War II developments, including the continued use of soy in small quantities in a variety of industries, is that today soy is found "wherever one looks," such as in "axle grease, beer and ale, wallboard, vitamins, dusting powder, putty, oilcloth, alcohol, varnish, bottle caps, caulking compounds, linoleum, cement, insecticides, nitroglycerin, [and] a dust-buster for grain elevators" (Kahn 1991, 221) as well as in diesel, waxes, plastics, paints, newspaper inks, paper, glues, cleaning products for circuit boards, animal feeds, alternative medicines and dietary supplements, hospital meals, vegetarian foods, sports drinks and snacks, pizza toppings, seafoods, diet products, infant formulas, frozen desserts, and myriad other ordinary grocery items.

Because of this prevalence in American society as well as complex issues surrounding soy's production, processing, financing, and consumption, in the years to come it will stand at the center of several controversies. In addition to debate over the effects of soy isoflavones on human health, other disputes are likely to remain in the foreseeable future. First, soy is a primary agricultural product in the polemic over genetic engineering, an intricate topic with a chapter of its own in this volume. Second, soy production is tangled up in arguments about federal agricultural policies. Third, like many other foods, soy is involved in a trend that some view with alarm: the increasing economic consolidation in agriculture and in American food industries. Fourth, soy is caught up in the altercations of capitalist competition. Despite economic consolidation, competition does remain among companies over soy's role in the U.S. diet, at times leading to intense struggles over U.S. food labeling requirements, institutional purchases, and interpretation of scientific findings. Each of these three latter arenas of controversy is dealt with below.

Agricultural policy disputes have arisen regarding the effects of the Freedom to Farm bill passed into federal law in 1996 and of the follow-up 2002 agricultural bill. Touted as a legal package that would gradually wean farmers and grain processors from federal subsidies, the 1996 bill failed to do so. Its provisions retained many controversial financial protections for farmers, such as "farm-program [aid], federal crop insurance, and disaster assistance" (Lee 1999). Farmers argue in favor of such safety nets as necessary for preserving rural communities and ensuring a stable food supply. Detractors contend that the subsidies are an unproductive use of taxpayers' money that mostly end up benefiting the richest landowners, many of whom do not even farm the land themselves (Skees 1999).

Whatever way one may view these issues, it is clear that despite the intentions behind the 1996 bill, in recent years government expenditures on agriculture have surged to record levels (Anonymous 2006a). In some years drought, the financial crisis in Asia (which reduced demand for U.S. agricultural exports, including soy), and lowered crop prices (including for soy) made farmers more dependent than ever on government assistance (Lee 1999). Illustrative of this situation were the lines that formed in February and March 2000 at offices of the U.S. Farm Service Agency as soy farmers signed up to receive their shares of $475 million in federal relief for oilseed growers (Keen 2000).

The effects of the Freedom to Farm bill on soy farming have also been contested in international trade negotiations, a nontrivial issue since, as previously stated, soy is America's number one agricultural export and, more broadly, the "most important oilseed in international trade" (Grayson 1983, 427; see also Golbitz 1999, 339). Although the 1996 bill continued many subsidies to farmers, it decoupled certain payments from the type and amount of crops that farmers were growing. After 1996, a farmer who previously received a subsidy only if he grew wheat still received the subsidy while having the freedom to farm a number of other crops instead, notably soy. Because for several years soy prices, while low, were nevertheless higher than those of other major crops, in this less restrictive subsidy context many farmers elected to grow soy instead of wheat or corn. Indeed, between 1996 and 1999 U.S. soy acreage increased 16 percent (Golbitz 1999, 362).

To America's international oil- and oilseed-producing competitors, this change in the law has looked suspiciously like a shift in government subsidies from other crops to soy. Moreover, the competitors are angry about U.S. government price supports for soy, protesting them at sessions of the World Trade Organization (Elliott 1999; Ash, Livezey, and Dohlman 2006, 26). These issues along with disagreements about whether and how to regulate global trade in genetically engineered products promise to keep soy at the center of international trade disputes for years to come.

Another controversial arena involving soy is the growing economic consolidation in farming, in agribusiness, and in food manufacturing (Ross 1980, 280–15; Ross 1987). Larger and larger and fewer and fewer farms now produce U.S. crops, including soy. Between 1950 and 1980 "the average size of [U.S.] farms grew from 87 to 182 hectares (215 to 450 acres), [and] the number of farms fell from 5.6 to 2.4 million" (Shideler 1993). Moreover, greater than 80 percent of U.S. crops are currently produced by only the largest five hundred thousand of these farms (at most) (Shideler 1993; Heffernan 1999b, 8).

This shift in the structure of agriculture is an offshoot of industrialization, since modern farming requires very costly equipment and economies of scale. The shift favors those with the capital to make such daunting investments: wealthy families and corporations, which purchase large tracts of farmland. Unless producing for a specialty niche market (such as organic soy or soy to be eaten in the pod as a green vegetable, also known as edamame), the small-scale farmer rarely can successfully compete in growing soy.

But even more consolidation among farmers has occurred in the crop-processing industries, so much so that the U.S. food system has been described as an hourglass, with farmers and consumers on either end and the narrowest part representing the processors (Heffernan 1999a; Hendrickson and Heffernan 2005). Consolidation among processors is well illustrated by the case of soy protein destined for human consumption. In 1950, there were at least twenty-four major manufacturers of edible soy protein, whereas by 1990 only five were left: ADM, Cargill, Central Soya, Protein Technology International (PTI), and the A. E. Staley Company (Johnson, Myers, and Burden 1992, 442). Since that time a notable addition has been the Solae company, a Dupont-Bunge alliance, that has taken on PTI's soy protein work. The resulting concentration in "the soy protein industry has followed and matched a similar trend in the principal industries that make up its client base. These include meat processing, nutritional supplements, baking, and food processing. The natural food products market has also increased significantly in scale" (LMC 1999, 3).

Indeed, the rate at which soy-processing companies are currently purchasing smaller firms, creating joint ventures, buying each other out, and combining with or selling off portions of their subsidiaries to other agribusiness enterprises (such as seed producers and distributors, manufacturers of herbicides and pesticides, and food manufacturers) is dizzying. In the past several years, Associated British Foods acquired Karlshamns, a midwestern soy-oil processor (Anonymous 1995); Dupont purchased Protein Technologies International (Kane 1999); Dupont and General Mills launched 8th Continent LLC, a joint venture producing a popular soymilk (Knox 2000); Cargill purchased Continental's grain marketing enterprises (Shean 1999); Michigan's organic food company, Eden Foods, joined with three Japanese companies to form American Soy Products, Inc. (Theodore 1999); Worthington Foods, a manufacturer of soy-based meat analogs, was purchased by cereal giant Kellogg (Kane 1999); and so on and on. As this tip-of-the-iceberg listing suggests, the restructuring is complex and has many international ramifications.

The end result of all this consolidation is that few Americans actually grow soy, and despite the many later steps needed to process, market, and export it, only a relatively small number of companies controls what happens to soy after it has left the field. Partly for this reason—belying soy's importance as a U.S. crop and ubiquitous presence in daily lives—most Americans know little about it. The average American's insight into the medical debates, biotechnological questions, pesticide and herbicide choices, environmental issues, and federal policies surrounding this product is limited. As consumers and in the voting booth, Americans can exercise choice about soy, but on many points they do not even know there is a choice to be made.

Intense awareness of these debates does exist among the big companies that process and sell soy and the advocacy groups that monitor them. Altercations between companies and advocacy groups and competition among the companies often lead to tremendous expenditures of effort to sway government policies (see Nestle 2002). One example is the struggle in recent years over the status of soymilk in USDA dietary guidelines. Some lobbyists contend that for the significant portion of the U.S. population who are lactose intolerant, soymilk should receive government endorsement as a valid source of calcium in lieu of dairy milk (Karlin 2000). The dairy industry has vigorously protested this argument. It has also petitioned the FDA to disallow soymilk containers from using the word "milk," pointing out that the nutritional profile of soymilk differs considerably from that of dairy milk (Skrzycki 2000; USDA 1999a). The dairy industry is clearly threatened by the still small but rapidly growing soymilk industry, especially by the relatively recent marketing of soymilk in refrigerated cartons in the dairy cases of major supermarkets. In fact, dairy companies felt threatened enough to buy out their competition: in 2002, dairy giant Dean Foods finalized the purchase of soymilk leader White Wave.

At the level of government policy, these arguments have resulted in compromise. In recent years the USDA has listed soymilk as a nutritional option without giving it the prominence that some wished for (USDA 2006b). The FDA, meanwhile, has continued to permit use of the word "milk" on soymilk containers.

Conclusion

To much of the dairy industry, then, soy is an unwanted competitor. To the larger food industry, soyfoods are a hot trend and a potential avenue to fresh profits. To farmers and policymakers in Washington, soy is a critical anchor in the agricultural economy. To biotechnology companies, soy in its genetically modified form is a herald of the future. To many medical researchers, it is an intriguing plant whose biochemical properties are only now beginning to be understood. To anthropologists of food, it is a rich topic through which to examine the interplay of ecological, political-economic, and cultural processes in the patterning of dietary preferences. This versatile "miracle bean" is undoubtedly the "ugly duckling" of U.S. agriculture (USDA 1993, 85) that grew into a powerful, contested, and startlingly valuable swan.

Notes

1. Many individuals assisted me during the research and writing of this essay; I am grateful to all. Special thanks go to Bill Hardin, Chris Novak, Laurence Buxbaum, Sidney Mintz, and above all to Theodore Hymowitz. In addition, Harriet Friedmann and Philip McMichael provided useful feedback on a very early version of this project. Any errors are, of course, entirely mine. The research was supported through grants from the Johns Hopkins University's Center for a Livable Future and the Salus Mundi Foundation.

2. By total value of wholesale production. The top crop is corn.

3. The case could even be made for coining a phrase: "the soy-farming-industrial complex" or, for short, "the soy-industrial complex."

4. I am indebted to Sidney Mintz for this insight.

5. For a spirited critique of functional foods, see Pollan (2008).

6. From a segment on soy diesel on National Public Radio's show *Morning Edition,* April 21, 2000.

7. Some trans fats can also be created by the repeated reuse of oil for deep-fat frying (Carter 2002).

8. Note that both of these new soybeans are genetically engineered to tolerate the herbicide Roundup. A soybean that has not been genetically engineered and that has a similarly non-trans fat profile is produced by the small Iowa Asoyia company, www.asoyia.com (Shelke 2005).

References

ADM (Archer, Daniels, Midland Company). n.d.a "The Magic Bean." Brochure. Decatur, IL: ADM.

———. n.d.b "Feeding the World and Feeding It Better." Decatur, IL: ADM.

Anonymous. 1916. "After More Soya Beans." *New York Times,* August 13, sec. 3, p. 3.

———. 1995. "A Radical Change. *Food Research & Development* 2(3): 22.

———. 2006a. "Harvesting Cash." Editorial. *Rocky Mountain News,* July 9, p. 5E.

———. 2006b. "Poultry Farming." *Encyclopedia Britannica.* http://www.eb.com/library/online/bol.html (available with subscription).

ASA (American Soybean Association). n.d. "ASA History Highlights." http://www.soygrowers.com/history/default.htm.

Ash, Mark, Janet Livezey, and Eric Dohlman. 2006. "Soybean Backgrounder." Outlook Report No. OCS-2006-1. Washington, DC: USDA. http://www.ers.usda.gov/publications/OCS/apr06/OCS200601/.

Barrionuevo, Alexei. 2005. "Kellogg Will Use New Soybean Oil to Cut Fat." *New York Times,* December 9, p. 3.

Berlan, Jean-Pierre. 1991. "Historical Roots of the Present Agricultural Crisis." In William Friedland, Lawrence Busch, Frederick Buttel, and Alan Rudy, eds., *Towards a New Political Economy of Agriculture,* 115–36. Boulder, CO: Westview.

Berlan, Jean-Pierre, Jean-Pierre Bertrand, and Laurence Lebas. 1999[1976]. "The Growth of the American 'Soybean Complex.'" *European Review of Agricultural Economics* 4(4): 395–416.

Borth, Christy. 1942. *Pioneers of Plenty: The Story of Chemurgy.* New York: Bobbs-Merrill.

Bowdidge, Elizabeth. 1935. *The Soya Bean.* Oxford: Oxford University.

Bryan, Ford R. 1990. *Beyond the Model T: The Other Ventures of Henry Ford.* Detroit: Wayne State University.

Burros, Marian. 2000. "Doubts Cloud Rosy News on Soy." *New York Times,* January 26, pp. F1, F11.

Carter, Janet L. Stein. 2002. "Lipids: Fats, Oils, Waxes, Etc." Batavia, OH: University of Cincinnati, Clermont College, Biology Department. http://biology.clc.uc.edu/courses/bio104/lipids.htm.

Du Bois, Christine M., and Sidney W. Mintz. 2003. "Soy." In Solomon W. Katz, ed., *Encyclopedia of Food and Culture,* 322–26. New York: Thomson/Gale.

Earley, Tom. 1995. "Domestic Soybean Oil Outlook." Alexandria, VA: PROMAR International.

Elliott, Ian. 1999. "U.S. Forced to Defend Soybean Subsidies before WTO." *Feedstuffs* 71: 4.

Fishman, Margie. 2000. "Meatless Entrees Go to the Prom." *Philadelphia Inquirer,* May 24, pp. B1, B2.

Forrestal, Dan. 1982. *Kernel and the Bean: The 75-Year Story of the Staley Company.* New York: Simon and Schuster.

Golbitz, Peter. 1998. *Tofu and Soyfoods Cookery.* Summertown, TN: Book Publishing Company.

———, ed. 1999. *Soya and Oilseed Bluebook 2000.* Bar Harbor, ME: Soyatech.

Grayson, Martin, ed. 1983. "Soybeans and Other Oilseeds." In *Kirk-Othmer Encyclopedia of Chemical Technology,* Vol. 21, 417–42. New York: Wiley.

Hapgood, Fred. 1987. "The Prodigious Soybean." *National Geographic* 172(1): 66–91.

Hayes, Keri. 1996. "Aquaculture Gets Hooked on Oilmeals." *Bluebook Update* 3(2): 4–5. Bar Harbor, ME: Soyatech.

Heffernan, William. 1999a. "Consolidation in the Food and Agriculture System." With Mary Hendrickson and Robert Gronski. Columbia: University of Missouri, Department of Rural Sociology. http://www.foodcircles.missouri.edu/consol.htm.

———. 1999b. "The Influence of the Big Three—ADM, Cargill, and ConAgra." Columbia: University of Missouri, Department of Rural Sociology. http://www.foodcircles.missouri.edu/consol.htm.

Hendrickson, Mary, and William Heffernan. 2005. "Concentration of Agricultural Markets." Columbia: University of Missouri, Department of Rural Sociology. http://www.foodcircles.missouri.edu/consol.htm.

Hesseltine, C. W. 1983. "The Future of Fermented Foods." *Nutrition Reviews* 41(10): 293–301.

Hymowitz, Theodore. 1984. "Dorsett-Morse Soybean Collection Trip to East Asia." *Economic Botany* 38(4): 378–88.

———. 1987. "Introduction of the Soybean to Illinois." *Economic Botany* 41(1): 28–32.

———. 1990. "Soybeans: The Success Story." In Jules Janick and James Simon, eds., *Soybeans: The Success Story, Advances in New Crops,* 159–63. Portland, OR: Timber Press.

Hymowitz, Theodore, and J. R. Harlan. 1983. "Introduction of Soybean to North America by Samuel Bowen in 1765." *Economic Botany* 39(4): 371–79.

Jenkins, Edward. 1975. "Percy L. Julian, Soybean Chemist." In Edward Jenkins, ed., *American Black Scientists and Inventors,* 27–36. Washington, DC: National Science Teachers' Association.

Johnson, L. A., D. J. Myers, and D. J. Burden. 1992. "Soy Protein's History, Prospects in Food, Feed." *International News on Fats, Oils, and Related Materials* 3(4): 429–44.

Johnson, Paul. 1978. *Farm Power in the Making of America.* Des Moines: Wallace-Homestead.

Kahn, E. J., Jr. 1991. *The Story of Dwayne Andreas, CEO of Archer Daniels Midland, Supermarketer to the World.* New York: Time Warner.

Kane, Janice. 1999. "Chemical Companies Fortify with Soy." *Chemical Market Reporter* 256: 14.

Karlin, Rick. 2000. "Soy Industry Targets Students with Government-Funded Nutrition Guides." *Times Union,* February 22.

Keen, Russ. 2000. "Federal Disaster Payments to Oilseed Growers Begin in Aberdeen, S.D." *Aberdeen American News,* February 28.

Knox, Andrea. 2000. "DuPont, General Mills Sign Deal to Develop, Sell Soy-Based Foods." *Philadelphia Inquirer,* January 14.

Lappé, Frances Moore. 1971. *Diet for a Small Planet.* New York: Ballantine.

Lee, Steven. 1999. "Pair of Texans Steers U.S. Agriculture Policy." *Dallas Morning News,* May 15.

Liu, KeShun. 1997. "Agronomic Characteristics, Production, and Marketing." In Ke-Shun Liu, ed., *Soybeans: Chemistry, Technology, and Utilization,* 1–24. New York: Chapman & Hall.

LMC International. 1999. "Soy Protein Market Analysis." New York: LMC International.

Lueck, Thomas J. 2006. "City Plans to Place Sharp Limits on Restaurants' Use of Trans Fats." *New York Times,* September 27, p. A1, B4.

Messina, Mark, Virginia Messina, and Ken Setchell. 1994. *The Simple Soybean and Your Health.* Garden City Park, NY: Avery.

Mindell, Earl. 1995. *Earl Mindell's Soy Miracle.* New York: Simon & Schuster.

Mounts, T. L., W. J. Wolf, and W. H. Martinez. 1987. "Processing and Utilization." In *Soybeans: Improvement, Production, and Uses.* Agronomy Monograph No. 16. Madison, WI: Agronomy Society of America.

National Biodiesel Board. 2005. "Biodiesel Backgrounder." http://www.biodiesel.org/resources/fuelfactsheets/.

Nestle, Marion. 2002. *Food Politics.* Berkeley: University of California Press.

Nevins, Allan, and Frank Hill. 1954. *Expansion and Challenge: 1915–1933,* Vol. 2. Ford Series. New York: Scribner.

Pimentel, David, O. Bailey, P. Kim, E. Mullaney, J. Calabrese, L. Walman, F. Nelson, and X. Yao. 1999. "Will Limits of the Earth's Resources Control Human Numbers?" Ithaca, NY: College of Agriculture and Life Sciences, Cornell University.

Pitchford, Paul. 1993. *Healing with Whole Foods: Oriental Traditions and Modern Nutrition.* Berkeley: North Atlantic.

Pollan, Michael. 2008. *In Defense of Food: An Eater's Manifesto.* New York: Penguin.

Powell, Lanny. 1971. "An Examination of Factors Influencing the Temporal-Spatial Diffusion of Soybean Production in Illinois, 1930–1968." Unpublished PhD dissertation, University of Illinois, Urbana-Champaign.

PROMAR International. 2000. "Soybean Product Segment Review: Outlook to 2004/05." Alexandria, VA: PROMAR International.

Rackis, J. J., D. J. Sessa, and D. H. Honig. 1979. "Flavor Problems of Vegetable Food Proteins." *Journal of the American Oil Chemists' Society* 56: 262–71.

Ross, Eric B. 1980. "Patterns of Diet and Forces of Production: An Economic and Ecological History of the Ascendancy of Beef in the United States Diet." In Eric B. Ross, ed., *Beyond the Myths of Culture: Essays in Cultural Materialism,* 181–225. New York: Academic Press.

———. 1987. "An Overview of Trends in Dietary Variation from Hunter-Gatherer to Modern Capitalist Societies." In Marvin Harris and Eric B. Ross, eds., *Food and*

Evolution: Toward a Theory of Human Food Habits, 7–55. Philadelphia: Temple University Press.

Sabatini, Patricia. 2000. "Heinz to Create Nutritional Unit to Capitalize on Sector's Growth." *Pittsburgh Post-Gazette,* February 24.

Sacks, Frank M., Alice Lichtenstein, Linda Van Horn, William Harris, Penny Kris-Etherton, and Mary Winston. 2006. "Soy Protein, Isoflavones, and Cardiovascular Health: An American Heart Association Science Advisory for Professionals from the Nutrition Committee." *Circulation,* February 21. Advanced Internet release in January 2006. http://circ.ahajournals.org/cgi/content/full/113/7/1034?maxtoshow=&HITS=10&hits=10&RESULTFORMAT=&fulltext=Soy+Protein%2C+Isoflavones%2C+and+Cardiovascular+Health&searchid=1&FIRSTINDEX=0&resourcetype=HWCIT.

Schaible, Philip J. 1970. *Poultry: Feeds and Nutrition.* Westport, CT: Avi.

Shean, Tom. 1999. "Government Restricts Commodities Trader from Buying Rival's Grain." *Virginian-Pilot,* July 15.

Shelke, Kantha. 2005. "Fear and Loathing over Trans Fats." http://www.foodprocessing.com/articles/2005/399.html.

Shideler, James. 1993. "Farms and Farming." In *Grolier Multimedia Encyclopedia.* CD-ROM, Release 6.

Shurtleff, William, and Akiko Aoyagi. 1975. *The Book of Tofu.* Berkeley: Ten Speed.

———. 2004a. "A. E. Staley Manufacturing Company (1922–1980s): Work With Soy." http://www.soyinfocenter.com/HSS/ae_staley_manufacturing.php.

———. 2004b. "Central Soya Company (1934–): Work with Soy." http://www.soyinfocenter.com/HSS/central_soya.php.

———. 2007a. "History of Soybean Crushing: Soy Oil and Soybean Meal." http://www.soyinfocenter.com/HSS/soybean_crushing1.php.

———. 2007b. "History of World Soybean Production and Trade." http://www.soyinfocenter.com/HSS/production_and_trade1.php.

Sigler, Josie. 2000. "Controversy over Soy and Health Builds." *Bluebook Update* 7(3): 4–5. Bar Habor, ME: Soyatech.

Skees, Jerry. 1999. "Agricultural Risk Management or Income Enhancement?" *Regulation* 22(1): 35–43. Washington, DC: Cato Institute.

Skrzycki, Cindy. 2000. "Dairy Group Has a Cow over 'Milk' That Doesn't." *Washington Post,* February 29, p. A1.

Smith, Allan, and Sidney Circle. 1972. *Soybeans: Chemistry and Technology,* Vol. 1, *Proteins.* Westport, CT: Avi.

Soyfoods Association of North America. 2006. "Sales and Trends." http://www.soyfoods.org/sales/sales.html.

Stahler, Charles. 2005. "How Many Youth Are Vegetarian?" *Vegetarian Journal* 4. http://www.vrg.org/journal/vj2005issue4/vj2005issue4youth.htm.

Theodore, Sarah. 1999. "Plant Expansion Fills Growing Product Niche." *Beverage Industry,* May, p. 32.

U.S. Census Bureau. 2006. "Fats and Oils: Production, Consumption, and Stocks 2005." M311-K(05)-13. June. http://www.census.gov/cir/www/311/m311k.html.

USDA (United States Department of Agriculture). 1937. *Yearbook of Agriculture.* Washington, DC: USDA.

———. 1945. "Final Report of the War Food Administrator." Washington, DC: USDA.

———. 1951. *Yearbook of Agriculture.* Washington, DC: USDA.

———. 1966. *U.S. Fats and Oils Statistics, 1909–1965.* Statistical Bulletin No. 376. Washington, DC: USDA.

———. 1975. *Yearbook of Agriculture.* Washington, DC: USDA.

———. 1993. *Always Something New: A Cavalcade of Scientific Discovery.* Miscellaneous Publication No. 1507. Washington, DC: USDA.

———. 1999a. "USDA Nutrient Database for Standard Reference, Release 13." www.nal.usda.gov/fnic.

———. 1999b. *Oil Crops Situation and Outlook.* Washington, DC: USDA.

———. 2005. "Briefing Room—Soybeans and Oil Crops." http://www.ers.usda.gov/Briefing/SoybeansOilCrops/.

———. 2006a. "U.S. and All States Data—Soybeans." http://www.nass.usda.gov:8080/QuickStats/.

———. 2006b. "Inside the Pyramid: Milk." http://www.mypyramid.gov/pyramid/milk.html.

———. 2006c. "U.S. Agricultural Trade Update." FAU-117. Washington, DC: USDA. http://usda.mannlib.cornell.edu/usda/ers/FAU/2000s/2006/FAU-09-13-2006.pdf.

———. 2008. "Oilseeds: World Market and Trade." Foreign Agricultural Service Circular Series FOP 1-08.

———. n.d. "Soybeans—Planted and Harvested Area, Yield and Production" 1924–97." Crops Production Data by States. http://usda.mannlib.cornell.edu/data-sets/crops/95111/.

Walsh, Robert. 1947. *Fats and Oils in World War II.* Washington, DC: USDA.

Whitton, Carol. 2004. "Processed Agricultural Exports Led Gains in U.S. Agricultural Exports between 1976 and 2002." FAU-85-01. Washington, DC: USDA. http://usda.mannlib.cornell.edu/reports/erssor/trade/fau-bb/text/2004/fau8501.pdf.

Wik, Reynold. 1972. *Henry Ford and Grass-Roots America.* Ann Arbor: University of Michigan.

Windish, Leo. 1981. *The Soybean Pioneers: Trailblazers, Crusaders, Missionaries.* Henry, IL: M & D Printing.

Wolf, Walter. 1973. "Processing Soybean into Protein Products." *Bulletin—Association of Operative Millers.* No. 3479.

Wright, Rebecca. 2005. "The Soy Slowdown." *Nutraceuticals World,* April.

Yates, Ronald. 1998. *The Kikkoman Chronicles: A Global Company with a Japanese Soul.* New York: McGraw-Hill.

12

Soybeans and Soyfoods in Brazil, with Notes on Argentina

Sketch of an Expanding World Commodity

IVAN SERGIO FREIRE DE SOUSA AND
RITA DE CÁSSIA MILAGRES TEIXEIRA VIEIRA

Introduction

In Latin America, the direct presence of soybeans in human nutrition is a recent development with uncharted growth ahead.[1] This growth, however, will probably not parallel their history in Asian cuisine. Ongoing changes in food technology alongside the creativity of local chefs will eventually bring the soybean into the Brazilian diet. Fortunately, technological advances, such as improvements in the product's taste and odor, have eliminated some of the soybean's less desirable qualities.

Thanks to its high protein content and to animal husbandry research in the United States and Europe, the soybean plays a role in Latin America today as a basic component of animal nutrition. Its insertion into the system of meat production has been clearest in Brazil and Argentina.

All kinds of interests (economic, political, social, and scientific) combine and interweave powerful global networks[2] of transformation and development where soybeans are concerned. The beans have generally been sold in three main forms: as whole soybeans, as soy meal,[3] and as soy oil. Derived from those original forms, there are now a multitude of products for humans, for animals, and for many industries (e.g., pharmaceuticals).

The soy network is tightly enmeshed with other strong networks such as those dealing with poultry, swine, cattle, and animal feed. The soybean, then, is not merely a cash crop but instead brings to Latin American agribusiness a new and powerful motor of change. In Brazil, agriculture found in the soybean a powerful force for the dissemination of inputs, machines, silos, and processing units. The crop is always associated with the use of research-generated technologies and agricultural expansion; its presence supports whole regions of the countryside.

Soy also plays a crucial role in the internal Brazilian food supply. Derivatives such as oil and other components for processed foods have extraordinary importance in the daily diet of the population of all classes.

In the 2003–2004 harvest, Brazil and Argentina together contributed about 47 percent of total world soybean production. The combined production of these countries surpassed production in the United States, the current global leader. The three countries produce 81 percent of the world's soybeans (USDA/FAS 2004).

North America's share of soybean production has recently declined due to increasing competition from Brazil and Argentina. Brazilian soybean production grew from 1.5 million metric tons in 1970 to 51 million metric tons in 2005, with an expected 52.4 million metric tons in 2006. In Argentina soybean production may have leveled off, with 38.3 million metric tons produced in the 2004–2005 harvest (Brazil 2004; SAGPyA 2006; IBGE 2006).

Factors such as the strength of the dollar relative to South American currencies as well as North American price support programs (which indirectly raise the price of land) have been limiting somewhat the competitiveness of the North American product. The expansion of soy agriculture in South America has also been spurred by favorable conditions in external markets, adaptation and generation of varieties, other agronomic research, increases in crushing capacity, rapid growth of the poultry sector, agricultural policy incentives, and technical support for farmers.

Evolution of Soybean Production in Brazil and Argentina

Until the mid-1960s, soybeans did not figure among the main crops of Brazil and Argentina. In the late 1960s and early 1970s, however, soybean production experienced extraordinary growth, altering its relative importance on the national and international scenes (Soskin 1988; Warnken 1999).

In the early 1960s the main motive for soybean production was to obtain vegetable oil, not protein meal. In the latter part of that decade, Brazil's increasing need for foreign exchange earnings prompted the government to encourage meal export. Domestic soybean processing was greatly stimulated. At the same time, soy oil began to be a more important consumer item.

Expansion was further stimulated by President Richard Nixon's decision in 1973 to restrict soy exports from the United States. This greatly upset the Japanese, who were quite dependent on U.S. soybeans and therefore turned to Brazil for soy. This event propelled Brazilian soy production to the world stage. In 1974 with Japanese financial support, a program was launched to transform Brazilian savannahs into areas suitable for a dynamic agriculture. The program known as PRODECER (short for Japanese-Brazilian Cooperation Program for Cerrado Development) began concrete actions in 1978. The pilot project was financed by the Japan International Cooperation Agency with monetary resources managed by Japan's Long Term Credit Bank. The later expansion project was funded by Japan's Overseas Economic Cooperation Fund.

Warnken (1999) has pointed out six key Brazilian policy objectives tied to soybean agriculture: saving foreign exchange, increasing foreign exchange earnings, improving the national diet, stimulating industrial development, holding down food price increases, and territorial occupation. These motivations led to such a rapid rise in production and crushing of soybeans during the 1970s that Brazil became the world's top exporter of soy meal, although the country has recently been supplanted by Argentina. While the emergence of soy production in Argentina followed Brazil's by about a decade, Argentina is now the world's largest exporter of oil and meal, with Brazil ranked second (USDA/FAS 2005c). The bulk of Brazilian soy oil is consumed internally.

In Brazil, the expansion of soybean production has occurred most notably in the southern and west-central regions. During the 1960s, soybean production was mainly located in the northern part of Rio Grande do Sul and in the state of Paraná. These southern lands lie principally within the same humid, warm semitropical latitudes as the northern portions of Argentina's agricultural region. Brazil's southern region has been for decades among the world's most productive agricultural zones.

In 1980 under a variety of government incentives, agriculture expanded into the *cerrado* (savannah) lands of Brazil's interior states. Today, the central-western region rivals the south as the main area of agricultural production within Brazil. The region lies entirely within South America's sprawling tropical zone. As a result, Brazil has had to develop crop varieties adapted to the lower variability of day length and to temperatures associated with tropical agriculture (figure 9).

By 2002, the traditional soybean-producing areas remained important, but less significant than before, as the central-western state of Mato Grosso

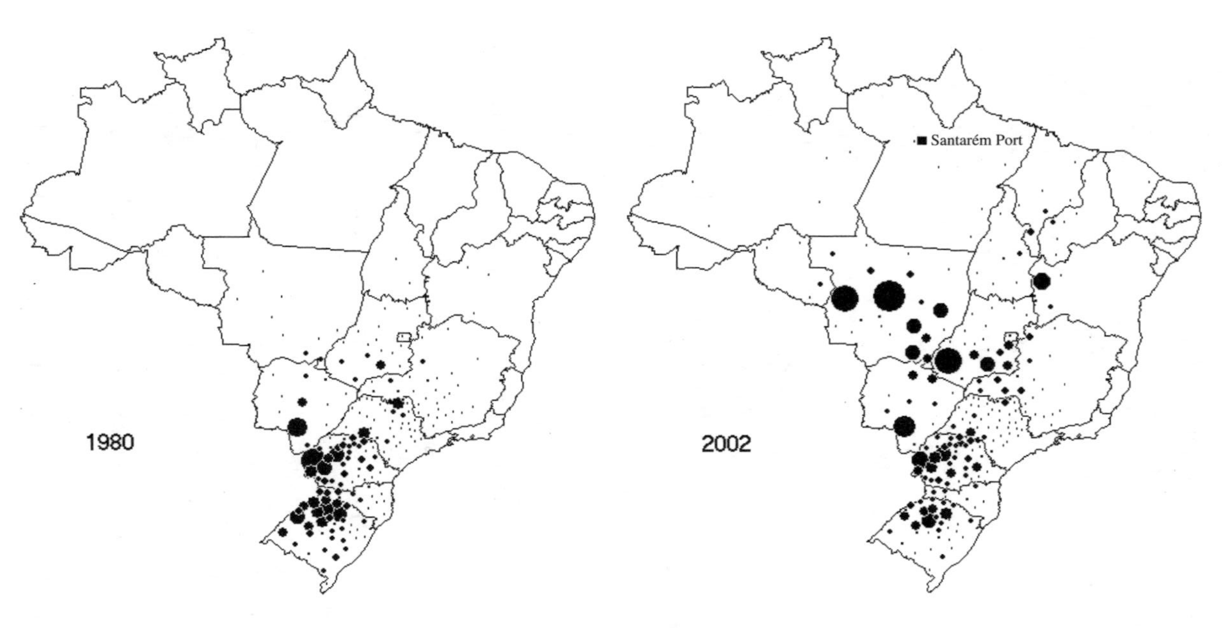

Figure 9. Geographical changes in Brazilian soybean production over time. (Data from IBGE [1980, 2002]. Figure was constructed by the authors.)

surpassed them in production. Increased production in the central-eastern states of Minas Gerais and Bahia is also noteworthy. In the 2003–2004 harvest, the central-western region contributed 49 percent to national soybean production, while the contribution of the south was 33 percent. The central-western area also presents the highest average yields in Brazil and is the area where the most spectacular growth in soy agriculture is occurring. In fact, Brazil's *cerrado* lands are the area of the globe most conducive to the expansion of soy agriculture. There are still about 66 million hectares of *cerrado* lands that could be converted to farmland, and soybeans are particularly suited to the agroecological and economic conditions of the area.

Brazil has the technical potential to increase its soybean production nearly tenfold. This will not occur without opposition, however (Ratter, Ribeiro, and Bridgewater 1997; Stedman-Edwards 1999). Some studies emphasize the environmental consequences of soybean expansion. The Brazilian savannahs are apparently the most species-diverse in the world (Fearnside 2001; Myers et al. 2000; Klink, Moreira, Solbrig 1993). Because soy is a basic export commodity with a strong economic network, its cultivation could lead to the destruction of natural habitats over wide areas.

Soybean cultivation could also entail significant social costs. Even in regions where soybeans generate visible economic benefits, factors conducive to inequality should be noted. In some places big firms dominate the soybean business, transferring inputs to producers and receiving the product back during harvest. Profits are concentrated in a relatively small number of hands. There is also excessive vertical integration of production, that is, a multiplicity of economic functions relating to soybeans (growing, transporting, processing, exporting) all controlled by the same firm.

In Argentina, nearly all field crop production occurs in the central and northern divisions of the eastern third of the country. This rich agricultural zone is centered on the fertile pampas—an area of slightly more than fifty million hectares—but extends into Argentina's northern tier of warm, semitropical provinces. The central provinces of Buenos Aires, Cordoba, Santa Fe, and western Entre Rios, located in the heart of the pampas, dominate row-crop production. More than 90 percent of Argentina's soybean farming takes place in these provinces.

Underlying Technical and Economic Reasons for the Expansion

Both Argentina and Brazil have made the most of cultivars produced and adapted in the United States. Because the soybean originated in East Asian regions situated between 40° and 50° latitude, the plant had to be modified by selective breeding in order to succeed as a crop in the United States (Sousa and Busch 1998; Warnken 1999, 46–52). Scientists of both the public and private sectors in the United States effected the needed modification. Much of their technology later set the pattern of development for scientific institutions and soybean farms in Argentina and Brazil.

Further technological advances were a more important challenge for Brazil than for Argentina. Unlike Argentina, most of Brazil's lands lie in the tropics, yet the major American cultivars imported into Brazil were bred for latitudes between 30° and 35°. The traditional or prototypic soybean plant inherently required long days to flourish properly, a function of its photoperiodism. The short days of tropical regions would induce precocious flowering, leading to low yields. But from 1980 on, Brazilian researchers developed soybean cultivars that were less and less dependent on latitude (Hartwig and Kiihl 1979; Kiihl and Garcia 1988), making soybean production possible across Brazil and in other low-latitude regions.

However, other limiting factors existed in Brazil. In addition to constraints stemming from their high photoperiodic sensitivity, soybeans were limited by aluminum toxicity in *cerrado* soils, low soil fertility in certain new lands, and the low capacity of some soils for retaining water (Souza and Goedert 1987). Technical solutions were found for each of these difficulties (Hartwig and Kiihl 1979; Kiihl and Garcia 1988; Döbereiner 1992; Souza and Goedert 1987).

The new agriculture in the *cerrado* is thus a product of modern mechanical, chemical, and biological technologies: the mechanical opens up the land, the chemical allows for correction of the soil, and the biological produces specific genetic material for local agroecological conditions. Production was also enhanced because the farmers came from parts of Brazil, such as Rio Grande do Sul, that already knew modern capitalist agriculture. Other factors including the availability of natural resources, conservationist practices such as no-till farming, and the existence of efficient financing, processing, and trading entrepreneurs were also important for soybean expansion in Brazil. The increase of installed processing capacity and the development of new export corridors through intermodal transport systems also played a role in the shifting of production areas.

New factors stimulating production include the reaction of European consumers to the risks of Bovine Spongiform Encephalopathy (BSE, or Mad Cow Disease), which forced greater use of plants in the composition of animal feed. At the same time, increasing consumer incomes within

Brazil have stimulated production. The income elasticity of demand for meat is high. That is, as consumer incomes increase so does the demand for meat, and those animals are frequently raised on soybeans. The market is also expanding due to economic growth in Asia, which has led Asians to increase their direct importing of both meal and meats.

Like Brazil, Argentina showed spectacular performance in agricultural production during the 1990s. During that decade, the production of major field crops nearly doubled. This performance was due to large-scale structural changes in Argentina's economy as well as in sectoral policies. Agriculture experienced the reduction of state interventionism, which in turn led to a friendly environment for private investments, targeted to increase the sector's competitiveness. Major changes have included removal of taxes on exports in 1991, reduction of tariffs and removal of import quotas for agricultural inputs, the breaking of the government's monopoly on commodity exports, privatization of the storage and transportation systems, enlargement and modernization of the industrial sector, the use of easy-to-farm genetically modified organisms (GMOs), and overall stabilization of the economy (Pessoa 2002).

But the great agricultural transformations in South America cannot be explained solely within national contexts. Soybeans demonstrate the internationalism of the process. In the first place, the soybean seed itself came from abroad, as did much of the initial technology surrounding it. In addition, there are Brazilian farmers producing soybeans in Paraguay (the *brasiguaios*), Brazilian-bred seeds being used in Bolivia, and North American farmers growing soybeans in places as unexpected as Barreiras and Luis Eduardo Magalhães in Bahia (in 2004, there were approximately 350 North American farmers producing soybeans in Brazil). The major soybean processors are multinational conglomerates, and the bulk of soybean demand comes from abroad.

Classification and Standardization

Soybeans provide a clear example of local production for the global consumer market. But soybeans differ from other Latin American export crops such as sugar and coffee. Unlike these far older agricultural products, soybeans arrived in Latin America as an already-modern crop. Built into the soy seeds came the necessity for more specific technological packages and standardization of production to satisfy both producer and consumer demands. Soybeans thus helped to fortify Brazilian and Argentine agribusiness and facilitated the integration of rural and urban interests.

Virtually all industrialized food contains soybean-derived components: oil, protein, stabilizers, and so on. In part for this reason, both governmental and private organizations strongly regulate soy production in the fields as well as the industrial processing of the beans and the further use of soy protein for feed and food. Two important instruments that make production in the field compatible with industrial processing are classification and standardization. Categories are created (for instance, soybean meal type 1, soybean meal type 2, and so on) based on standards.

Standards shape and define both physical objects and social structures, reflecting the outcomes of political processes of negotiation, persuasion, and coercion. Standards thereby embody fundamental ethical decisions and worldviews (Busch 2000; Bowker and Star 2000). The standardization of things moreover implies the standardization of persons. What is considered a good soybean plantation, following the rules and standards, similarly defines a good soybean farmer. Good soy meal is linked to good whole soybeans, to a good processing unit, and to a good processor. Such value judgments facilitate network formation and in capitalist countries the power of capital to establish and expand itself. Yet standardization can also serve consumer interests. Food safety crises (see, for instance, Juska, Gouveia, and Koneck 2000) have increased popular awareness of food risks, leading to an increased strategic use of agrifood standards.

Historically, the central issue in standardization has been the tension between the state and the market in the determination of classifications and standards; soybeans brought added complexity. This state-market dichotomy has gradually been superseded by the entry of other agents, for the expansion of Brazilian soybean production coincided with the rising influence of other organizations. The most important of these new agents are the standards organizations. In addition to the governmental standards organizations, private ones emerged nationally as well. Internationally, other standards organizations were formed, including the International Organization for Standardization, the World Trade Organization, the Codex Alimentarius Commission, and entities such as Mercosul (the South American common market).

Brazil did not develop a comprehensive legal instrument for the standardization, classification, and commercialization of soybeans until 1983 (Regulation 262 of the Ministry of Agriculture). But this laggardness did not hold back Brazil's export of soybeans. Norms and international patterns guided this trade from the first and determined the shape of domestic production. State standardization was always a step behind what was common practice in the international domain. Thus, Regulation 262 simply provided a domestic legal footing for inspections based on the presence or absence of undesirable qualities: excess humidity, broken beans, impurities or foreign materials, damaged beans, and unripe beans.

Regulations have also established an operational sequence to be followed in order to determine the classification of an analyzed sample (for a history of these regulations, see Sousa 2001). This happens at the time the soybean enters the processing unit. Further official norms—of identity, quality, packaging, labeling, and presentation of oil and meal—came into existence in 1993.

Modern standardization is not only present in the functioning of markets and the wording of contracts (see Krislov 1997); it also invades the private space of individuals. For this reason, among others, it does not occur without the resistance of traditional standardization. Traditional standards of taste and seasoning, for example, are historically and informally constructed and can serve as a locus of resistance to modernizing processes.

Factors connected to resistance against technological standardization are numerous: physical, chemical, economic, social, cultural, climatic, and others. Note that among those factors are elements of the so-called natural world (see Latour 1993). Soil and climate, for instance, can influence the appearance, smell, and taste of a specific agricultural product. When technology intervenes in this process (e.g., by altering soils and plant varieties), it can change not only the appearance but also the taste and odor of that product. In such a context, the previous appearance, odor, and taste can be called a traditional standard. Concealed within traditional standards are the sensory attributes of identity, important indices of belonging to some particular culture and society. Such standards are mediated by sociality, and they are not easily changed.

Manioc, corn, rice, and common beans are examples of crops with strong ties to the fundamentals of Brazilian culture and history (Ferreira, Sousa, and del Villar 2004). Largely because of such ties, Brazilians have often resisted change in how these crops are produced, sold, and consumed with regard to taste, color, smell, texture, and so on. By contrast, soybean standards in Latin America are more linked to new technologies than to tradition. Soybeans arrived in Latin America already standardized, mediated not by sociality but by money.[4] Moreover, in Brazil and Argentina the soybean commodity system mostly has its origins in the global capitalist system, which is heavily supported by science and technology. In other words, until recently the soybean was merely pasted onto Brazilian culture, taste, attachments, nutrition, and history.

By contrast with soybeans, the commercialization process of other products such as rice does not happen with the same intensity or ease, even though rice is consumed worldwide. The appearance and flavor of rice, especially after cooking, vary as functions of the physical and chemical traits of the grain, which in turn depend on the variety. These peculiarities do not turn up in soybeans with this intensity; when they do, they are less commercially important than is the case with rice (since most soy is fed to animals). Hence, soybeans have more easily become a standardized, global commodity.

Soybean Competitiveness in Brazil and Argentina

Both Brazil and Argentina show great competitiveness in soybean production. In particular, Brazil's west-central region has low production costs, partly due to the cheapness of land there. Yet Brazil does struggle to maintain soy competitiveness. The main difficulties arise from the lack of an efficient infrastructure (enough highways, railroads, ports, and warehouses). In Brazil, the average distance from the soy-processing units to the closest port is between 900 and 1,000 kilometers, while in Argentina the processing region is closer to the shipment zones, in a 250- to 300-kilometer radius. The transport costs are a burden to Brazilian exports. Each transported ton of Brazilian soybean registers a US$12 disadvantage compared to U.S. soybeans and a US$4 disadvantage when compared to Argentine soy (Espírito Santo 2001). These expenses reduce the competitive advantage that low production costs provide to Brazil.

In the United States, the distances are similar to those of Brazil. However, about 60 percent of North American soybeans are transported on waterways, which are much cheaper to operate than road transportation. By contrast, as late as 2001 about 67 percent of the Brazilian soy was transported via the highway system and only 5 percent via waterways (Espírito Santo 2001).

But the logistics of Brazil's agricultural transportation are changing, albeit slowly (Caixeta-Filho and Gameiro 2001). A series of government and private initiatives is beginning to reduce transport costs. According to Espírito Santo (2001), railroad transportation volumes increased 144 percent from 1997 to 2001 versus only a 77 percent increase over the highway system. In addition, in 2003 soybean transport through the Amazon and Madeira rivers took 1 million tons of soybeans away from the highway system. Another 1.5 million tons that would otherwise have occupied fifty-five thousand trucks were transported from Mato Grosso to the Atlantic port of Santos through the Ferronorte railroad. Moreover, in that same year the Tietê-Parapanema waterway transported 1.5 million tons of soybeans from the southwest of Goiás and the Triângulo Mineiro area to São Paulo (Loureiro and Cade 2003). Recently, a port was constructed in Santarém, a town on the Amazon River in the state of Pará, to deal exclusively with field crops. The port was built by Cargill, a private transnational enterprise, and is expected to handle around 800,000 tons of soybean exports this year:

> It has been reported that the governments of Mato Grosso and Rondônia are actively seeking federal funds to improve the main highway (BR-364) linking the soybean production regions of western Mato Grosso and southern Rondônia to the barge facility at Porto Velho on the Madeira River. Barge facilities are maintained by both Grupo Maggi [now Amaggi] and Cargill here, with roughly 1.7 million tons of soybeans transshipped to their respective floating ports at Itacoatiara and Santarém in 2002/03. With the completion of paving the other primary Amazonian artery, BR-163, in the next [few] years, Cargill estimates 2–3 million tons of soybeans will be transported to its port facility at Santarém from Mato Grosso (Shean 2004).

The costs of transportation through Santarém are approximately US$30 cheaper per metric ton of soybeans than the costs through southerly Atlantic ports such as Santos and Paranaguá. The lower costs are due primarily to geography, as the port in Santarém is closer to soybean-producing areas in the northern states as well as to ports in Europe and, because of the Panama Canal, even to ports in Asia.

The competitive advantages that this transportation system will offer should be taken into account, but so too should the system's potential for environmental harm. Improving roads almost inevitably leads to habitat destruction, and intensive use of waterways can lead to pollution and the destruction of wildlife.

Society must also try to ensure that the existence of the port at Santarém does not encourage large-scale soybean production in the Amazon. It is estimated that within a radius of two hundred kilometers from the port, approximately one million hectares of land can be used for agricultural purposes. According to Shean (2004), "This land is primarily pasture or small-scale permanent agricultural fields. With appropriate fertility, technology, and management the soybean crop yield potential in this region is estimated to be 3.6 tons per hectare, while the production capacity could reach between 5–7 million tons." Although the government is not providing direct financial incentives for soy expansion in this region, private investors are interested in its potential profitability.

But modernization of agriculture in the Amazon could cause environmental and social problems. Soybeans are different from the livestock already in the area in their capacity to stimulate the local economies. In livestock areas demand for services and products is low, whereas in soybean areas demand is high for cooperatives, mechanical services, banks, medical services, and so on. Changes in the economy and population of the region—an area with little previous contact with the modern world—could be abrupt. They could, for example, change local eating habits that are currently based on regional products. Local diets could become less nutritious. Hence, despite the port's huge economic potential, caution is needed in developing it further.

In addition, vigilance is needed to protect virgin Amazonian jungle. Unfortunately, not only Amazonian pasture lands and small farms may be affected by the soybean boom: there are already reports that virgin forest south of Santarém is being cleared for soy production (Hall 2004a) and that the rate of deforestation for crop land correlates with the yearly average price of soybeans (Harder 2006). In late 2004, Brazil enacted a law to protect a small portion of the jungle from illegal squatters who were forcibly evicting residents for the purpose of growing soy (Hall 2004a, 2004b). Also helpful was the August 2006 pledge by all of the major soy processors in Brazil—Cargill, Archer Daniels Midland (ADM), Bunge, Dreyfus, and Amaggi—to refuse to buy soybeans from newly deforested lands (Muello 2006). The effectiveness of the 2004 law and the 2006 corporate pledge depends on government actions and resources, however, and is questionable. More extensive studies of this complex issue are necessary to grasp all the environmental, political, economic, and social variables within a global context of conflicting interests.

By contrast with Brazil, in Argentina soy industries invested in new processing units—at the level of about US$1 billion from 1997 to 2001 (Espírito Santo 2001)—rather than so heavily in transportation. In consequence, Argentina's modern units have twice the crushing capacity and earn US$3 per ton more than Brazil's units. This Argentine advantage should change as investments in Brazilian processing grow, however. The same international agricultural companies that operate in Argentina also operate in Brazil and can transfer useful insights and business models from country to country as conditions warrant. In addition, dynamic companies such as El Tejar in Argentina and Amaggi in Brazil have shown the importance of large grower and grower-processor soy companies that are privately owned by a country's own citizens.

Nevertheless, despite the positive future outlook for soy industries in Brazil, the fiscal difficulties present there should be emphasized. The industries are burdened by a 12 percent interstate transport tax (ICMS, or Services and Commodity Circulation Tax). Fortunately, since September 1996 the Kandir Law has exempted from the tax whole and semiprocessed soybeans destined for export. This law has, of course, spurred Brazil's soy exports. Unfortunately, at the same time the cost of whole soybeans to Brazil's internal processing industry increased as the international price rose.

We have seen that Brazil's soybean industries benefit from cheap and plentiful land but suffer from internal transportation problems and, for internally consumed soy, from significant taxation. Argentina's soy industries enjoy a modern processing system and less arduous internal transportation, but they suffer from Argentina's distance from ultimate ports of destination. Each of these countries has thus benefited from certain aspects of competitive advantage.

Soyfoods in Brazil

The crushing of soybeans yields 70 percent protein meal and 20 percent edible oil. No other oilseed has such a valuable performance when oil and meal are jointly analyzed. The soybean represents more than 60 percent and 30 percent, respectively, of world production of protein meal and vegetable oil (Bonato, Bertagnolli, Lange, and Rubin 1999).

In contemporary Brazil, about 90 percent of consumed oil comes from soybeans. First, during the 1950s and early 1960s, vegetable oils—mostly cotton and peanut—began replacing animal fat in the Brazilian diet. Later, soy oil not only replaced the cotton and peanut oils but also eliminated the use of animal fat almost entirely. Whereas in 1960 soy oil represented only 14 percent of the vegetable oil market, by 1974 it had captured 80 percent.

The 1980s were marked by serious economic challenges, and although soy oil consumption was still rising, the rate of increase had dropped. It was only in 1994 that economic conditions started to improve. Since 2000, soy oil consumption has seen an average annual growth of 2.23 percent (USDA/FAS 2005b).

The substitution of soy oil for animal fat was encouraged by competitive pricing and by increased consumer attention to nutrition. Before the soybean era, no vegetable oil had really been able to overcome the supremacy of animal fat in the Brazilian kitchen. Yet now about three-fourths of the soy oil that Brazil consumes is used as cooking oil in the kitchen; the remaining fourth is used mostly in margarine, mayonnaise, and other foods.

Beyond this crop's oil, the other nutritional values are unquestionable. Soy flour contains approximately 47 percent protein, wheat flour is only around 13 percent protein, and corn meal about 8 percent protein (Miyasaka and Medina 1981). However, soy protein has mostly been used for animal feed. In other words, humans eat soy protein indirectly by eating animal protein. Thus, although soy meal is not largely used for human food in Brazil, it is a vital intermediate product for animal protein in the human alimentary chain.

In the last three decades, the expansion of soy meal sales made fast growth of the poultry industry possible. About 65 percent of the soy-based feed in Brazil is consumed by the poultry industry, 10 percent by the dairy products industry, and 20 percent by the swine industry. The production of inexpensive soy thus had a direct and positive impact on the national diet by containing the prices for meat, especially chicken.

Until recently, poultry was of secondary importance as a source of animal protein in the Brazilian diet. Due to its considerably higher unitary price relative to the bovine and swine meats, poultry was consumed as a Sunday delicacy, mainly by higher-income families (see Camara Cascudo 2004). In Brazil, beef has always been the most important source of animal protein; however, because of its relatively high unitary cost, only a small part of the population consumes it regularly. The meat consumption of the poor varies with the region and the price of meat. Since the 1990s, however, chicken has nationally become much less expensive than it had been. Between 1970 and 2002, Brazilian per capita consumption of poultry grew more than 1,400 percent (from 2.3 kg to 33.8 kg a year) (USDA/FAS 2005a). Undoubtedly, the advent of soy agriculture made meat in the form of chicken accessible to the urban poor on a regular basis. It is not without reason that in Brazil chicken has been called soybeans with wings.

From 1991 to 2001, Brazilian poultry production increased 130 percent while exports quadrupled. Now Brazil is the world's second-largest producer and exporter (Pessoa and Jank 2002). The production of pork doubled during the same period, and pork exports had a magnificent performance with a 1,576 percent increase, making the country the fourth-largest pork exporter. These trends were intensified with the devaluation of the Brazilian real and the European meat-production crises (e.g., BSE and foot-and-mouth disease). This excellent performance of meat production in Brazil has further positively impacted the domestic demand for feedstuffs (Pessoa and Jank 2002).

Soybean processors are increasingly determining the geography of the poultry industry. New poultry operations are being developed in the vicinity of the new agricultural borders, close to the soybean processors. Beyond the benefit of proximity with new and dynamic soybean production areas, there has been an environmental benefit to this shift. Because of the topography and farming practices of the new agricultural areas, the serious pollution problems found, for instance, with the production of swine in the state of Santa Catarina have not occurred in Brazil's central-western region (Goiás and Mato Grosso) (see Santos Filho et al. 1999).

In Brazil, among the several factors slowing down the direct use of soybeans as food is the widespread consumption of another crop, the common bean (*Phaseolus vulgaris* L.). Common beans contain roughly 22 percent protein and are an important source of this essential nutrient. Unlike soybeans, common beans are embedded in Brazilian culture and history; indeed, Brazil is the largest per capita consumer of common beans in the world (see Yokoyama and Stone 2000). This bean along with rice (*Oriza sativa* L.)—also a traditional crop—is a basic staple for Brazilians. The combination of the two is quite powerful even from a nutritional perspective, as the proteins from beans are rich in lysine, offsetting the poor profile of rice for that amino acid. The joining of rice and beans has been characterized as traditional food wisdom (Castro and Peliano 1985), or what Ishige (2006) calls the meal pattern specific to a society.

The taste and odor of soybeans were the initial major obstacles to their widespread acceptance as food (see Carrão-Panizzi 1998). During the 1940s and 1950s several attempts were made to incorporate soybeans in the Brazilian diet, including an effort by the famous sociologist and constitutional representative Gilberto Freyre. The stimulus for these efforts was twofold: the suffering of many undernourished people, mainly in rural areas, and the knowledge of soy's nutritional content (in addition to the protein and oil, soybeans contain vitamins and minerals). Unfortunately, however, soy became known as a legume "for the pigs and the poor" (see Hasse and Bueno 1996, 249).

Pigs are much more inclined to ingest nutritious preparations recommended by food science than are poor people, however. In addition to showing strong preferences for certain tastes, textures, and smells, in eating a person reveals himself or herself, identifying the self with a group that the person not only accepts but also wants to be accepted by. Humans thereby give the acts of cooking and eating a whole range of social and cultural meanings. The label "food for the poor and animals" caused soyfoods to encounter great resistance in Brazil during the 1970s and 1980s. Even the favorable nutrition to price ratio for soybeans did not convince the poor to eat them. As Castro and Peliano (1985) point out, the poor eat with neither optimal nutrition nor optimal expense. Not only do sensory preferences play a role in food choices, so also do the many social meanings at stake.

Soy-oil margarine, for instance, was always cheaper than butter. But for many years, poor people preferred to buy expensive butter rather than margarine. Only when margarine began to be associated with good health and became a product for all (middle and upper classes included) did its consumption among the poor exceed their consumption of butter.

As milk, soy had a troubled but ultimately successful journey in Brazil. In the early 1970s Brazil's Food Technology Institute (ITAL) began soymilk extraction in Campinas, São Paulo. The extraction machine was developed there and was known as the mechanical cow. A 1979 model of the machine could process two hundred liters of soymilk per hour. According to Hasse and Bueno (1996, 251), "Its main components were a sink used for heating the soy; a basket from a *Brastemp* washing machine for centrifugation; and at the end of the line, devices to pasteurize the soymilk, add flavors, and pack the milk into plastic bags. One kilogram of soy yielded eight liters of milk."

In 1975 soymilk was introduced to five hundred schoolchildren (aged six to fourteen years). For this first test, the soymilk had seven different flavors: chocolate, vanilla, banana, raspberry, strawberry, coconut, and pineapple. At the end of the trial period, 72 percent of the children approved of the soymilk (Hasse and Bueno 1996). In fact, after flavoring the use of soymilk in public schools has enjoyed ample acceptance. The major problem has been with the adult population and its traditional attachment to cow's milk. Problems with the taste of soymilk have taken time to overcome.

During the second half of the 1970s, experiments in marketing soymilk to the general public were numerous but with no great success. The basic buyer was always the government. Schoolchildren and, during a certain period, pregnant women under the care of the State of São Paulo Department of Health were the principal consumers. As Hasse and Bueno (1996) note, the Coca-Cola Company also tried to develop a nourishing soy drink during that decade, but the beverage did not win public acceptance.

During the 1980s, use of the mechanical cow spread to more Brazilian states. In one of several official ceremonies introducing the machine, an unexpected setback occurred: after tasting the soymilk, Brazil's president João Batista Figueiredo (1980–85) qualified it as "disgusting." The remark cannot be totally explained by Figueiredo's bluntness. As Hasse and Bueno (1996, 251) explain, "The 'cow' had been assembled in a hurry at a meeting place of the Brazilian Legion of Assistance (LBA). Two hours before the ceremony, it was put in operation, but the engine was working backwards. The people from LBA had no operational training. Soy industrialists suspected that this turn of events had been planned by the dairy industry to blemish the image of its supposed opponent." Fortunately, today the complexity and size of soymilk extractors permit large skilled food companies to sell a variety of soymilks, even in regular supermarkets.

The use of soymilk and other soyfoods in schools remains more significant, however, than grocery sales. In the 1970s texturized soy protein was prepared by untrained school chefs and usually ended up in soups that children would not eagerly eat. Today, after more than thirty years, food science has vastly improved the palatability of soyfoods. Soyfoods have been used in the schools of several Brazilian states with the aim of improving the children's nutrition. Soy products do not tend to replace other foods but are instead being added to various recipes (cookies, cakes, banana pie, bread, sweets, milk, and others). More than thirty-seven million students are affected, making Brazil's National School Food Program one of the biggest in the world.

Fortunately, during the 1990s the barriers against the larger public's direct soybean consumption began to be knocked down. Several institutions and companies have contributed to make soyfoods attractive to Brazilian tastes, eyes, and odor preferences. Among those institutions are the Federal University of Viçosa, the ITAL, and the government's Brazilian Agricultural Research Corporation (EMBRAPA).

The endeavors focus not only on the use of soy derivatives in various recipes but also, since the 1952 pioneering work of Murilio Moreira, on the creation of new so-called flavorless soybean varieties. These are whole soybeans without the off-tastes produced by the oxidation of linolenic acid. In 2000 EMBRAPA announced that it had developed two new varieties, BRS 213 and BRS 216, specific for human consumption. BRS 213 has a mild taste and requires no special treatment to make it palatable. It also provides good yields in the fields (Carrão-Panizzi et al. 2002a). BRS 216, by contrast, has a higher-than-usual protein content of 43 percent, but it still requires industrial treatment to improve the taste (Carrão-Panizzi 2000; Carrão-Panizzi et al. 2002b; Carrão-Panizzi and Erhan 2002).

Extensive bibliographies in Portuguese have been dedicated to soybeans in human food. Two useful examples are Mandarino and Carrão-Panizzi (1999) and Bordignon, Carrão-Panizzi, and Mandarino (2000). In addition to providing recipes, these publications argue that soy tastes good when the balance of ingredients in a recipe is correct. For this reason, in fact, defatted soy flour and soymilk are finding a growing acceptance among those interested in a healthy diet.

Tofu is another source of soy protein available in Brazil. Popular among Japanese and Chinese immigrants and their descendants, it has also attracted other Brazilians wanting to eat healthy food. It is widely marketed in large supermarkets or in Japanese and Chinese delicatessens. In Asian-style cuisine in Brazil, soybeans and soy derivatives are found in sauces as well as in pasta and stew dishes. Asian cuisine has become popular among the general population although mainly in big urban centers.

The use of soy in Brazilian cuisine still has a long way to go. As a secondary ingredient, however, soybeans have already been integrated firmly within Brazilian cuisine. Soy products (defatted flour, isolated and concentrated protein, texturized protein, and soymilk) appear—although often in small quantities—in industrial baked products, hamburgers, soups, sausages, canned foods, sweets and snacks, cereals, chocolate powders, sauces, mayonnaise, cake toppings and fillings, yogurt, and frozen foods.

Conclusion

Soybeans have contributed decisively to Brazil's modernization process of the 1970s; to the development of wide economic and social networks in Brazil and Argentina, involving people, objects, and animals; to the opening and occupation of new agricultural frontiers in Brazil; and to the integration of Brazilian territory. Occupation of the *cerrado* is the most visible aspect of this process, which began some thirty-five years ago.

This *cerrado* occupation has had characteristics that are striking (although by no means unique), such as the development of technologies that allowed for agricultural exploration of the ecosystem and the strong presence of government as well as its offers of incentives in all stages of the process. Unfortunately, there has been a lack of planning regarding the conservation of biodiversity and proper socioeconomic development for all populations involved. The economic difficulties that small farmers have faced were made very public during protests in the spring of 2006. Squeezed by "rising production costs and a strong Brazilian *real* that affect[ed] profitability, [for several weeks] Brazilian farmers . . . block[ed] key roads and railway routes along which grains are shipped to port" (Heller 2006). In consequence, multinational companies such as Bunge reported financial losses in Brazil during that period.

The soybean expansion has contributed to dietary change as well. By the end of the 1960s, the majority of Brazil's population lived in urban areas. In big cities such as São Paulo, Rio de Janeiro, Belo Horizonte, and Recife, the urban mode of life brought great shifts in food habits, notably the introduction of prepared food. The expansion of Brazil's soybean network coincided with this urbanization, making the supremacy of soy oil in Brazilian cooking and the presence of soy protein as a minor yet important functional ingredient in processed foods both economical and logical. Some have rightly called soybeans used in this manner "an invisible friend"; their presence in a large variety of foods goes unnoticed by most people. Except for soymilk in schools and occasional tofu consumption among typical urban dwellers when they enjoy Asian cuisine, foods that are rich in soy protein have not yet had a significant impact on the Brazilian diet.

Argentina has gone through similar changes and a dramatic economic liberalization. These circumstances have promoted the flourishing of Argentina's soybean industries. Argentina has thus made choices parallel to those of Brazil in embracing the soybean, this ancient and yet most modern of crops.

Notes

1. We thank Edward G. Singer, William H. Fisher, Carlos Magri Ferreira, Mercedes C. Carrão-Panizzi, and Christine Du Bois for their critical comments and suggestions on an early draft of this essay.

2. "The word network indicates that resources are concentrated in a few places—the knots and the nodes [whose] . . . connections transform the scattered resources into a net that may seem to extend everywhere" (Latour 1987, 180).

3. Soy meal is the product left after the oil has been removed from the beans. It is high in protein.

4. In his *Philosophie des Geldes* (*The Philosophy of Money*), published for the first time in 1900, Simmel (2001) identifies as the cultural tragedy of modernity the separation between subjective and objective cultures. The cultural productions created by humans to serve them assume (with their objectification) a logic independent from the original intentions of their creation. To Simmel, the most important structural factor of modernity is the rise of the monetary economy. Money has a central role in the constitution of both modern liberty and modern tragedy.

References

Bonato, E. R., P. F. Bertagnolli, C. E. Lange, and S. A. L. Rubin. 1999. "Teores do Óleo e de Proteína em Cultivares do Soja Desenvolvidas em Diferentes Períodos." *Anais Congresso Brasileiro de Soja.* Documentos, 124. Londrina, Paraná: Embrapa Soja.

Bordignon, J. R., M. C. Carrão-Panizzi, and J. M. G. Mandarino. 2000. *Mais Saúde em Sua Vida—Cozinhando com Tofu.* Circular Técnica 29. Londrina: Embrapa Soja.

Bowker, Geoffrey C., and Susan Leigh Star. 2000. *Sorting Things Out: Classification and Its Consequences.* Cambridge, MA: MIT Press.

Brazil—Secretaria de Produção e Comercialização. 2004. *Agronegócio Brasileiro: Desempenho do Comércio Exterior.* Brasília, DF: Ministério da Agricultura, Pecuária e Abastecimento. Secretaria de Produção e Comercialização (MAPA/SPC).

Busch, Lawrence. 2000. "The Moral Economy of Grades and Standards." *Journal of Rural Studies* 16: 273–83.

Caixeta-Filho, J. V., and A. H. Gameiro, eds. 2001. *Transporte e Logística em Sistemas Agroindustriais.* São Paulo: Editora Atlas S. A.

Camara Cascudo, Luis da. 2004. *História da Alimentação no Brasil,* 3rd ed. São Paulo: Global Editora.

Carrão-Panizzi, Mercedes C. 1998. "Potential Uses of Soybeans As Food in South America." JIRCAS Working Report No. 13, pp. 89–96. Tokyo: Japan International Research Center for Agricultural Sciences (JIRCAS), Ministry of Agriculture, Forestry and Fisheries.

———. 2000. "Melhoramento Genético da Soja Para a Obtenção de Cultivares Mais Adequadas ao Consumo Humano." *Revista Brasileira de Nutrição Clínica* 15(2): 330–40.

Carrão-Panizzi, M. C., L. A. Almeida, L. C. Miranda, R. A. S. Kiihl, J. M. G. Mandarino, C. A. A. Arias, J. T. Yorinori, A. M. R. Almeida, and J. F. F. Toledo. 2002a. "BRS 213—Nova Cultivar de Soja Para Alimentação Humana." *Resumos do II Congresso Brasileiro de Soja e Mercosoja.* Documentos 181, p. 201. Londrina: Embrapa Soja.

———. 2002b. "BRS 216—Nova Cultivar de Soja Para Alimentação Humana." *Resumos do II Congresso Brasileiro de Soja e Mercosoja.* Documentos 181, p. 202. Londrina: Embrapa Soja.

Carrão-Panizzi, M. C., and S. Erhan. 2002. "Chemical Composition of Specialty Soybean Genotypes." In J. P. Cherry and A. E. Pavlath, eds., *Proceedings of the 31st U.S. and Japan Natural Resources (UJNR) Protein Resources Panel Meeting*, pp. UU1–UU8. December 1–6, Monterey, California.

Castro, Cláudio de Moura, and Anna Medeiros Peliano. 1985. "Novos Alimentos, Velhos Hábitos e o Espaço para Ações Educativas." In C. de M. Castro and M. Coimbra, eds., *O Problema Alimentar no Brasil*, 195–213. São Paulo: Editora da Unicamp, ALMED.

Döbereiner, J. 1992. "Recent Changes in Concepts of Plant Bacteria Interactions: Endophytic N_2 Fixing Bacteria." *Ciência e Cultura* 44: 310–13.

Espírito Santo, B. R. do. 2001. *Os Caminhos da Agricultura Brasileira*, 2nd ed. São Paulo: Evoluir.

Fearnside, Philip M. 2001. "Soybean Cultivation As a Threat to the Environment in Brazil." *Environmental Conservation* 28(1): 23–38.

Ferreira, Carlos Magri, Ivan Sergio Freire de Sousa, and Patricio Méndez del Villar. 2004. *Desenvolvimento Tecnológico e Dinâmica da Produção de Arroz de Terras Altas no Brasil*. Goiânia: Embrapa Arroz e Feijão.

Hall, Kevin G. 2004a. "Armed Land-Grabbers Set Sights on Amazon Jungle Settlement." Knight Ridder/Tribune News Service, August 15.

———. 2004b. "Brazil Creates Rainforest Preserves." *Pittsburgh Post-Gazette*, November 12, p. A-4.

Harder, B. 2006. "Plowing Down the Amazon." *Science News* 170 (September 9): 166.

Hartwig, Edgar E., and Romeu Afonso de Souza Kiihl. 1979. "Identification and Utilization of a Delayed Flowering Character in Soybeans for Short-Day Conditions." *Field Crop Research* 2: 145–51.

Hasse, Geraldo, and Fernando Bueno. 1996. *O Brasil da Soja: Abrindo Fronteiras, Semeando Cidades*. Porto Alegre: CEVAL Alimentos/L&P.

Heller, Lorraine. 2006. "Bunge Soybean Supply Disrupted in Brazil." Decision News Media, May 19. http://www.foodnavigator-usa.com/news/ng.asp?n=67840-bunge-soybeans-brazil.

IBGE (Instituto Brasileiro de Geografia e Estatística). 1980. *Levantamento Sistemático da Produção Agrícola*. Rio de Janeiro: IBGE. www.sidra.ibge.gov.br.

———. 2002. *Levantamento Sistemático da Produção Agrícola*. Rio de Janeiro: IBGE. www.sidra.ibge.gov.br.

———. 2006. *Levantamento Sistemático da Produção Agrícola*. Rio de Janeiro: IBGE. www.sidra.ibge.gov.br.

Ishige, Naomichi. 2006. "East Asian Families and the Dining Table." *Journal of Chinese Dietary Culture* 2(2): 1–26.

Juska, Arunas, L. Gouveia, J. Gabriel, and S. Koneck. 2000. "Negotiating Bacteriological Meat Contamination Standards in the US: The Case of E. coli O157:H7." *Sociologia Ruralis* 40 (April): 249–71.

Kiihl, Romeu Afonso de Souza, and Antonio Garcia. 1988. "The Use of the Long-Juvenile Trait in Breeding Soybean Cultivars." In *World Soybean Research Conference IV*, 994–1000. Buenos Aires, Argentina.

Klink, C. A., A. G. Moreira, and O. T. Solbrig. 1993. "Ecological Impacts of Agricultural Development in Brazilian Cerrados." In M. D. Young and O. T. Solbrig, eds., *The World's Savannas: Economic Driving Forces, Ecological Constraints, and Policy Options for Sustainable Land Use*, 259–82. Man and the Biosphere Series, Vol. 12. Paris: UNESCO.

Krislov, S. 1997. *How Nations Choose Product Standards and Standards Change Nations*. Pittsburgh: University of Pittsburgh Press.

Latour, Bruno. 1987. *Science in Action*. Cambridge: Harvard University Press.

———. 1993. *We Have Never Been Modern*. Cambridge: Harvard University Press.

Loureiro, E. N., and D. E. Cade. 2003. "Experiência da Companhia Vale do Rio Doce nas Novas Fronteiras de Produção e o Intermodal de Transporte." In *Anais Comgresso de Soja*, 182–96. Londrina, Paraná: Embrapa Soja.

Mandarino, J. M. G., and M. C. Carrão-Panizzi. 1999. *A Soja na Cozinha*. Documentos 136. Londrina: Embrapa Soja.

Miyasaka, Shiro, and Júlio César Medina, eds. 1981. *A Soja no Brasil*. Campinas, SP: Instituto de Tecnologia de Alimentos (ITAL).

Muello, Peter. 2006. "Greenpeace: Soy Ban Helping Amazon." Associated Press, July 25.

Myers, N., R. A. Mittermeier, C. G. Mittermeier, G. A. B. da Fonseca, and J. Kent. 2000. "Biodiversity Hotspots for Conservation Priorities." *Nature* 403: 853–58.

Pessoa, A. S. M., and M. S. Jank. 2002. "How Brazilians View the Soybean Market." Presentation to the Agricultural Outlook Forum, Arlington, Virginia, February 21–22. http://www.agweb.com/get_article.asp?pageid=89407&newscat=GN&src=gennews.

Ratter, J. A., J. F. Ribeiro, and S. Bridgewater. 1997. "The Brazilian Cerrado Vegetation and Threats to Its Biodiversity." *Annals of Botany* 80: 223–30.

SAGPyA (Secretaria de Agricultura, Ganadería, Pesca y Alimentos). 2006. www.sagpya.mecon.gov.ar.

Santos Filho, J. I. dos, N. A. dos Santos, M. D. Canaver, I. S. F. de Sousa, and L. F. Vieira. 1999. "O Cluster Suinícola do Oeste de Santa Catarina." In Paulo R. Haddad, ed., *A Competitividade do Agronegócio e o Desenvolvimento Regional no Brasil*, 125–80. Brasilia: CNPq—Embrapa.

Shean, Michael. 2004. "The Amazon: Brazil's Final Soybean Frontier." January 13. Washington: USDA/Foreign Agricultural Service. http://www.fas.usda.gov/pecad/highlights/2004/01/Amazon/Amazon_soybeans.htm.

Simmel, Georg. 2001. *The Philosophy of Money*. Reprint. New York: Routledge.

Soskin, Anthony B. 1988. *Non-Traditional Agriculture and Economic Development: The Brazilian Soybean Expansion, 1964–1982*. New York: Praeger.

Sousa, Ivan Sergio Freire de. 2001. *Classificação e Padronização de Produtos, com Ênfase na Agropecuária: Uma Análise Histórico-Conceitual.* Texto para Discussão, no. 10. Brasilia, DF.: Embrapa Informação Tecnológica.

Sousa, Ivan Sergio Freire de, and Lawrence Busch. 1998. "Networks and Agricultural Development: The Case of Soybean Production and Consumption in Brazil." *Rural Sociology* 63(3) (September): 349–71.

Souza, Plinio I. de M., and Wenceslay J. Goedert. 1987. *Soybeans in the Brazilian Cerrados: Soil Fertility and Management.* Brasilia, DF: Embrapa/CPAC.

Stedman-Edwards, P. A. 1999. "Root Causes of Biodiversity Loss: Case Study of the Brazilian Cerrado." Unpublished report. Washington, DC: World Wildlife Fund.

USDA/Foreign Agricultural Service. 2004. Raw data on soybeans. http://www.fas.usda.gov/psdonline/psdDownload.aspx. Click on "Oilseeds."

———. 2005a. Raw data on poultry production. http://www.fas.usda.gov/psdonline/psdDownload.aspx.

———. 2005b. Raw data on soy oil. http://www.fas.usda.gov/psdonline/psdDownload.aspx. Click on "Oilseeds."

———. 2005c. "Table 8: Soybean and Products: World Trade." http://www.fas.usda.gov/oilseeds/circular/2005/05-11/toc.htm.

Warnken, Philip F. 1999. *The Development and Growth of the Soybean Industry in Brazil.* Ames: Iowa State University Press.

Yokoyama, Lidia Pacheco, and Luis Fernando Stone. 2000. *Cultura do Feijoeiro no Brasil: Características da Produção.* Santo Antonio de Goiás: Embrapa Arroz e Feijão.

13

Soy in Bangladesh

History and Prospects

CHRISTINE M. DU BOIS

Introduction

Previous chapters have delineated the history of soy in countries where it is deemed either an essential food or an economically crucial crop.[1] But soy's history in other countries, where it is less known, should not be neglected. Many governments, nongovernmental organizations (NGOs), the United Nations, and even businesses have worked hard to raise the profile of soy in such places. The example of one such country, Bangladesh, demonstrates both the difficulties and the successes that these endeavors often entail. The present essay explores the history of soy in Bangladesh, contrasting it with that of the soy superpower, the United States.

The overall pictures of soy in Bangladesh and the United States differ sharply. Although Bangladeshis, like Americans, consume soy oil, they consume much less oil per capita than Americans, and what they eat they import.[2] The country as a whole eats very little soy protein. Despite several decades of effort by NGOs in Bangladesh as well as more recent government involvement, soy agriculture in that country is tiny. A few thousand poor farmers grow soy on small plots of land using very simple tools. These near-subsistence farmers themselves eat between 5 percent and 40 percent of the soy they produce (MCC 1989, 23; MCC 1996, 71–72).[3]

Yet the contrasts between the two countries' situations belie the connections between them. In fact, the story of soy in Bangladesh begins with America's Food for Peace program. It continues with the research and agricultural extension services of U.S.-trained agronomists and marketers working in Bangladesh. The history of soy in Bangladesh makes these connections abundantly clear. It also illuminates a variety of factors that impede the widespread consumption of soy protein among Bangladeshis, despite their severe need for high-quality protein.

Contemporary and Historical Soy in Bangladesh

Accurate statistics about present-day Bangladeshi soy agriculture are difficult to obtain, but according to expert observers production in 2003 was likely in the range of a mere seven thousand to ten thousand metric tons, and the situation has not changed much since (personal communications with Emerson Nafziger, Crop Sciences Department, University of Illinois, 2003, 2005; USDA 2006b).[4] All of the local beans are used domestically for poultry feed, seed, and some human consumption; there are no documented exports. Almost none of the local beans are processed into separate oil and protein products, as the first modern soybean extraction plant only came into operation in December of 2005 and relies heavily on imported beans (USDA 2006b, 2–3).[5]

Bangladesh's soy farmers and their attitudes toward their crop also contrast with the U.S. situation. While not the poorest of the poor in Bangladesh, these farmers are nevertheless quite impoverished based on world standards.[6] Their farming techniques are not mechanized. Oxen are the main source of power, and wooden plows are the primary implements (personal communication with Stout, 2003; see note 6). The crop is chosen for places and seasons where the preferred crop, rice, is not successful. Soybeans are treated as a secondary low-input, low-risk, and often low-yield crop that, when the weather is good, sometimes provides a bountiful harvest (personal communication with Nafziger, 2003).

Soy utilization in Bangladesh differs from the U.S. case as well. Rather than grow and process all they need, Bangladeshis import soy meal from India for their chickens; while domestic soybeans are mostly used for chickens too, the supply is much too small to be adequate (USDA 1998). As for human consumption, in Bangladesh the only soy protein products that have a popular market are soy-fortified biscuits and the roasted whole beans eaten as a snack. The population also consumes soybean oil imported from South America. Yet although soy oil was for years clearly the most popular oil on the market, per capita consumption is low. This is partly because poverty forces Bangladeshis to have one of the lowest edible oil consumption rates in the world (USDA 1998).

Bangladeshi consumption of soy oil is a relatively recent culinary habit. The oil became popular in the 1960s and 1970s when the U.S. government's PL 480 program, also known as Food for Peace (USDA 1998) provided the Bangladeshi government with large quantities of semiprocessed soy oil that it could then sell cheaply to local refiners. The program relieved the United States of some of its excess soy oil, provided the Bangladeshi government with a revenue source, and made cheap oil available to Bangladeshi consumers (personal communication with Stout, 2003). At first consumers did not accept the oil (USDA 1998; personal communication with Nafziger, 2003), but fairly soon its price made it popular.

The program's continuation through 1991 (USDA 1997, 6) imparted to the population the price and taste expectations that fit with soybean oil. Particularly after the PL 480 shipments stopped, Brazilian and Argentine exporters found a market in Bangladesh (USDA 2001).[7] Unfortunately, this chain of events hurt Bangladesh's traditional oilseed markets and farmers, especially producers of mustard oil (USDA 1998). However, in recent years higher yields in mustard seed agriculture have increased availability of that oil within Bangladesh, and the very low price of palm oil has led Bangladeshis to import more palm than soy. The palm oil is mixed with the preferred soy oil (USDA 2006b, 3).

Unfortunately, Food for Peace did little to encourage the much-needed consumption of soy protein in Bangladesh.[8] Yet the low levels of soy production and human consumption of soy protein are not, in general, from want of trying. Soy has probably been grown on a very, very small scale in Bangladesh for several centuries (Shurtleff and Aoyagi 2007, 2). In the late twentieth century, several NGOs and foreign governments endeavored, with varying degrees of success, to encourage soy cultivation and the eating of protein-rich soyfoods among Bangladeshis. For example, in 1987 a German-Bangladeshi project introduced soybeans to the Ghatail and Madhupur forest regions of northwestern Bangladesh (Xinhua General Overseas News Service 1990), and in 1988 the Japan Overseas Cooperation Volunteers distributed soybeans to twenty-eight hundred farmers in Comilla Province in the south (Sato 1990). The Seventh-day Adventist World Service, the International Soybean Program at the University of Illinois (INTSOY), the Canadian International Development Agency, and the Canadian Foodgrains Bank also figure among the numerous organizations that have assisted in promoting soy in Bangladesh (MCC 1982, 17; MCC 1986, 35; MCC 1990b, 28; MCC 1991, 4–12; MCC 1993, 59).

The government of Bangladesh has at times participated in such projects, eventually developing a sustained interest in soy. Government interest was initially strong during 1975–81 (see Shurtleff and Aoyagi 2007, 2), but due to agronomic difficulties this first government campaign to introduce soybeans was not continued. The campaign had unfortunately promoted varieties of soy that were not very successful in Bangladesh's climate and ecosystems (MCC 1990a, 1). Later, from 1990 forward, the government tried again with a more suitable variety. In that year the government adopted a five-year national soybean action plan (MCC 1990b, iv, 30).

By far the most consistent and active promoter of soy in Bangladesh has been the Mennonite Central Committee (MCC). The MCC is a North American Christian development organization that operated a soybean program between 1972 and 1999 in various parts of Bangladesh, especially the Noakhali region in the southern part of the country (Khokan and Horlings 1987, 3).[9] The MCC first came to Bangladesh to assist people in that district who had survived the great tidal bore disaster of 1970 (MCC 1994, vi). The MCC then initiated a soybean program, motivated both by the general Mennonite commitment to feeding the hungry and by the chronic deficiency of high-quality protein among the Bangladeshi population. Declining per capita cultivation of protein-providing pulse crops since the mid-1970s and particularly in the 1980s had contributed to this deficiency (Mahmud, Rahman, and Zohir 2000, 233; Alauddin and Hossain 2001, 94; Alauddin and Tisdell 1991, 92, 94–95, 98, 286). Unfortunately, despite the MCC's and others' efforts to encourage crop diversification, this problem has persisted. For example, in a society that often depends on pulses for protein, all pulses produced in 1997 made up only about 5 percent of the agricultural sector (USDA 1997, 3).

The MCC's program included research specific to Bangladesh on a broad array of agronomic concerns: appropriate soybean varieties, fungicides, inoculation regimens, fertilization, land preparation, intercropping, date of planting, irrigation, seed production, and seed storage. A breakthrough came in the early 1980s when MCC staff identified a variety known as Punjab-1 (Pb-1, also called Shohag) that flourished in some of Bangladesh's southern ecosystems, producing good yields and seed quality superior to that of other varieties, all within an acceptable duration so that other crops could also be grown (MCC 1983, 32; MCC 1985, 23). Years of MCC extension work imparted what was learned to Bangladeshi farmers, and training sessions for workers of other NGOs transferred the MCC's intellectual capital about soybeans to like-minded development organizations

(MCC 1993, vi, 56–59; MCC 1994, 40, 45; MCC 1995, 55–56). The MCC also operated a marketing program that guaranteed the farmers a minimum buy-back price for their soy. The buy-back program was a crucial support until the private market for soybeans was somewhat stabilized in the 1980s (MCC 1982, 9; MCC 1983, 22).

Meanwhile, staff members focusing on soy utilization developed culturally familiar recipes. Seeking a locally effective marketing technique, they trained and paid Bangladeshi women to conduct soy-cooking demonstrations in their home villages. An MCC survey with a variety of farmers later indicated two separate significant factors that spurred men to eat soybeans: farming soybeans themselves and their wives having attended one of the cooking demonstrations (MCC 1983, 44–47). The MCC continued with the demonstrations, which eventually numbered in the many thousands (MCC 1990b, 29; MCC 1992, 54; MCC 1994, 45). A later evaluation confirmed that the cooking demonstrations had had a positive impact on soy utilization as human food (Verhoef 1996).[10] In addition, landless men working as daily laborers were introduced to soyfoods by employers who offered soy as part of the daily meal (MCC 1983, 43).

The MCC also provided training in soyfoods preparation to workers in institutions such as schools, prisons, and hospitals (MCC 1994, 40, 45). A cookbook, leaflets, and various promotional materials were created and mass distributed (MCC 1981, 31; MCC 1989, 24; MCC 1990b, 28–29; MCC 1991, 4–14, 4–15; MCC 1994, 45). Moreover, since 1999 when the MCC's soybean program in Bangladesh formally ended, former MCC staff members and the MCC itself have continued to play a limited but appreciated role in Bangladesh's increasing soy production, such as in varietal trials and inoculant production (MCC 2001, 59, 73; MCC 2002, 10–13; personal communication with Ramont Schrock, inoculant specialist with MCC in Bangladesh, 2003). The MCC and its former soy specialists have also continued their decades of consultancy work with the government of Bangladesh and other development organizations (MCC 1991, 4–16; personal communication with Nafziger, 2003; personal communication with Schrock, 2003).

Today the only region in Bangladesh where thousands of hectares of soybeans are consistently grown is the south, where the MCC worked.[11] Due in large measure to the MCC's quarter century of effort, soy is now accepted as a viable crop in Bangladesh, and the central government is actively seeking ways to expand its production. The MCC thus provided a critical link between the soybean expertise of the scientific and marketing communities in North America and the impoverished farmers and consumers of Bangladesh. Their agronomic work particularly demonstrates that in the modern world, even cultivators using very rudimentary farming systems may actually have benefited from a great deal of contemporary science and technology. The science is not obvious to the untrained eye observing only a hand plow or an ox and a wooden plow, but it is there nonetheless.

Recently the market for soy in Bangladesh has received a modest but helpful boost from the World Food Programme (WFP) of the United Nations. In July 2002 the WFP began a program to feed fortified biscuits to nine hundred thousand Bangladeshi schoolchildren. The biscuits are formulated with 5 percent soy flour as well as other nutrients; 5 percent is typically the maximum amount of soy that can be added to biscuits without noticeably changing their taste, odor, or texture (MCC 1990a, 6). The WFP's plan calls for the periodic laboratory testing of the biscuits to verify that they have been manufactured with the specified proportions of ingredients (WFP 2003).

The objectives of this school feeding program, one of the largest in the world, are to improve the children's nutritional status and to encourage them to stay in school. But it also has two side benefits: it provides business for small-scale Bangladeshi entrepreneurs such as biscuit factories and soy flour producers, and it strengthens demand for the beans grown by Bangladeshi farmers (personal communication with Nafziger, 2003; WFP 2003). The program is expected to need more than two thousand metric tons of full fat soy flour during its planned five years (WFP 2003) and to purchase all of this soy locally.

Whether the program will be renewed, thereby maintaining the increased demand for soy, remains to be seen. Equally important, it is an open question whether cheaply imported soy meal from the United States could undercut demand for local soy, if not in the WFP program then in other areas of utilization. The U.S. Department of Agriculture (USDA) has suggested that although India is a strong competitor in the Bangladeshi market for soy meal, "PL 480 supplies could play an effective role in establishing a market for US soybean meal in the longer term" (USDA 1998, 4). Moreover, the American Soybean Association has an active program in Bangladesh[12] that promotes consumption of U.S. soy oil as well as the use of U.S. soy protein in the nascent Bangladeshi health-foods market (personal communication with the Regional Directorship of the Asia Subcontinent Office of the American Soybean Association, 2005).[13] Thus, while there are promising signs for local soy agriculture, there is also continual commercial competition.

Given the history of enthusiasm for soy in Bangladesh and the efforts of multiple parties, why does the Bangladeshi population still eat so little soy protein? This pressing question, silently reflected in the weak, stunted bodies of far too many Bangladeshis, compels further scrutiny.

Why Do Bangladeshis Eat So Little Soy Protein?

Before turning to this question we must first ask, why should they eat soy protein? The deficiency in high-quality protein of some 60 percent of the population (MCC 1996, 56) has already been noted. Although the Green Revolution significantly reduced the risk of famine in Bangladesh, allowing more people to survive (Alauddin and Hossain 2001, 73), it has not kept sufficient pace with population growth to eradicate malnutrition (Ahmed 2000, 115; Bangladesh Ministry of Food 2002). Moreover, although the Green Revolution greatly increased the production of rice and wheat, this expansion was too often at the expense of other crops (Alauddin and Tisdell 1991, 91–99; Mahmud, Rahman, and Zohir 2000). True, Bangladeshis now die from starvation less often, and per capita Bangladeshis eat more calories than prior to 1980 (Ahmed and Haggblade 2000, 5; Ahmed 2000, 106), all quite remarkable given the near-doubling of the population in thirty years to some 153 million (U.S. Bureau of the Census 2008). But the poor still consume too few calories (Ahmed 2000; USDA 1997), and most Bangladeshis have a less varied, less healthy diet than they did in nonfamine times prior to the Green Revolution (Alauddin and Tisdell 1991, 91–99).[14] Among Bangladeshis' nutritional problems, the frequent lack of good protein leads to poor growth, lassitude, and impaired immune function (MCC 1990a, 16).

An analysis by Bangladesh's Ministry of Food has found that although the country does not have a protein deficiency in terms of quantity, the rate of meat and pulse consumption is so low that the quality of the protein is inadequate for human health (Bangladesh Ministry of Food 2002, 5). In other words, much of the population does not receive a complete set of essential amino acids. Soybeans would be particularly helpful in ameliorating this situation, because of all crops, soy's amino acid profile is closest to the high-quality profiles of eggs and meat. Yet soy is much less expensive than meat in Bangladesh, as it is elsewhere. Whole soybeans are also rich in important vitamins and minerals, and although they contain less carbohydrate than many other beans, their high fat content ensures that they actually provide more calories. This difference is helpful in Bangladesh, where the diets are already skewed excessively toward carbohydrates. Soy's advantages become clear when one compares the nutritional profile of soybeans with those of traditional Bangladeshi pulses as they are utilized in local cooking (table 1).

But these nutritional advantages are not the only good reason for cultivating soy in Bangladesh. Soy's nitrogen-fixing qualities are helpful in renewing the fertility of the soil and potentially reducing the need for imported fertilizer. Soy agriculture could also reduce Bangladesh's $2.5 billion balance-of-trade problem (Bangladesh Export Promotion Bureau 2000).[15] If Bangladesh were to obtain sufficient crushing and extracting equipment, the production of oil from local soy could reduce the country's dependence on yearly imports of approximately a quarter million metric tons of mostly Brazilian soy oil, almost 200,000 tons of whole Argentine soybeans, and about 150,000 tons of soy meal from India (USDA 2001; USDA 2006b, 3–4).

Unfortunately, the spread of soy agriculture and soy protein consumption in Bangladesh has been slowed by a variety of agronomic, economic, and consumer difficulties. The agronomic struggles have been numerous. Moisture extremes in Bangladeshi soils, the need to find the best inoculant strain for each locality, the photoperiod sensitivity of the otherwise successful Shohag variety, and low pH in nearly 40 percent of Bangladeshi soils are among the most significant issues (Woodruff 1998, 3, 5–19). But the impediment that current and former MCC personnel have most consistently pointed to has been the difficulty in producing high-quality soy seed in Bangladesh (MCC 1994, 38; personal communication with Nafziger, 2003). Bangladesh's climate is hot and humid during the period when most soy farmers are harvesting their crop; these conditions impair the capacity of saved seed to germinate later (personal communication with Nafziger, 2003).

Economic troubles have included the paucity of soy-processing facilities (Woodruff 1998, 3–4, 36) and the continued partial instability of soy markets (Woodruff 1998, 33–34; personal communication with Nafziger, 2003). Soy is also insufficiently competitive with other crops from the farmer's point of view (Woodruff 1998, 3, 35; personal communication with Nafziger, 2003). The traditional staple, rice, always finds a market, and in recent decades has produced high yields, so farmers choose to plant rice whenever they can. Finding ways to increase soy's yield per hectare could ameliorate this problem (Woodruff 1998, 3).

Table 1. Nutrients in 100 Grams of Common Pulses

Pulse	*Energy (Kilo Calories)*	*Protein (Grams)*	*Oil (G)*	*Calcium (MG)*	*Iron (MG)*	*Carotene (MG)*	*Vitamin B1 (MG)*	*Vitamin B2 (MG)*
Soybean (whole)	432	43.2	19.5	240	11.5	426	0.73	0.39
Chickpea (dhal—i.e., split)	372	20.4	5.6	56	9.1	129	0.48	0.18
Blackgram (dhal)	347	24.0	1.4	154	9.1	38	0.42	0.37
Mungbean (i.e., green gram) (dhal)	348	24.5	1.2	75	8.5	49	0.72	0.15
Kesari (i.e., Bengal gram or grass pea) (dhal)	345	28.2	0.6	90	6.3	120	0.39	0.17
Lentil (dhal)	343	25.1	0.7	69	4.8	270	0.45	0.20
Fieldpea (whole)	315	19.7	1.1	45	5.1	39	0.47	0.19
Pigeonpea (dhal)	335	22.3	1.7	73	5.8	132	0.45	0.19

Sources: Khokan and Horlings (1987, 43) and personal communication with Nafziger (2003). Reprinted by permission of MCC.

In addition, consumer needs and preferences have created dilemmas. The MCC has encouraged the poor to eat soybeans in the less-processed ways that this target group can afford, for example as a substitute for other pulses in traditional recipes, prepared in the home as soymilk, or roasted as a snack (MCC 1996, 58–59). Yet at the same time, MCC staff have recognized that a wider array of successful soyfoods on the market, including more processed ones, would provide more stable incomes for soy farmers. An array of soyfoods with appeal to higher classes could also help prevent soy from developing the stigma of "poor man's food" (MCC 1987, 40), a stereotype that can inhibit even the poor from eating a food as soon as they obtain a little cash to eat alternatives. The promotion of more processed soyfoods such as tofu, soy-fortified bread, or noodles made with soy flour also has the advantage of showcasing soy in its more palatable forms; whole soy is difficult to cook and digest (Huang 2000, 292–378).

Indeed, a study of the effectiveness of the MCC's cooking demonstrations found that although the demonstrations were helpful, Bangladeshi consumers still had reservations about eating soy as it was presented to them (Verhoef 1996). Among most of the impoverished women questioned in group and individual sessions, soy had developed a reputation for causing digestive problems and flatulence, which in fact it probably had due to incorrect preparation (Verhoef 1996, 14; see also Khokan and Horlings 1987, 40–41). For this reason, some of the women declined to feed soy to their children (even though preschool children are among the most malnourished of Bangladeshis); moreover, some did not express enthusiasm for soy consumption even among other members of their families.

Many of the women interviewed also stated that to make soy taste acceptable to their families, they must use more spices than with other pulses (Verhoef 1996); the unpleasant taste may also be due in part to incorrect preparation (see Khokan and Horlings 1987, 40; MCC 1990a, 3). The greater spice expense offsets the cheaper price of soy compared with those pulses, making soy no more attractive from an economic standpoint than more traditional foods. Taste tests comparing soy with more traditional pulses (in which some participants were told that they were eating soy and some were not) confirmed that Bangladeshis find soy less palatable than those pulses (Verhoef 1996).

But these are the very sorts of consumer difficulties with soy that American companies are gradually overcoming, even as farmers and the industries that supply them have already overcome many agronomic obstacles to the expansion of soy agriculture in the United States. In contemporary

America, the presence of a large and generally vigorous market for soy animal feed provides the underlying support to farmers that in turn facilitates further developments. This comparatively secure market for and therefore abundance of soy encourages farmers and nonfarmers to invest, experiment, and innovate in soy agriculture, markets, processing, and food preparation. By contrast, although the poultry feed market in Bangladesh has grown at a rate of 20 percent per year (USDA 2001; see also USDA 2004), it is still small.[16] Most Bangladeshis are simply too poor to eat very much chicken or eggs, if they can afford them at all. Thus, ironically, much of the population has been too poor to demand the meat that would encourage a large feed market, which would then support the agriculture of a food ideal for the poor in place of meat.

The plight of Bangladesh's poor has historical and contemporary roots in a deeply inequitable distribution of wealth, whose brief examination will make clear the difficulty in spurring meat consumption in that country. In 1793 when Bangladesh was part of Bengal Province in the British Empire, the British introduced a tax-collection system called the Permanent Settlement. The Permanent Settlement allowed a small class of nonfarmer landlords and moneylenders (who were sometimes the same people) to squeeze every bit of profit from the land. It left the actual cultivators "destined to live in perpetual poverty, which more often than not forced [them] into bondage of indebtedness" (Alauddin and Hossain 2001, 158).

Although the disruptions of World War II along with a series of peasant movements and the shift away from British colonial power all shook up the power structure, the changes did not last. The governments of Pakistan and, later, independent Bangladesh made efforts to redistribute land, but the efforts were feeble or halfhearted and hence thwarted (Alauddin and Hossain 2001, 159–78).

The dangers of such social inequalities were starkly revealed in the famines of 1943 and 1974. Although these disasters were triggered by events outside Bangladesh (World War II in 1943 and the cutoff of U.S. food aid in 1974), their effects on the poor showed just how vulnerable the lower classes were within Bangladesh's social system. Considered together, the two famines killed millions of impoverished Bangladeshis (Ahmed, Chowdhury, and Haggblade 2000; Atwood, Jahangir, Smith, and Kabir 2000; Haggblade and Ahmed 2000).

Currently, in a country where land ownership is a major key to power and wealth, some two-thirds of all Bangladeshis are functionally landless (Dasgupta 1994, 45). The distribution of land is highly skewed and becoming even more so (Alauddin and Hossain 2001, 157, 167, 175, 237; Alauddin and Tisdell 1991, 160–62). In recent decades the poor have suffered from the loss of access to natural resources (Alauddin and Tisdell 1991, 161–63; Lappé, Collins, and Kinley 1981, 56–60), the unequal distribution of development credit (Dasgupta 1994, 38), and unequal benefits from the Green Revolution (Dasgupta 1994, 44–45; Lappé, Collins, and Kinley 1981). Over and over again, the poor have been left out of the development process, such that the bottom 25 percent of the population lives an existence so precarious (Haggblade and Ahmed 2000, 285) that it "straddles the outer limits of human survival" (Ahmed 2000, 112).

Unfortunately, whatever gains the poor have managed to make have been eroded by severe population pressures, which lead to the further fragmenting of already tiny landholdings. Even those who are better off face this problem, as the decline in landholding sizes among the higher classes demonstrates (Alauddin and Hossain 2001, 166, 170–71). Present-day Bangladesh must cope with "population pressure on arable land twice as high as in the late 1960s" (Alauddin and Hossain 2001, 252; see also Alauddin and Tisdell 1991, 290). It is within this historically and demographically shaped context that most Bangladeshis infrequently eat chicken, eggs, or other animal protein.

Yet despite these many difficult and sometimes agonizing factors impeding the spread of soy cultivation and soy protein consumption in Bangladesh, in the long run soy may still play a prominent role in Bangladeshi nutrition. The agronomic, marketing, and consumer difficulties with soy—as well as the social inequities, population pressures, and attendant grinding poverty that make robust support for soy farmers hard to achieve—will all certainly slow progress. But in the agricultural and culinary histories of East Asia, neither an animal feed market nor the eradication of severe poverty were necessary preconditions for the spread of soy cultivation and consumption. Soy gained acceptance without either condition within a wide variety of Asian climates and ecosystems.

Perhaps the most important difference between the East Asian cases and that of Bangladesh is time. Soy became popular in East Asia over the course of centuries, the time needed for a great deal of farmer and processor experimentation (Huang 2000). Soy has only seriously been pursued in Bangladesh for thirty years. We can, of course, expect greater speed in the present than in ancient times, but even in the resource-rich United States, some fifty years were necessary between the beginnings of the USDA's soy research to the rise of soy as a major crop, and soy is still not a major human food there.

Hope therefore remains for a vital link between soy protein and Bangladeshi nutrition in the future (if not, perhaps, for very many Bangladeshis in this generation). There is genuine reason to continue to be diligent in the many arenas related to soy farming and consumption, including equitable distribution of resources.[17] For Bangladeshi soy farmers and those who have put so much time and effort into helping them, there is even reason to be proud. The story of soy as a protein source in Bangladesh is really only just beginning, but it is a credibly good beginning.

Conclusion

The histories of soy in the United States and Bangladesh demonstrate the agronomic, trade, and culinary links that tie the food destinies of the two countries together. The capacities of each to affect the other are very unequal, however, as the 1974 famine in Bangladesh made tragically clear. With respect to soy, the main consequence of Bangladeshi food choices for the United States has been the small indirect support for U.S. soy prices that Bangladesh's willingness to accept surplus American oil has provided. But Bangladesh was only one of many countries receiving soy oil (Friedmann 1994, 182), and if it had not accepted the oil, another country would have done so in its place. Bangladesh's impact on the history and prospects for soy in the United States has therefore been minimal.

In contrast, by making available to consumers an oil that was both foreign and more affordable, the United States offer did lead to a change in the everyday cuisine of Bangladeshis. This dietary shift had a negative effect on the cultivation and processing of indigenous mustard oil. On a more positive note, the training that development workers received in the United States and the years of American science that informed that training have helped soy to become a minor yet finally viable and officially encouraged crop in Bangladesh. This advancement of soy in Bangladesh has come about in part because of the persistent labors of a North American service organization, the MCC. The MCC's success provides hope for the future improvement of Bangladeshi diets based on local agriculture. This success also indicates that the actions of the soybean superpower's government (in supporting scientific research on soy) and citizens (in undertaking soy development work abroad) have not all been problematic for vulnerable Bangladesh.

But a danger in the U.S.-Bangladeshi soy connection lurks on the horizon: if Bangladesh were to become more dependent on imports of soy meal from the United States (or India), as some would like, local soy farmers could be seriously undercut, and indigenous soy farming could disappear. Since the very poor would not then find soy in their local markets, they could become less likely to consume soy protein. The prospects for adding soy protein to the diets of impoverished Bangladeshis are thus subject to global trade and politics and are precarious.

The world agrifood system has become so complicated (Friedmann 2000), with so many variables and so many different countries interacting, that the twenty-first-century trajectory of soy in Bangladesh is quite uncertain. Huge complex questions loom behind the soy story. For one, it is not clear that the Green Revolution, with its reliance on agricultural chemicals and its toll on the environment, is sustainable in Bangladesh (see Alauddin and Hossain 2001; Friedmann 2000). If the techniques of the Green Revolution must be restructured or abandoned there, soil-renewing soy could be an important crop for agricultural researchers to consider. Crop scientists could put more effort into creating varieties of soy adapted to Bangladesh's diverse ecosystems, whether through genetic engineering or conventional breeding. But such painstaking effort is unlikely to be financially remunerative, and the private companies that currently fund so much of agricultural biotechnology would have little interest in it. Whether, instead, enough public or charitable funding will become available for soy research within (or on behalf of) poor countries such as Bangladesh remains to be seen.

A second uncertainty is how the trend in meat prices will affect the future of soy in Bangladesh. As demand for meat increases in China's enormous population, world meat production is expected to rise (USDA 2006a). The price of soy meal to feed farm animals may therefore also rise unless increased world soy production keeps the price down. It is unclear how shifts in world prices could affect soy farming in Bangladesh. The farmers would find higher soy prices an incentive for more production, but the higher price of soy meal could cause the local chicken industry financial difficulties. Such difficulties could make the soy-for-meal market unstable or even unsustainable within Bangladesh.

A starker question remains. In the long run, will population pressures, maldistribution of wealth, global warming, and the apathy of rich nations lead to famine in Bangladesh as existed in decades past? Mass intense hunger would make Bangladesh vulnerable to dislocations, violence, and desperate choices that could ultimately disrupt soy agriculture there.

The answers to these varied questions are not known. What we do know is that soy can provide a lens with which to view these larger issues as well as a source of hope for better nutrition among the world's poorest peoples.

Notes

1. Many individuals assisted me during the research and writing of this essay; I am grateful to all. Special thanks go to Laurence Buxbaum, Sidney Mintz, and above all to Emerson Nafziger and Kevin Stout. Any errors are, of course, entirely mine. The research was supported through grants from the Johns Hopkins University's Center for a Livable Future and the Salus Mundi Foundation.

2. They import either the oil itself or, more recently, the whole soybeans to crush within Bangladesh.

3. Their consumption rate has depended on the strength of the market for soy from year to year. Bangladesh's debt-ridden farmers generally prefer to sell their soy, if they can, rather than eat it.

4. The difficulty in obtaining accurate statistics is reflected in the contradictions among expert reports. Woodruff (1998, 3) lists a higher figure for 1997 (12,500 metric tons) even though production then was actually lower than now. By contrast, the USDA lists a significantly smaller figure of 3,000 metric tons for the relatively recent 2000–2001 harvest (USDA 2001, 1). Dr. Nafziger's observations on his research-consulting trip to Bangladesh in 2003 suggest the in-between figure of 7,000–10,000 metric tons.

5. However, a second plant is expected to be commissioned (USDA 2006b, 3).

6. See MCC (1991, 4–7), MCC (1996, 71), and Alauddin and Hossain (2001, 166). This was confirmed in personal communications in 2003 with Kevin Stout, former soybean agronomist and marketing/utilization specialist in Bangladesh with the Mennonite Central Committee, and Emerson Nafziger.

7. The U.S. government's donor shipments of soy oil to Bangladesh resumed in 2001 (USDA 2001; Anonymous 2001).

8. Some revenues from the program have, however, occasionally been used to promote soy farming in Bangladesh (Anonymous 2001; personal communication with Nafziger, 2003).

9. The MCC does not focus on converting non-Christians to Christianity. Although its workers will discuss their faith if asked about it and are active in local churches, their primary tasks are relief, development, and peace work.

10. Other organizations interested in encouraging consumption of a particular food—for example, the Malaysian Palm Oil Promotion Council—have also found cooking demonstrations to be an especially effective marketing tool in Bangladesh (Ismail 2002).

11. The government of Bangladesh is about three years behind in releasing official statistics on soy production. The unofficial estimate for the winter of 2005 lists a bit over eighteen thousand hectares devoted to soy (Stout, personal communication, 2005).

12. The ASA's program also includes some work with NGOs and the WFP to provide technical expertise or to make U.S. soy protein available to protein-deficient segments of the population (ASA, personal communication, 2005).

13. The U.S.-based Solae Company recently announced a collaboration in Bangladesh with Jayson Natural Products to produce nutritional products for mid- to higher-income consumers using U.S. soy protein. The collaboration may eventually have charitable components as well through the Bangladesh Red Crescent's Mother and Child Health Program (Solae Company, personal communication, 2005).

14. The Green Revolution's effects of at times increasing the skew of wealth distribution—and the power of the better-off to exploit the poor (see Lappé and Collins 1978)—does not seem to have been paralleled by any changes in the distribution of wealth or power attendant upon soybean cultivation as it is currently practiced in Bangladesh (personal communication with Nafziger, 2003).

15. The current accounts deficit is not so high once adjustments have been made for the remittances that Bangladeshi emigrants send home. For example, in 1997 a trade deficit of $2.7 billion was adjusted to $0.9 billion after taking remittances into account (FAO 1998).

16. Some soy meal is also used in Bangladesh to raise fish, but the quantities are even smaller than for chicken (personal communication with Nafziger, 2003).

17. The soy farming that the MCC promoted in Bangladesh does not appear to have caused any worsening of the distribution of land in that country.

References

Ahmed, A. W. Nuruddin, Lutful Hoque Chowdhury, and Steven Haggblade. 2000. "History of Public Food Interventions in Bangladesh." In Raisuddin Ahmed, Steven Haggblade, and Tawfiq-e-Elahi Chowdhury, eds., *Out of the Shadow of Famine: Evolving Food Markets and Food Policy in Bangladesh,* 121–36. Baltimore: Johns Hopkins University Press.

Ahmed, Akhter U. 2000. "Trends in Consumption, Nutrition, and Poverty." In Raisuddin Ahmed, Steven Haggblade, and Tawfiq-e-Elahi Chowdhury, eds., *Out of the Shadow of Famine: Evolving Food Markets and Food Policy in Bangladesh,* 101–17. Baltimore: Johns Hopkins University Press.

Ahmed, Raisuddin, and Steven Haggblade. 2000. "Introduction." In Raisuddin Ahmed, Steven Haggblade, and Tawfiq-e-Elahi Chowdhury, eds., *Out of the Shadow of Famine: Evolving Food Markets and Food Policy in Bangladesh,* 1–17. Baltimore: Johns Hopkins University Press.

Alauddin, Mohammad, and Mosharaff Hossain. 2001. *Environment and Agriculture in a Developing Economy: Problems and Prospects for Bangladesh.* Cheltenham, UK, and Northampton, MA: Edward Elgar.

Alauddin, Mohammad, and Clement Tisdell. 1991. *The "Green Revolution" and Economic Development: The Process and Its Impact in Bangladesh.* New York: St. Martin's.

Anonymous. 2001. "US—Soybean." *United News of Bangladesh* (Dhaka), December 4.

Atwood, David A., A. S. M. Jahangir, Herbie Smith, and Golam Kabir. 2000. "Food Aid in Bangladesh: From Relief to Development." In Raisuddin Ahmed, Steven Haggblade, and Tawfiq-e-Elahi Chowdhury, eds., *Out of the Shadow of Famine: Evolving Food Markets and Food Policy in Bangladesh,* 148–64. Baltimore: Johns Hopkins University Press.

Bangladesh Export Promotion Bureau of Bangladesh Bureau of Statistics. 2000. "Balance of Trade of Bangladesh." Dhaka: Bangladesh Export Promotion Bureau. Available through the Bangladeshi Embassy in Washington, DC.

Bangladesh Ministry of Food. 2002. "Bangladesh Food Situation Report." July. Dhaka, Bangladesh: Government of Bangladesh. http://www.mofdm.gov.bd/Bangladesh%20Food%20Situation%20Report.htm.

Dasgupta, Swapan Kumar. 1994. *Poverty and Food Insecurity: The Case of Bangladesh.* Kotbari, Comilla, Bangladesh: Bangladesh Academy for Rural Development.

FAO (Food and Agriculture Organization of the United Nations). 1998. "Special Report: FAO/WFP Crop and Food Supply Assessment Mission to Bangladesh." November 13. Rome, Italy: FAO. http://www.fao.org/docrep/004/x0619e/x0619e00.htm.

Friedmann, Harriet. 1994. "The International Relations of Food: The Unfolding Crisis of National Regulation." In Barbara Harriss-White and Sir Raymond Hoffenberg, eds., *Food: Multidisciplinary Perspectives,* 174–204. Oxford, UK: Blackwell.

———. 2000. "What on Earth Is the Modern World-System? Foodgetting and Territory in the Modern Era and Beyond." *Journal of World-Systems Research* 1(2) (Summer/Fall): 480–515.

Haggblade, Steven, and Raisuddin Ahmed. 2000. "Conclusion: Old Lessons and New Directions in Food Policy." In Raisuddin Ahmed, Steven Haggblade, and Tawfiq-e-Elahi Chowdhury, eds., *Out of the Shadow of Famine: Evolving Food Markets and Food Policy in Bangladesh,* 278–93. Baltimore: Johns Hopkins University Press.

Huang, H. T. 2000. *Science and Civilization in China,* Vol. 6, *Biology and Technology,* Pt. 5, *Fermentations and Food Science.* Cambridge: Cambridge University Press.

Ismail, Zaidi Isham. 2002. "Palm Oil Consumption Increasing, Says Council." *Business Times* (Malaysia), January 4, p. 4.

Khokan, K. I., and G. Horlings. 1987. "Soybean Production and Utilization in Bangladesh." Akron, PA: Mennonite Central Committee.

Lappé, Frances Moore, and Joseph Collins. 1978. *Food First: Beyond the Myth of Scarcity,* rev. ed. New York: Ballantine.

Lappé, Frances Moore, Joseph Collins, and David Kinley. 1981. *Aid As Obstacle: Twenty Questions about Our Foreign Aid and the Hungry.* San Francisco: Institute for Food and Development Policy.

Mahmud, Wahiduddin, Sultan Hafeez Rahman, and Sajjad Zohir. 2000. "Agricultural Diversification: A Strategic Factor for Growth." In Raisuddin Ahmed, Steven

Haggblade, and Tawfiq-e-Elahi Chowdhury, eds., *Out of the Shadow of Famine: Evolving Food Markets and Food Policy in Bangladesh,* 232–60. Baltimore: Johns Hopkins University Press.

MCC (Mennonite Central Committee). 1981. "A Summary of MCC's Soybean Research and Extension Activities 1975–1981 Bangladesh." Akron, PA: Mennonite Central Committee.

———. 1982. *Agriculture Program Bangladesh,* Vol. 9. Akron, PA: Mennonite Central Committee.

———.1983. *Agriculture Program Bangladesh,* Vol. 10. Akron, PA: Mennonite Central Committee.

———.1985. *Agriculture Program Bangladesh,* Vol. 12. Akron, PA: Mennonite Central Committee.

———.1986. *Agriculture Program Bangladesh,* Vol. 13. Akron, PA: Mennonite Central Committee.

———.1987. *Agriculture Program Bangladesh,* Vol. 14. Akron, PA: Mennonite Central Committee.

———.1989. *Agriculture Program Bangladesh,* Vol. 16. Akron, PA: Mennonite Central Committee.

———. 1990a. *Soybeans for Institutional, Commercial, Village and Home Level Use in Bangladesh.* Akron, PA: Mennonite Central Committee.

———.1990b. *Agriculture Program Bangladesh,* Vol. 17. Akron, PA: Mennonite Central Committee.

———. 1991. *Agriculture Program Bangladesh,* Vol. 18. Akron, PA: Mennonite Central Committee.

———.1992. *Agriculture Program Bangladesh,* Vol. 19. Akron, PA: Mennonite Central Committee.

———.1993. *Agriculture Program Bangladesh,* Vol. 20. Akron, PA: Mennonite Central Committee.

———.1994. *Agriculture Program Bangladesh,* Vol. 21. Akron, PA: Mennonite Central Committee.

———.1995. *Agriculture Program Bangladesh,* Vol. 22. Akron, PA: Mennonite Central Committee.

———.1996. *Agriculture Program Bangladesh,* Vol. 23. Akron, PA: Mennonite Central Committee.

———.2001. *Agriculture Program Research Results 1999 to 2000 Bangladesh,* Vol. 26. Akron, PA: Mennonite Central Committee.

———.2002. *Agriculture Program Research Results 2001 Bangladesh,* Vol. 27. Akron, PA: Mennonite Central Committee.

Sato, Noriaki. 1990. "JOCV Volunteers: Introducing Soybeans to Bangladesh Farmers." *Daily Yomiuri,* April 27, p. 3.

Shurtleff, William, and Akiko Aoyagi. 2007. "History of Soybeans and Soyfoods in the Indian Subcontinent." http://www.soyinfocenter.com/HSS/indian_subcon1.php.

U.S. Bureau of the Census. 2008. International Data Base. http://www.census.gov/ipc/www/idb/country/bgportal.html. See IDB Table Access for Bangladesh at bottom of page.

USDA (United States Department of Agriculture). 1997. "Bangladesh Annual." Report from the American Embassy, Delhi, India. Washington, DC: U.S. Department of Agriculture. September 15.

———. 1998. "Bangladesh Oilseed & Products, Annual Report." Washington, DC: United States Department of Agriculture.

———. 2001. *Bangladesh Oilseeds and Products Annual 2001*. Washington, DC: United States Department of Agriculture. www.fas.usda.gov/gainfiles/200105/90680505.pdf.

———. 2004. *Bangladesh Oilseeds and Products Annual 2004*. Washington, DC: United States Department of Agriculture. www.fas.usda.gov/gainfiles/200404/146106190.pdf.

———. 2006a. "Briefing Room: Corn Market Outlook." http://www.ers.usda.gov/Briefing/corn/2005baseline.htm.

———. 2006b. *Bangladesh Oilseeds and Products Annual 2006*. May 1. Washington, DC: United States Department of Agriculture. www.fas.usda.gov/gainfiles/200605/146187616.pdf.

Verhoef, Linda. 1996. "Impact Study of Cooking Demonstrations in Soybean Programme MCC." Unpublished report available from the Mennonite Central Committee, Akron, Pennsylvania.

WFP (World Food Programme of the United Nations). 2003. "Soybean and School Feeding Programme in Bangladesh." Paper available from the World Food Programme Bangladesh, Dhaka.

Woodruff, John M. 1998. "Report on the Soybean: Its Status and Potential for Bangladesh." A report prepared for the Ministry of Agriculture for the Government of the People's Republic of Bangladesh, by RONCO Consultancy/Winrock International.

Xinhua General Overseas News Service. 1990. "Soybean Farming Suitable in Northwest Bangladesh." August 14.

14

Soybeans and Soybean Products in West Africa

Adoption by Farmers and Adaptation to Foodways

DONALD Z. OSBORN

Introduction

Soybeans are a historically recent introduction to Africa, with the first systematic, if episodic, experiments beginning about a century ago.[1] Long a minor crop destined mainly for export and a focus of development programs, it has gradually been finding a place in local agriculture and cuisine.

The process of introduction of this new crop in West Africa, its adoption by farmers, and its adaptation to foodways merit attention for several reasons. First, soybeans represent, as even early researchers suggested, both an excellent source of protein for a continent too often facing malnutrition and hunger and a crop well suited to most agroecological conditions there. Second, the specific case of the spread of bean curd making in eastern West Africa is interesting in part for the insights it may give into endogenous mechanisms for accepting, transforming, and transferring new technology. Finally, and partly related to the previous reason, the gradual acceptance of soybeans in agriculture and foodways in parts of Africa may offer insights into the historical spread of new crops introduced to the continent from the Americas a half millennium ago.

History

The first introductions of soybeans in West Africa were made early in the last century (table 2). Europeans were interested in introducing species of various sorts in their newly acquired African colonies, and among food crops soybeans seemed to hold particular promise.[2]

Introduction of and experimentation with soybeans in Africa was, especially in the early years, undertaken through individual (European) initiative, and the source of the beans was northeastern China. These efforts were often not sustained, and it may actually be that in many parts of the continent, soybeans were reintroduced on separate occasions, perhaps years apart, by different people or organizations. A number of sources trace parts of this history in greater detail (Root, Oyekan, and Dashiell 1987; Smith, Woodworth, and Dashiell 1993; Shannon and Kalala 1994; Shurtleff and Aoyagi 1997).

Although introduction of soybeans into many areas did not occur until the latter half of the twentieth century and although experimentation continues today, there are several periods that can be tentatively identified in the history of soybeans across the continent. The first period would encompass the early introductions in a few localities, mainly in some British possessions before World War I. Although there had been some attempts to grow soybeans in French-ruled Algeria as early as the late nineteenth century, the French apparently did not try introducing them to their West African territories until later.

Table 2. Earliest Documentation of Soybeans in West African Countries

Country	*Year First Noted*	*Source*
Benin	1935 or 1939	Portères 1946; Matagrin 1939
Burkina Faso (former Upper Volta)	1942	Chevalier 1948
Cameroon	1924	Numfor 1983
Côte d'Ivoire	1939	Matagrin 1939; Chevalier 1948
Gambia	1909	Pynaert 1920
Ghana	1909	Snow 1961
Guinea	1935	Portères 1946
Guinea-Bissau	1981	Jackobs, Smyth, and Erickson 1984
Liberia	1974	Wenger 1976
Mali	1923	Vuillet 1924
Niger	1975	Whigham and Judy 1978
Nigeria	1908	Ezendinma 1964
Senegal	1963	IRAT/CNRA 1964
Sierra Leone	1913	IIA 1936
Togo	1939	Matagrin 1939

Between the wars there were more systematic efforts to introduce and experiment with soybeans over much of the continent (see, e.g., Morse 1939; Matagrin 1939), and even to produce them commercially. There was interest in growing the crop as an oilseed to supply growing European demand for edible oils.

This incremental progress continued after World War II until the period when most African countries gained independence (ca. 1960). However, Englebeen (1948) estimated that at midcentury soybeans were still in an experimental stage in Africa, and Morse (1950; cf. Morse 1939) repeated his earlier assessment that although experiments had been conducted in most regions of the continent, the crop was unfamiliar to African farmers.

Since the 1970s there seems to have been a new impetus for work on soybeans with the founding of the International Institute of Tropical Agriculture (IITA) in Ibadan, Nigeria, in 1967 and of the International Soybean Program (INTSOY) based at the University of Illinois in the United States in 1973. These institutions, in collaboration with others, facilitated more systematic research and exchange of information on soybeans in African cropping systems and on uses of soybeans in Africa.

Growing Soybeans in Africa

Promotion of the soybean as a crop in Africa has encountered two main types of problems. First, there has been a need to get the crop to perform well in local conditions, which has mainly been a matter of plant characteristics. The plant features cited as limiting optimal growth and yields of soybeans have included growth characteristics, seed germination, pod shattering, photoperiodicity, and the need for Bradyrhizobia.[3] Ultimately, problems of this kind have been overcome through variety selection and plant breeding.

The second challenge has been to give farmers a reason to plant soy, with limited land and labor already devoted to other crops. The early years of soybean agriculture involved low levels of overall production. Farmers in various parts of the continent grew soybeans in response to colonial policies. In some cases cultivation began and stopped when farmers found little benefit. For instance, Chevalier (1948) noted that farmers in one region of Côte d'Ivoire simply refused to grow the crop due to low yields and prices.

Generally there was not a lot of reason for African farmers to grow soybeans at all, let alone in the place of traditional crops, unless it was for a sufficient price. In particular, smallholder farmers, who account for the vast majority of African agriculture even today, would not be likely to take risks with a crop that was either unfamiliar or for which there was no commonly accepted food use. Nevertheless, introduction and cultivation of the soybean continued such that by the 1970s, although it was not a major crop anywhere in the region, it was more widely known.[4]

In Nigeria, for example, soybean production was most notable in the Benue state, where it had been introduced in the mid-twentieth century (Shannon and Kalala 1994). Before the Biafra War, all soybeans produced there were exported (Root, Oyekan, and Dashiell 1987). However, after the war, presumably because of the conflict's disruption to the previous export trade, soybeans were sold to *daddawa* producers in the Kaduna region (Shannon and Kalala 1994).

The IITA's work to promote soybeans since the latter part of the 1970s has served to significantly increase farmer adoption of this crop, especially in Nigeria. In 2000 after a little more than two decades, Nigerian annual production of the crop had risen twentyfold to half a million tons, the largest for any country in Africa (FutureHarvest 2001).

Outside of West Africa, soybean production has been notable in Zimbabwe, which for some years was Africa's major producer (until Nigeria surpassed it), and the Democratic Republic of the Congo (formerly Zaire), where efforts to introduce it by missionaries led to its adoption by some farmers (Root, Oyekan, and Dashiell 1987) and incorporation into some foods (Shannon and Kalala 1994).

Soybeans As Food

Various efforts to expand the use of soybeans as food naturally followed or accompanied its promotion as a crop. Some of these efforts were associated with research on cultivating the crop; some with the work of missionaries, development projects, or foreign volunteers; and some with the food processing industry.

Early on, preparation of the unfamiliar soybean and its incorporation into local foodways posed various problems. Portères (1945, 1946) mentions cases in West Africa where local people did not know how to cook soybeans, the assumption being to treat them as other beans and the question arising as to how long to boil them. In another case, in East Africa, Maidment (1946) noted that people ate soybeans green or after roasting. It is not clear that such uses were of sufficient interest for people to continue cultivation.

Later efforts, generally foreign sponsored, focused on different ways to process and incorporate soybeans into other foods.[5] Some of these efforts were primarily concerned with nutritional benefits (for example, within hospitals dealing with malnutrition). In general, however, at least during the colonial period, the main focus of interest in soybeans was as a crop for export.

The processing of soybeans on an industrial scale into cooking oil and for incorporation into various processed foods was and is significant in certain countries such as Nigeria and Zimbabwe, but consideration of this goes beyond the scope of the present essay. Instead, the focus here is on nonindustrial production and on the consumption of soy protein, rather than soy oil.

Soybeans for *Daddawa*

One relatively early and by now fairly common adaptation of soybeans to local foodways in West Africa has been its use as a substitute for seeds of the *nèrè*, or African locust bean tree (*Parkia biglobosa*), in the making of the fermented condiment known by various names, notably *daddawa* (or *dawa-dawa*) in Hausa, *sumbala* in Mande languages, and *iru* in Yoruba. Chevalier (1947) noted this use in the 1940s in an area of Guinea where soybean cultivation was being tried, although it is not clear either whether the practice continued there in the ensuing years or whether it spread to other areas from there. Mention of soybeans for *daddawa* surfaces in some literature later on, for instance in what is now Burkina Faso (Kay 1974b), where at first the darker varieties were preferred (Picasso 1986), and in Nigeria in the 1960s (Yuwa 1963–64; Shannon and Kalala 1994). By the mid-1980s soybeans had become the main ingredient for *daddawa* in Nigeria (INTSOY 1987), and *daddawa* had become the most widely consumed food made with soybeans in rural West Africa (Weingartner, Dashiell, and Nelson 1987).

Daddawa is a commonly used seasoning, generally cooked in sauces for eating with grain-based staples. It is sometimes dried and crumbled on certain dishes. The physical form of the product may vary slightly, appearing as a small ball, patty, or cluster of ripened beans, but it is always black in color and has a very pungent odor. It is produced locally or traded widely from certain areas known for production.[6] Vendors in local markets may sell it along with other condiments and ingredients used in local cuisine.

Traditionally a woman's activity, the making of *daddawa* is somewhat labor-intensive, consumes significant amounts of firewood, and has the inconvenience of producing a strong odor. The process, which may vary slightly by region and among producers, is described in the following way (using the Yoruba term *iru*):

> The traditional process for producing *iru* begins with the manual removal of the pod's outer layer. The yellow pulp inside the pod, in which the seed is embedded, is then soaked in water and strained through a sieve or basket to remove the seeds. The clean seeds are boiled in water for about 24 hours to soften the hard seed coat. When the seeds are cool, the seed coats are loosened through abrasion. They float to the top of the water while the clean beans settle to the bottom of the container. The next stage is fermentation. The clean beans are wrapped in leaves or plastic and placed in an air-tight container. This is kept at room temperature for three to seven days depending on the type of *iru* to be produced. Usually charcoal is placed on top to aid fermentation. After fermentation the product is ready for use. For storage, common salt is added and the product is then dried in the sun. The salted, dried *iru* can be kept for months (IKWW 2002).

The fermentation process involves bacteria belonging to the genus *Bacillus,* typically *B. subtilis* (Steinkraus 2002). No inoculum is used. The production and fermentation processes are similar for locust beans and soybeans. Also, the nutritional profiles of the end products—high in protein (particularly the amino acid lysine) and a good source of B-group vitamins (Sakyi-Dawson, Nartey, Amoa-Awuah 2001; Diawara et al. 2000; Baccus-Taylor and Gail n.d.)—are similar.

Locust beans and soybeans have different advantages in the making of *daddawa,* but trends seem to favor expanded soybean use. Locust beans, aside from being the traditional ingredient familiar to *daddawa* makers, are relatively easily gathered when the trees come into fruit, whereas soybeans require cultivation. Also, the sweet yellow pulp in the locust bean pod can be eaten raw or processed into a snack. The African locust bean tree is "about 10 to 25m in height and may produce 25 to 100 kg of fruit (pods) containing about 30% seeds in a year" (Diawara et al. 2000), so in areas where the tree is plentiful it is possible to obtain surpluses for surplus production or sale to producers elsewhere. In fact, the ripe pods are often sold in local markets across the region.

Soybeans, on the other hand, are easier to prepare and, being smaller, take as little as a quarter as long to cook (Waters-Bayer 1988). Also, the product made with soybeans has no disadvantage with consumers compared to the locust bean *daddawa.* A significant advantage of soybeans is that as an annual crop, it can be produced readily to respond to increased demand, whereas African locust bean trees begin fruiting at eight years and take that many more years to reach peak production (Von Maydell 1990). Indeed, rapid population growth in the region (around 3 percent) would seem to predict both less potential for the tree to regenerate (it is not the object of significant replanting efforts) and ever-greater demand for *daddawa* than what can be produced from existing locust bean harvest levels. Gutierrez (1999), in the case of Benin, and Shao (2002) in Ghana note this fact as well as the increased substitution of soybeans for locust beans in making *daddawa*.[7]

In addition to these longer-term trends, it is likely that specific events have given added impetus to the use of soybeans in particular places. For instance, Smith, Woodworth, and Dashiell (1993) note that substitution of soybeans for locust beans in Nigeria increased as a result of the severe drought in 1984 (since low rainfall affects locust pod yields). In that same year, also in Nigeria, an IITA survey estimated that 60 percent of *daddawa* was made from soybeans and another 20 percent made from a combination of locust beans and soybeans (INTSOY 1987).

As production of soybeans has become more common in certain areas, it has been increasingly easy and accepted to use them to make *daddawa* in place of scarce or expensive locust beans. I am not aware of any survey of production of *daddawa* region-wide, but anecdotal evidence suggests that even where soybeans are not a significant crop, the needs of *daddawa* producers make alternatives a necessary option, and this has encouraged small-scale cultivation of soybeans.[8] An interesting question is whether producers who have switched to using soybeans will ever return to using the traditional ingredient.

The use of other alternatives to locust bean in the making of *daddawa* is not unknown. In some areas the seeds of roselle or red sorrel (*Hibiscus sabdariffa*) are used,[9] and groundnuts can also be used. However, soybeans have clearly achieved a rapid and wide acceptance as a preferred ingredient for this condiment.

In this role, soybeans may be considered to have become an African crop, but it is with the spread of locally made bean curd that it is achieving a higher level of impact on African foodways.

Bean Curd

Although bean curd is well known in much of the world outside its region of origin, it is not frequently made in Africa,[10] and efforts to introduce it and the techniques to make it have generally fared no better than efforts to promote other local uses of soybeans for food there.

However, the IITA's program of research on and promotion of soybean products in Nigeria did achieve significant success. A turning point in this effort was the work of Osamu Nakayama, a soyfoods expert brought by the Japanese International Cooperation Agency (JICA) to work with the IITA in Ibadan during 1989–91. Working with local people, he noted the potential to adapt a traditional technique for making an unripened dairy cheese, commonly called *wagashi,* to the making of bean curd (IITA 1998; JICA 2001). The technique involved the sap of the giant milkweed or Sodom apple tree (*Calotropis procera*) to curdle cow's milk. Although the idea of making a soy-based substitute for the cheese was not new (see, e.g., Kay 1974a), apparently adapting this curdling ingredient had not been tried successfully.

The process for making *wagashi* cheese is fairly well known, at least in some parts of eastern West Africa.[11] The Calotropis sap can be extracted from every part of the plant except the roots.[12] A common way of obtaining the sap involves crushing the leaves, which are rather thick. The cleaned leaves and soft stems are crushed on a grinding stone and then either placed in water or mixed with some milk. This liquid is then strained or poured off the top and then added to fresh milk that is being heated up. The curds and whey separate, and the mixture can easily be poured through a strainer. The curds are then pressed together with something heavy so that they will stick together and the residual whey will drain out. The pressed curd is then turned over so that the other side can drain. A round patty is thus produced (Amanda Rawls, former Peace Corps volunteer in Togo, personal communication, 2002; Kees n.d.).

This product, also known as *wara* (in Yoruba), is a firm white cheese with very small holes. It is commonly cut up and deep-fried to eat with spices or cooked in a sauce for eating with a grain-based staple.

According to Nakayama, it took six months of research to determine how best to use this curdling ingredient to solidify soymilk (JICA 2001). The resultant bean curd, resembling more the local dairy cheese than Asian tofu, readily found a role as a substitute for the former. It compared well with the cheese in flavor and texture and had the important advantage of being much less expensive to produce.[13]

In the ensuing decade, the making of bean curd spread largely on its own through the north of Nigeria and across the border into Niger, becoming an important income-earning activity for many women. As it spread, other ingredients for solidifying soymilk were identified by local producers, notably water in which tamarind fruit had been left to soak and the water from rinsing pounded pearl millet, left overnight (JICA 2001).

Soybeans and Bean Curd in Niger

Soybeans have been the subject of a limited amount of agronomic research in Niger and are not produced in any significant amount. In part this is due to the dry climate, but even in areas where it could be grown in the south, it has not yet been cultivated in any notable way.[14] Nevertheless, since at least the year 2000 the making and marketing of bean curd made with soybeans from Nigeria has begun in many villages, towns, and markets, mainly in the Hausa-speaking south-central part of the country.

The earliest instances of bean curd making were apparently in southern parts of the Zinder and Maradi regions in about 2000.[15] In 2001 it was possible to find it in local villages' weekly markets in these areas, fried and sold with red pepper (capsicum) spice, much as other snacks common in such gathering places. By 2002 it was more readily available in the cities of Zinder and Maradi and was produced in Birnin'Konni in the Tahoua region. By 2003 it was available in Gaya, and by midyear it was also available in Dosso town in the Dosso region.

Bean curd making, like the soybeans used, clearly spread along Hausa networks that cross the border.[16] It would seem significant that the Hausa names used for bean curd differ between Zinder and Maradi on the one hand, where a loanword from Yoruba—*awara*—is used, and Birnin'Konni on the other hand, where the term used is *ƙwai-da-ƙwai,* which implies a comparison with the texture of eggs. This suggests that different networks within the larger Hausaphone area were involved in transmitting the bean curd technique.[17] It will be of significant interest, therefore, to follow this evolution in the western predominately ethnically Zarma region of Niger.

The making of bean curd in Niger is a small-scale home activity. Women who make it generally do so to coincide with weekly markets or, if in larger towns, perhaps two or three times a week or even daily in response to demand. Three curdling agents are used, generally depending on the area. The two innovations indicated above—pearl millet washing water and water with tamarind—are used in the Zinder and Maradi areas, with the former innovation more frequent in villages and the latter more frequent in towns. In Birnin'Konni, the women use a potassium salt that is left behind in shallow, evaporated ponds; it is known locally as *dalas.* It is added directly into the soymilk in which it dissolves, solidifying it (personal communication with Amanda Ree, former Peace Corps volunteer in Niger, 2004).

The typical process as observed or related in several locations in Niger[18] begins with grinding dry soybeans into flour at a local mill. This is different from the common technique elsewhere, which involves soaking the beans before making the curd. The bean flour is soaked in water, with any clumps broken up by hand, before filtering and mixing with a larger quantity of water for heating. The mixture is heated in a large pot over a wood fire. Once it reaches boiling, the coagulant is added. The coagulated mixture is ladled onto a cloth used as a filter, and the curds are then pressed using weights (generally as simple as a pot lid with rocks) long enough for the whey to be separated out. The resulting product is generally cut into cubes for sale as is or after frying (figures 10–13).

Although the process involves more work for women than some other kinds of food preparation for small-income generation, if all the bean curd is sold the profits are more than twice what is invested in the soybeans and other materials.[19] An additional benefit of bean curd making is access to the by-products. Typically a liquid by-product, such as the water used to wash pearl millet or the whey from making bean curd, would be given to animals to drink. The solids left from the initial filtering of the soyflour and water mixture can find a number of uses including addition to other foods.

Other Local Uses

Soybeans have also been incorporated into other traditional dishes on the local level in West Africa, although this practice is not widespread. As indicated above, this approach has been encouraged by various foreign individuals, projects, and agencies as a way of fortifying local foods. A partial list from Nigeria and Cameroon follows:

1. *gari*—grated fermented dried cassava with soybean added (Egounlety 1997)
2. *fufu*—doughlike dish made from yams or cassava with soy flour added (Numfor and Noubi 1995)
3. *ogi*—fermented maize-based stiff-porridge in which soy flour is included
4. *moimoi*—steamed cowpea flour, with soy flour as a partial substitute (Shannon 1992)

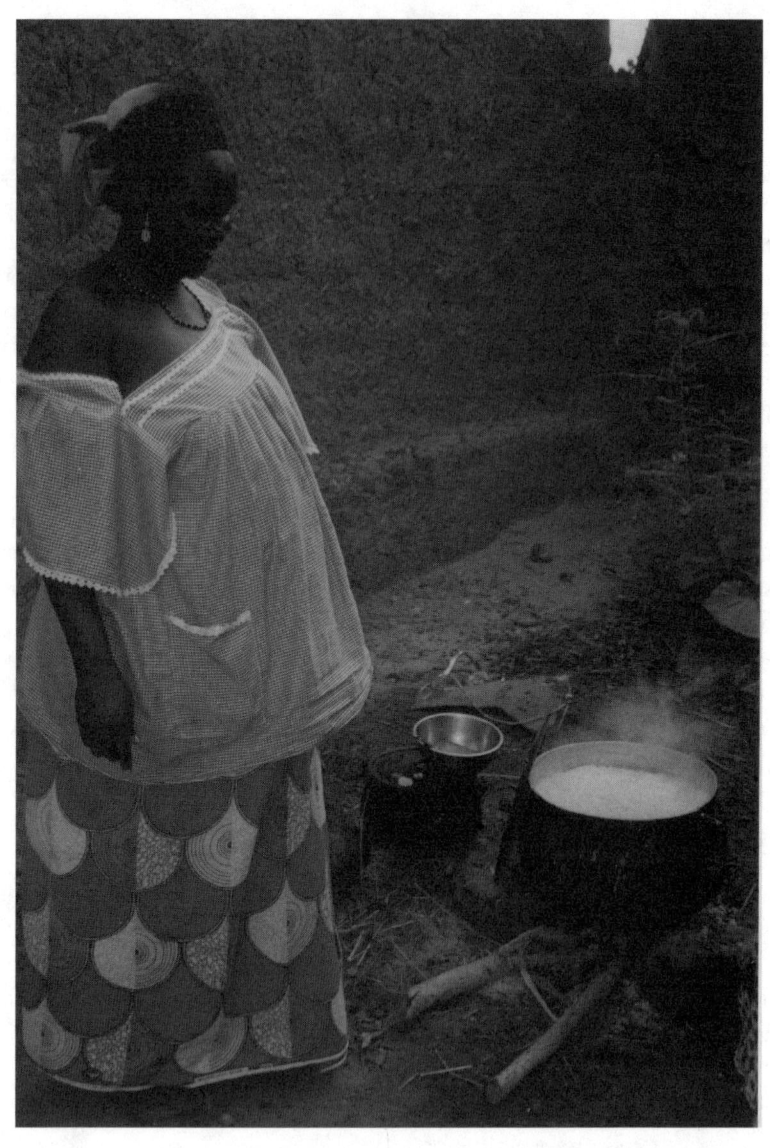

Figure 10. Heating water and a soy flour mixture to make bean curd in the village of Guiddan Iddar, Niger, West Africa. (Photo by Amanda Ree, 2004)

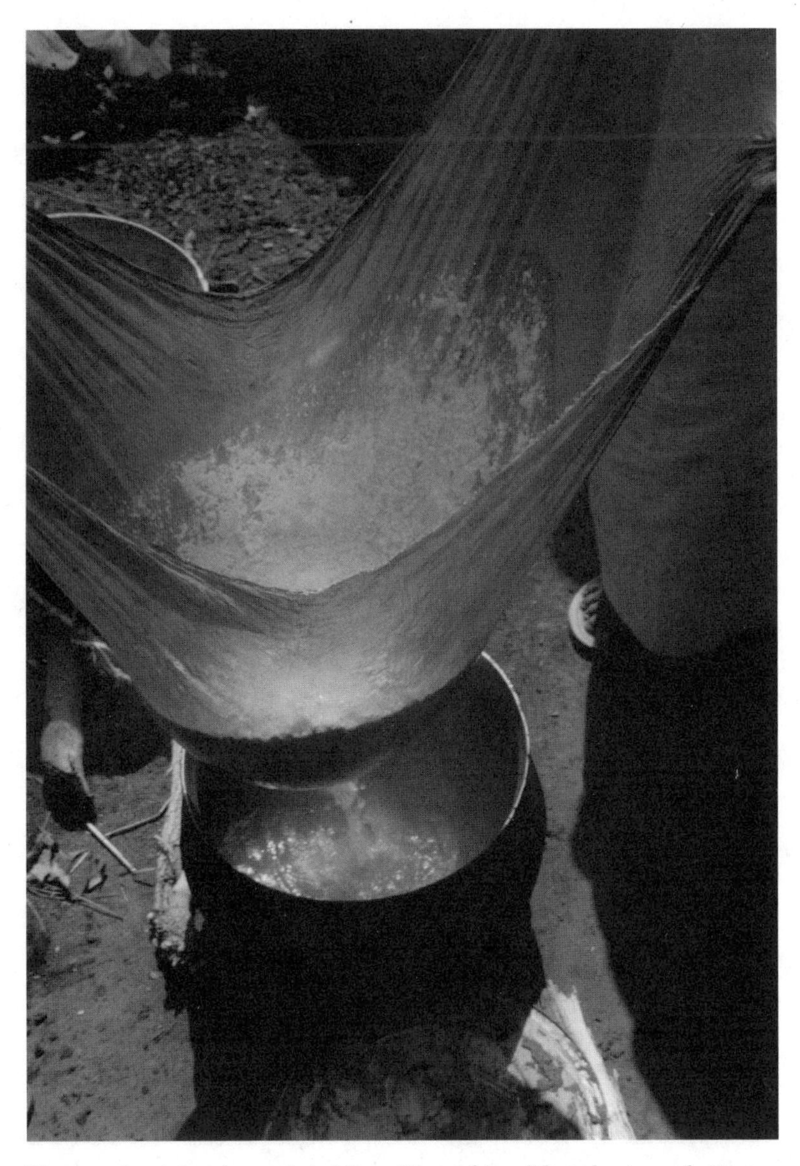

Figure 11. Straining the curds in Niger, West Africa. (Photo by Amanda Ree, 2004)

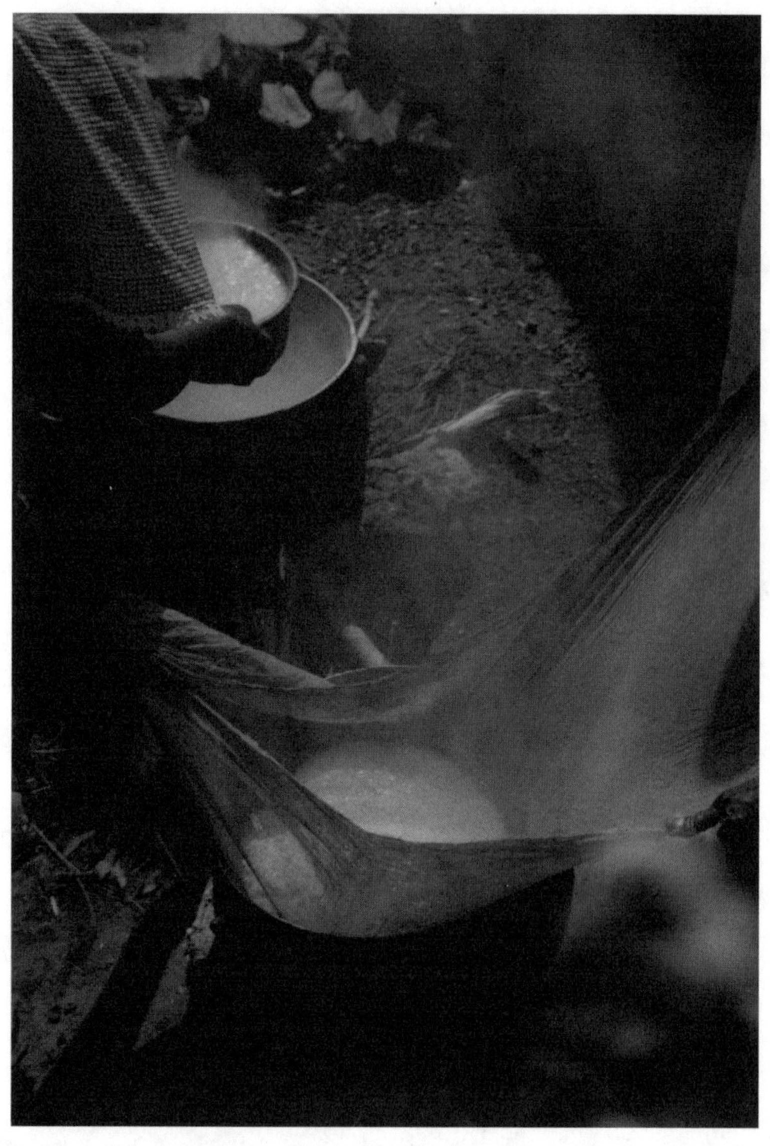

Figure 12. Straining one batch of curds while cooking the soy mixture for another batch. (Photo by Amanda Ree, 2004)

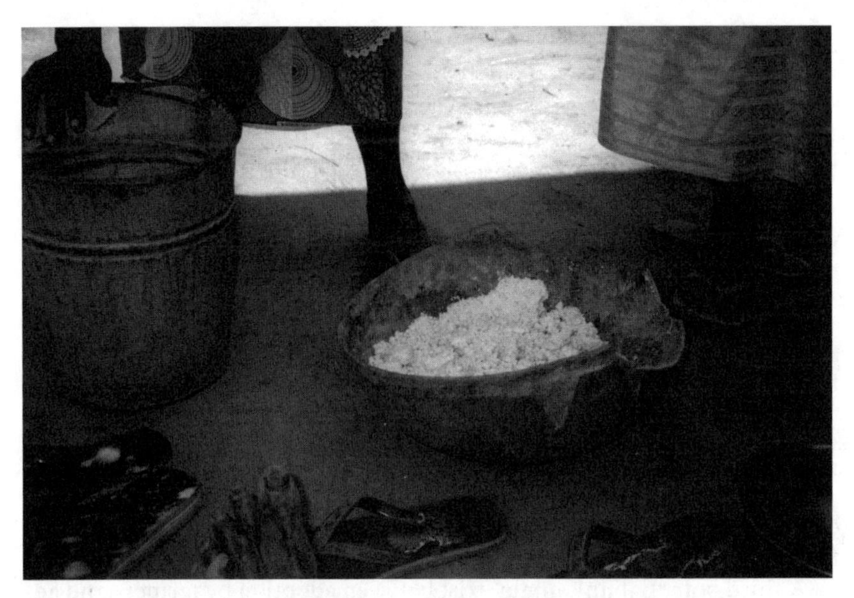

Figure 13. Finished curds awaiting pressing. (Photo by Amanda Ree, 2004)

5. *akara*—fritters made with cowpea flour, with soy flour as a partial substitute (Shannon 1992)

In such cases, which involve a partial substitution that is largely a matter of choice, the soy element would always be nonessential from the production or consumption points of view, however beneficial it might be from nutritional or even economic points of view.

Soybeans have been readily adopted as a main ingredient or as a complete substitute for various other foods, including for an oilseed such as peanuts,[20] for locust beans in *daddawa,* and for milk in *wagashi* cheese. The question remains as to whether, by contrast, the soybean in combination with (i.e., as an additive to) traditional ingredients has become or will become the general rule in local preferences, whether it will remain merely an option, or whether it will eventually be abandoned.

Conclusion

There can be two sorts of links between the farmers growing a new crop and the local people making use of it. The first arises when farmers grow it for a reason other than local consumption (such as cash crops), and local people come to find uses for it (unless it cannot easily be processed locally, as is the case with cocoa, or unless belief systems discourage this sort of experimentation). The second is when people have a use for it and thus seek to grow it. Of course, the two are often linked, sometimes in complex ways, but the more we observe the second (demand-driven) link, the more we can say that the crop is indigenized.

In the case of soybeans in West Africa, there are areas—especially in Nigeria—where soybeans were a cash crop for export, and the first link mentioned above was likely preeminent. This has facilitated people's trying out local uses for soybeans, such as making soy *daddawa* or partially substituting soy for other ingredients in various products.

There are also areas where people have more recently been seeking to grow soybeans to supply the demand for making *daddawa* because of a scarcity of locust beans. There the second link is more important. In other words, soybeans in this kind of situation have recently found a ready niche in local food systems.

A third potential link might exist between adoption by farmers and adaptation to foodways, and that link is the role of an outside agency, whether national or foreign. In the case of soybeans there have been many efforts to encourage their cultivation and utilization. For farmers to grow it there needs to be some incentive, and for a nonstaple crop grown for cash, this can come and go with changes in the market. For people to take it into their eating habits is another matter. A lot of promotion of soybean consumption in Africa seems to have sought to teach lessons about its nutritional value, which, however true, are no more likely to prompt widespread adoption there than anywhere else in the world.

Nakayama's remarkable summing up of why previous attempts to introduce soybean products in Nigeria failed, while his succeeded, imparts a lesson for other such efforts: "It's not true that soybean products have not been eaten in Nigeria in the past because they have a peculiar smell. It is because of how we tried to make the Nigerians eat soybeans. We pushed Japanese eating styles on the locals, which only made them reject soybeans. I showed Nigerians how to make tofu, but I left how to eat it up to them" (JICA 2001). In effect, Nakayama, the JICA, and the IITA were able to successfully make a connection between, on the one hand, familiar techniques and foods and, on the other hand, a crop not previously associated with those and then to give the initiative to the intended beneficiaries.

Bean curd spread quickly in Nigeria and into Niger once presented as a substitute for a traditional cheese, but will it spread to other parts of West

Africa where the cheese, and indeed soybeans, are not as well known? In looking at this question and the potential for other soy products, it may help to better understand the local networks that have spread innovations as well as the way that preparation techniques relate to existing food practices.

This spread of bean curd making seems to be mainly a matter of women learning from other women, with very little if any outside involvement (other than some instances of outsiders such as Peace Corps volunteers in Niger facilitating local women's learning from each other). Indeed, transfer of the technique across the border from Nigeria into south-central Niger did not involve any outside agency. Part of the reason that the recent appearance of bean curd making in non-Hausa areas of western Niger is interesting is that the network is being expanded across cultural boundaries.

The spread of soybeans for *daddawa* must also involve women's networks, but the as yet little-documented story of this diffusion across West Africa is likely to be found to be more complicated than the spread of bean curd since it happened over a longer period in a larger region and may even have involved independent development of the technique in different places.

As for techniques, the substitution of soybeans for locust beans in *daddawa* involves little change to existing production methods. In this case, production techniques for soy dovetail very well with local food practices.

In the case of bean curd, it seems that unlike women in Nigeria where the technique was first introduced by the IITA and the JICA, many of the women (perhaps all) who are making it in Niger have not previously made *wagashi* cheese. There could be several reasons for this (e.g., women in sedentary communities may not have access to sufficient milk, and knowledge of the *wagashi* processing technique may not have spread that far), but the important thing is that they are successfully learning and practicing a technique that has previously unfamiliar elements, notably those related to coagulation and pressing. On the other hand, other elements of the process are very routine, and ways of handling and consuming the end product fit local foodways.

This may be a key lesson for understanding the spread of preparation techniques for and consumption of new foods. Once a new crop and a new way of processing it are established in a local system—which may be facilitated to the extent that familiar techniques are used—then transfer to other local systems may not be so much of a challenge, even where the crop and process are less familiar. This certainly seems to be the case among Hausa communities from northern Nigeria into Niger. The spread of the bean curd making to other ethnic communities and parts of the region will offer further information on mechanisms and the success of such transfer.

Given the central role of women in the spread of bean curd making and the making of *daddawa* with soybeans and the effect that these have had on the local value of soybeans as a crop, another question concerns what can be inferred about the past roles of women in the spread of new crops and ways of consuming them. In the rural economy, the value of a food crop is in its consumption or in one's ability to trade it to other areas. Since the cash crop economy is relatively new in this region, in the past any newly introduced crop such as maize or groundnuts would have had to find a use in local foodways before being accepted. In other words, a new crop would have been likely to find a niche only as a food, and since women traditionally have responsibility in households for food preparation, their ability to find ways to use the crop would seem to have been critical to its spread.

In the case of soybeans in West Africa, although there are other factors in the spread of the crop, it seems that the techniques for *daddawa* and bean curd have been passed on mainly among women, from those who know it to those who learn. The role of cultivation of the crop—whether done by men or women—is of course essential. But the question is whether in the case of historically introduced crops their adoption by farmers followed their adaptation to foodways, as appears to be the case today with soybean in Niger, which in turn implies a primary role for women in the process, or whether there were other dynamics in the spread of the crops and incorporation into local eating habits.

In any event, it is clear that soybeans have gained a solid niche in both the agriculture of West Africa as an export crop and increasingly for local use and in its foodways, particularly as an ingredient for *daddawa* and for the making of bean curd. They also play a dynamic role in some household economies and in food consumption in the eastern part of the region, including the continent's most populous country, Nigeria. Although Africa still accounts for a tiny proportion of world soy production,[21] soybeans are now as never before an African crop and food.

Notes

1. I am indebted to Kit O'Connor, Amanda Ree, Stephanie Sandford, Yacouba Sangaré, Leah Smith, and Nakamura H. Sule for their help. The content of this essay is of course my responsibility alone.

2. One particular source seems as prophetic as it does premature: "Some people maintain that there is a great future before growers of the [soy]beans in West and

South Africa, and experiments go to prove this theory perfectly sound" (African World, April 1910, as quoted in Shurtleff and Aoyagi 1997).

3. Rhizobia—soil bacteria that can live in symbiosis with legume species such as soybeans and give the plants their ability to fix nitrogen—exist in many different genera and strains, not all of which are compatible with every variety of legume. Early introductions of soybean varieties encountered soils without compatible Bradyrhizobia, which meant low yields and a consequent need to add small quantities of appropriate strains when planting in order to achieve optimal performance.

4. I had the experience in the plateau region of Togo in 1980 of being able to obtain a small quantity of soybeans through local connections for a demonstration field in Amlamé. Some other farmers on hearing of this inquired about making soymilk, which they had learned about some years earlier from Taiwanese working on a small rice project in nearby Amou-Oblo.

5. I encountered discussions of this approach in West Africa in the 1980s. In some ways this partial-substitution approach resembled the then relatively novel technique in the Western world of incorporating soybeans into ground meat, except that in this case the objective was something that could boost protein in grain-based staples.

6. Some of the *daddawa* sold in markets in Niger originates from Nigeria.

7. Gutierrez and Juhé-Beaulaton (2002) also note increased prices for locust beans in markets, citing a tripling of their price over a ten-year period in Abomey, Benin.

8. I have heard that soybeans are being used by women making *daddawa* (*sumbala* as it is known locally) in the Sikasso region of Mali and also that soybeans were being grown in small quantities to meet this new demand.

9. This is common in the predominately ethnically Zarma areas of western Niger and yields a product with a characteristic taste.

10. It is not even made where one might expect to find it. Up until at least 2000, tofu was not available in any of the several Chinese restaurants in the Malian capital of Bamako. I was told by one restaurant owner that tofu could not be made there because of the high temperatures.

11. This cheese, commonly associated with the Fulani ethnic group that has traditionally specialized in cattle herding across West Africa, is apparently not commonly made farther west in the region by them or any others. Kees, Guiwa, and Ouali (1995) note it only in Benin, but in addition to being common in at least some parts of Nigeria (per the discussion in this essay), it is known in Togo and Ghana. I never noted it while living in parts of Mali and Guinea that have large Fulani populations.

12. An enzyme in the sap, calotropin, is what causes the coagulation (Egounlety 1997). The sap is toxic, and cooking does not break down the toxic elements. Apparently, however, the low concentration used to achieve the desired result causes no ill effects in people consuming the cheese.

13. FutureHarvest (2001) indicates that the costs for bean curd were about one-third of those for the dairy cheese.

14. There have been some ongoing experiments in the southern part of the Dosso region. The government of Niger recently decided to encourage production of soybeans on a wider scale in other suitable parts of the country.

15. This information came from American Peace Corps volunteers working in these areas.

16. An excellent perspective on these cross-border ties in a general context is William F. S. Miles's *Hausaland Divided: Colonialism and Independence in Nigeria and Niger* (Ithaca, NY: Cornell University Press, 1994).

17. Nakamura Sule (2004) notes use of the word *ƙwaidaƙwai* in Sokoto, Nigeria, and indeed the same dialect of Hausa is used from Sokoto north to Birnin'Konni and Tahoua in Niger.

18. The sites are Matameye and Kada Zaki in the Matameye district of the Zinder region, the city of Maradi in Maradi region, and Karaye in the Illela district of Tahoua region (north of Birnin'Konni). This description benefited in particular from input by Amanda Ree, a Peace Corps volunteer in Karaye who has worked to facilitate Nigerien women's learning of bean curd making from other Nigerien women in the Birnin'Konni area.

19. Ree (personal communication, 2004) reports that a *tiya* of soybeans (a market measure totaling about a kilogram) costing 600 CFA (franc of the Communauté Financière Africaine) plus additional supplies totaling 200 CFA can yield a gross return of 2500 CFA (approximately 550 CFA = US$1). Other conversations indicated similar returns.

20. Shannon and Kalala (1994) note the roasting of soybeans as a snack (like peanuts) in the Democratic Republic of Congo (formerly Zaire). This is apparently not a common food in West Africa.

21. Smit (1995) puts African production of soybeans at less than 1 percent of world production.

References

Baccus-Taylor, S. H. Gail. n.d. "Health and Nutritive Benefits of Soy and Soy-Based Products." http://www.rmco.com/study.html.

Chevalier, Auguste. 1947. "Cultures Nouvelles et Cultures Qui Disparaissent en Afrique Occidentale." *Revue Internationale de Botanique Appliquée et d'Agriculture Tropicale* 27(293): 134–38.

———. 1948. "La Culture du Soja en Afrique Occidentale." *Revue Internationale de Botanique Appliquée et d'Agriculture Tropicale* 28(307–8): 259–60.

Diawara, Brehima, et al. 2000. *HACCP System for Traditional African Fermented Foods: Soumbala.* Ouagadougou, Burkina Faso: Département de Technologie Alimentaire, Centre National de la Recherche Scientifique et Technologique; and World Association of Industrial and Technological Research Organizations.

Egounlety, Moutairou. 1997. "Contribution de l'Artisanat à l'Approvisionnement Alimentaire des Villes en Afrique." Programme FAO Approvisionnement et Distribution Alimentaires des Villes. Document DT/17-97F.

Engelbeen, M. 1948. *Le Soja au Congo Belge.* Brussels: Ministère des Colonies.

Ezendinma, F. O. C. 1964. "The Soybean in Nigeria." *Proceedings of the Agricultural Society of Nigeria* 3: 13–16.

FutureHarvest. 2001. "Research Gives Birth to Nigerian Soybean Industry." http://go.worldbank.org/RAJVLB1XJ1.

Gutierrez, Marie-Laure. 1999. "Dynamique de Production et de Commercialisation de l'Afitin Fon dans la Région d'Abomey-Bohicon (Bénin)." Mémoire Esat 2/M.Sc. Dat. Montpelier, France: Centre National d'Etudes Agronomiques des Régions Chaudes.

Gutierrez, Marie-Laure, and Dominique Juhé-Beaulaton. 2002. "Histoire du Parc à Néré (Parkia biglobosa) sur le Plateau d'Abomey (Bénin): de sa Conservation pour la Production et la Commercialisation d'un Condiment, l'Afitin." *Les Cahiers d'Outre-Mer* 55(220): 453–74.

IDRC (International Development Research Center). 1998. "An Effort to Promote the Production and Consumption of Soybeans As a Means of Improving Nutrition in Nigeria." http://www.solutions-site.org/cat11_sol101.htm.

IIA (International Institute of Agriculture). 1936. *Use of Leguminous Plants in Tropical Countries As Green Manure, As Cover and As Shade.* Rome: IIA.

IITA (International Institute for Tropical Agriculture). 1998. "IITA and Japan Bring Tofu to Sub-Saharan Africa." IITA Annual Report 1998. Croydon, UK: IITA. http://web.archive.org/web/20031224210706/http://www.iita.org/info/ar98/9-10.htm.

IKWW (Indigenous Knowledge Worldwide). 2002. "Traditional Methods for Processing Locust Beans." *IKWW* (May issue). Silang, Cavite, Philippines: International Institute of Rural Reconstruction.

INTSOY (International Soybean Program). 1987. "Cooperative Efforts in Nigeria Aim to Increase Soybean Use across Africa." *INTSOY Newsletter* 37: 3–4.

IRAT/CNRA (Institut de Recherches Agronomiques Tropicales/Centre National de Recherches Agronomiques). 1964. "Collection de Soja." In *Division d'Amélioration des Plantes. Section d'Amélioration des Cultures de Diversification. Compte Rendu d'Activité, 1963.* Senegal: IRAT-CNRA.

Jackobs, Joseph A., C. A. Smyth, and D. R. Erickson. 1984. "International Soybean Variety Experiment: Eighth Report of Results, 1980–81." *INTSOY Series* No. 26. Urbana-Champaign, Illinois: International Soybean Program.

JICA (Japanese International Cooperation Agency). 2001. "Tofu Production in Nigeria." *Japan Close-Up* (May issue). Php International Ptd, Ltd.

Kay, Theodore. 1974a. "Soybeans in the Nigerian Diet." *Samaru Agricultural Newsletter* 16(1): 18–22.

———. 1974b. "Le Soja dans le Régime Alimentaire Nigerian." Unpublished ms.

Kees, Marlis. n.d. "Production on Marketing Cheese: Good Income for Women." ALIN-EA. http://web.archive.org/web/20051222192700/http://www.alin.or.ke/tech-note/data/pro_che.html.

Kees, Marlis, Clairisse Guiwa, and Alice Massim Ouali. 1995. "Fabrication Artisanale de Fromage au Bénin: Un Exemple à Suivre en Zone Tropicale." *Bulletin du Réseau TPA* 11 (December): 15–16.

Maidment, W. T. O. 1946. "Report of the Provincial Agricultural Officer, Western Province." Uganda Protectorate Department of Agriculture, Annual Report (July 1, 1944–June 30, 1945), 13–23.

Matagrin, A. 1939. *Le Soja et Les Industries du Soja.* Paris: Gauthier-Villars.

Morse, W. J. 1939. "Soybeans the World Round." *Proceedings of the American Soybean Association* (ASA). Nineteenth Annual Meeting, September 11–12. Madison, WI: ASA.

———. 1950. "History of Soybean Production." In K. S. Markley, ed., *Soybeans and Soybean Products,* Vol. 1, 3–59. New York: Interscience Publishers and Wiley.

Numfor, Festus A. 1983. "Soybean Utilization in Cameroon (a Country Report)." Paper prepared for a symposium on utilization of soybeans in Africa, December 5–9. Ibadan, Nigeria: International Institute for Tropical Agriculture.

Numfor, Festus A., and L. Noubi. 1995. "Effect of Full-Fat Soya Bean Flour on the Quality and Acceptability of Fermented Cassava Flour." *Food and Nutrition Bulletin* 16(3): 241–44.

Picasso, Christian. 1986. "Soybean in Burkina Faso: Agronomic Studies and Development Prospects." In S. Shanmugasundaram and E. W. Sulzberger, eds., *Soybeans in Tropical and Subtropical Cropping Systems,* 421–25. Shanhua, Taiwan: Asian Vegetable Research and Development Center.

Portères, Roland. 1945. "Introduction du Soja dans L'alimentation des Populations Indigènes de la Region Forestière de la Guinée Française." *Agriculture* 57: 62–63.

———. 1946. "Observations sur les Possibilités de la Culture du Soja en Guinée Forestière." *Bulletin Agronomique* 1.

Pynaert, L. 1920. "Le Soja." *Bulletin Agricole du Congo Belge et du Ruanda-Urundi* 11(1–2): 151–86.

Root, W. R., P. O. Oyekan, and K. E. Dashiell. 1987. "West and Central Africa: Nigeria Sets the Example for Expansion of Soybeans." In S. R. Singh et al., eds., *Soybeans for the Tropics,* 81–85. New York: Wiley.

Sakyi-Dawson, E. O., N. N. Nartey, and W. K. Amoa-Awuah. 2001. *Feasibility of the Use of Starter Cultures in the Production of Soydawadawa.* Abstract of presentation, IFT Annual Meeting, June 23–27. http://ift.confex.com/ift/2001/techprogram/paper_8633.htm.

Shannon, Dennis A. 1992. "Work with Soybeans in Nigeria." Interview conducted by William Shurtleff, October 9. *SoyaScan Notes.* Lafayette, CA: Soyfoods Center.

Shannon, Dennis A., and M. Mwamba Kalala. 1994. "Adoption of Soybean in Sub-Saharan Africa: A Comparative Analysis of Production and Utilization in Zaire and Nigeria." *Agricultural Systems* 46(4): 369–84.

Shao, Margaret. 2002. "Parkia biglobosa: Changes in Resource Allocation in Kandiga, Ghana." Master's thesis, Michigan Technological University. http://peace corps.mtu.edu/people/1998/shao.pdf.

Shurtleff, William, and Akiko Aoyagi. 1997. "Soy in Africa: Bibliography and Sourcebook, 1857 to 1997." Lafayette, CA: Soyfoods Center.

Smith, Joyotee, J. B. Woodworth, and K. E. Dashiell. 1993. "Government Policy and Farm Level Technologies: The Expansion of Soya Bean in Nigeria." *Agricultural Systems in Africa* 3(1): 20–32.

Snow, O. W. 1961. "Soya Bean in Ghana, a Preliminary Note Based on Annual Reports." Special Report, Ministry of Agriculture, Accra, Ghana.

Steinkraus, K. H. 2002. "Fermentations in World Food Processing." *Comprehensive Reviews in Food Science and Food Safety* 1(1): 23–32.

Von Maydell, H.-J. 1990. *Trees and Shrubs of the Sahel, Their Characteristics and Uses.* Produced with GTZ. Weikersheim, Germany: Verlag Josef Margraf Scientific Books.

Vuillet, J. 1924. "Essais de Légumineuses Fourragères Poursuivis dans la Vallée du Niger en 1923." *Revue de Botanique Appliquée et d'Agriculture Coloniale* 4: 690–92.

Waters-Bayer, Ann. 1988. "Soybean Daddawa: An Innovation by Nigerian Women." *ILEIA Newsletter* 4(3): 8–9.

Weingartner, Karl E., K. E. Dashiell, and A. I. Nelson. 1987. "Soybean Utilization in Africa: Making Place for a New Food." *Food and Nutrition* (FAO) 13(2): 21–28.

Wenger, O. E. 1976. "Performance of Some Soybean Varieties in Liberia." *Tropical Grain Legume Bulletin* 3: 8–9.

Whigham, D. K., and W. H. Judy. 1978. "International Soybean Variety Experiment: Third Report of Results, 1975." INTSOY Series No. 15. Urbana-Champaign, IL: International Soybean Program.

Yuwa, J. A. 1963–64. "Introduction of Soyabeans into Abuja." *Samaru Agricultural Newsletter* 5: 100–101.

CONCLUSION

Soy's Dominance and Destiny

CHRISTINE M. DU BOIS
AND SIDNEY W. MINTZ

Soy through Time

This volume helps us to trace the history of soy from its ancient Asian origins to its ongoing adoption into the economies and cuisines of new lands.[1] Our authors have provided detailed examinations of diverse local uses for this exceptional plant. In what follows we try to make sense of these many pieces of the soy puzzle by projecting them against a wider background through time, one that uncovers soy's special significance in global terms.

The ancient Chinese first learned to overcome the difficulties that raw soybeans pose for human digestion. Their processing techniques consisted of lengthy cooking, fermentation, sprouting, grinding, and the transformation of soy into tofu. Over time and under varying local conditions, the preparation of that amazing product, tofu, became highly differentiated, both regionally within China and in the Chinese diaspora.

Gradually, soy agriculture and processing methods spread to other Asian societies through migration, Buddhist missionary activity, trade, government exchanges, and war. In new societies, soy preparation techniques were creatively readapted to different conditions and preferences. Throughout Asia, myths, rituals, folklore, proverbs, and medical treatments came to incorporate soy.

Specifically, fermented soy products took on a central role in the standard taste of the cuisines of Korea and Japan (for a discussion of standard tastes, see the Ozeki, Mintz, and Cwiertka and Moriya essays in this volume). This was probably due, at least in part, to the preservability of the fermented products but also to the varying organoleptic qualities of those products.

In the twentieth century, the center of soybean production shifted to the New World. In the United States, fresh experimentation with soy has led to new analog products imitating meat and dairy products. These products are reminiscent of Buddhists' mock meat and seafood formulations of soy, which have an ancient history in Asia. Nevertheless, the production and marketing of the new analogs are decidedly modern. In addition, in recent decades many initiatives have helped nutritionally deprived populations with innovative recipes that incorporate soy. These include governments' and development agencies' fortification of school lunches with soy protein.

Beyond these initiatives, indigenous creativity applied to soybeans in areas of the world not traditionally associated with the crop has protected or improved the protein levels in local diets. Nonetheless, the worldwide consumption of legumes such as soy actually appears to be declining. Instead of legumes, in developing countries the well-off are eating meat increasingly, while the poor remain protein-deficient. Most notably, in China people are eating more pork instead of soy products (Geissler 1999). There is significant variation in soy consumption among countries and social groups, however.

Soy in the Contemporary World

Despite the worldwide decline in legume consumption, soy is an enormously important crop, although the paucity of social-scientific literature about soy has helped to obscure that significance. In terms of the calories it provides, soy is the fourth most important food source in the world (FAO 2005a) and the first in importance among legumes. In money equivalents, only wheat outranks soy as an imported crop (FAO 2005b), and it has already surpassed wheat and all other crops in tonnage of whole, semiprocessed, and processed beans traded across the globe. Increased demand in developing countries for vegetable oil and for protein meal to nourish livestock—especially in China—is expected to stimulate the trade in soy even further, to perhaps some 170 million metric tons by 2015 (USDA 2006). Once called the "Cinderella crop" because of its dazzling rise in U.S. agriculture after World War II, soy is no longer merely a newcomer upon which the potentates have smiled. Now soy is a potentate in its own right.

Some of the essays in this volume have touched on the serious agricultural issues with which soy is inextricably entangled. This now-powerful food source plays a key part in the global trend—many centuries old but ever more worrisome today—toward supplanting the vast biodiversity of plant life on our planet with relatively few species and varieties of cultivated crops (Friedmann 2000; Bruinsma 2003, 104, 106). Such monoculture radically diminishes the richness of natural ecosystems, with grave moral and aesthetic implications. Through extinctions, it can also deprive us of life forms potentially useful in medicine, industry, or agriculture itself. This is a disturbing possibility, for instance, for lands converted to soy agriculture in Brazil's *cerrado* region (Kneen 2002, 125–29).

Single-species and variety concentrations also make the global food system more vulnerable to catastrophic loss in the event of a serious plant disease or pest invasion. Ireland's nineteenth-century potato blight cruelly demonstrated that danger. Fungal diseases of the popular Cavendish variety of banana threaten to repeat this scenario in the near future with a less essential yet still important food and basis of livelihood. Lack of genetic diversity could also eventually limit growth in crop yields. Most of the soy grown in the Western Hemisphere (where more than 80 percent of soy production now occurs) rests on a rather limited genetic base (see Nelson 2002; GRAIN 1997). Despite efforts to improve access to, analyze, and preserve the many varieties of Asian soy, excessive concentration of relatively few soy varieties in the West remains a genuine concern.[2]

Another very serious agricultural issue involving soy is the difficulty for many poor farmers in developing countries of making a viable living. Soy could provide at least some of these farmers with increased incomes and calories, yet both in soy agriculture and in the food trade worldwide, the needs of the poor have all too frequently been ignored. This neglect is apparent when one considers the production of soy for animal feed. Surely if the efficient nourishment of humanity were the goal of commerce in soy, then the ratio of feed versus food uses of the bean would be entirely different today. Of the world's 2004 soybean production, some 93 percent of the protein was processed into animal feed rather than human food (Brown 2004, 50).

The cycling of soy through animals is a spectacularly inefficient means of providing human populations with protein no matter how profitable it may be to the producers. For example, less than half of the feed that a pig eats ends up on a dinner table as pork; much of it is "irretrievably lost in the process of animal metabolism" (Shurtleff and Aoyagi 1979, 5).[3] The production of meat is also prodigal in its waste of fossil fuels and water (see Lappé 1991, 10), and it requires the application of many more chemicals to the land than does the production of plant foods for direct human consumption.

Not surprisingly, soy has played a huge role in the spread of American-style meat production (Berlan, Bertrand, and Lebas 1999 [1976]; Friedmann

1994a). As Friedmann (1994b, 268) explains, "Soybeans are by far the fastest-growing crop in world agriculture since 1945. From an Asian food crop, soybeans became the basis for a global transformation of livestock production, linking field crops with intensive, scientific animal production, through giant agri-food corporations, across many national boundaries." This transformation even occurred in Asian countries where soy was traditionally an important human food, both culturally and nutritively, and still is. For example, in Korea in the 1970s and early 1980s, human consumption of animal protein rose dramatically. The associated "expansion of the South Korean livestock industry relied heavily on imported feed grains from the United States, imports of corn and soybean increasing roughly tenfold from 1970 to 1984" (McMichael and Kim 1994, 33).

It may be simplistic to argue that the mass adoption of vegetarian diets (including soy protein) in wealthy countries would lead to major improvements in the diets of the poor in developing countries. Mass vegetarianism in the West—whatever collateral benefits it might have—probably would not lower the price of foodstuffs sufficiently to really help the poor elsewhere (see Rosegrant, Leach, and Gerpacio 1999; Leathers and Foster 2004, 335–42).

But this observation does not magically turn soybean agriculture to feed livestock into a benign enterprise. The expansion of such agriculture has sometimes had a direct negative effect on the nutrition of the poor in those very countries where the soy is grown. Barkin, Batt, and DeWalt (1990) detail how production of animal feed frequently replaces production of food for local consumption. Countries that switch to export-oriented agriculture must compensate by importing more food. While this economic strategy can enrich individual large farmers and businessmen and increase a nation's foreign exchange earnings, it can also result in a rise in the price of basic foodstuffs. In Brazil's "poorest region . . . cassava and bean prices registered the greatest increases. Low income families in the northeast have been the hardest hit by the soybean revolution" in that country (Barkin, Batt, and DeWalt 1990, 48).[4] Far better than a soybean revolution that hurts the poor would be one that helped them. More—or enhanced—soy agriculture in developing countries tied directly to supplying economically priced, culturally desirable soyfoods could be part of a concerted effort to reduce global malnutrition.

The feed-versus-food imbalance in the uses of soy is part of what motivated the writing of this book. Our authors document the gradual emergence of remarkable culinary diversity in the preparation and consumption of soyfoods by and for humans rather than the preparation of soy protein for animal feed. Although the meat industry has learned to disparage soy protein as merely an inferior substitute for meat, the history of soyfoods tells a different and much richer story. Parts of that story are the many steps that make up the long, inventive history of soy processing and culinary experimentation.

What do this history and these trends bode for the future? How will humanity feed its ever-burgeoning ranks? What role will soy play? We turn now to several possible scenarios.

The Once and Future Soy

Although there is no consensus among scholars in regard to this century's food trends, virtually everyone agrees that the planet's human population will grow much larger within a few decades. The United Nations' middle-of-the-road prediction for world population in the year 2050 is more than nine billion (United Nations 2004). If this is correct, it means that in only forty-four years there will be nearly three billion more people in the world to feed than there are right now.

We see five major perspectives among scholars, policymakers, corporate officials, and political activists about how to approach the provision of food for so many extra hungry mouths. Writers and thinkers can be grouped into five (admittedly rather inexact) categories: steadfast optimists, cautious optimists, social-justice advocates, resource pessimists, and a group that Stone (2005) has called the neo-Malthusian biotechnologists.

The steadfast optimists are confident that human ingenuity will meet the challenge through rapid technological growth and cultural adaptation. Their view is that in 2050 humans will be able to produce enough food and other needed resources (such as energy with which to transport and distribute the food) so as to satisfy everyone's basic needs (see Simon 1996). Because this outlook emphasizes human technical creativity, the possibilities that one can imagine for soy are practically limitless. Perhaps soy biodiesel will become more efficient and environmentally sound, strengthening economies. Perhaps breakthroughs in genetic engineering will make soy easier to grow in difficult climates, thereby jump-starting more protein production for needy populations. Perhaps a startling revolution in yields per hectare will make soy-and-grain–fed meat cheaper to produce and far more accessible worldwide.[5] Soy could eventually even be grown in outer space (d'Arcier 2005). In this (somewhat fanciful) rendering of the optimistic scenario, the human potential for making good use of soy is open-ended.

Other scholars are more cautiously optimistic (e.g., Bruinsma 2003). They argue that our rate of population growth must continue to decline, that we must give farmers adequate support, that we must devise technologies to sustainably improve yields or expand cropland, and that we must boost the incomes of the world's poorest, all in order to prevent yet more pressure from the problems that humans already face (serious inequality, malnutrition, ill health, pollution, a shrinking resource base, etc.). In other words, appropriate steps must be taken within the world's currently dominant scientific and economic contexts: conventional farming along with emerging biotechnologies and a partly regulated global capitalism. While cautious, such scholars do not view the coming century with a sense of alarm. For the most part they perceive trends as moving in the right directions, albeit more slowly than one would wish (see Leathers and Foster 2004, 385–93, for a discussion of this outlook). From this perspective, soy will most likely continue to play the roles it does today, only more so. The most obvious shift in relation to soy will be that much of Brazil's vast remaining *cerrado* lands will have been plowed over and devoted to soy agriculture by 2050.

The third viewpoint, that of social-justice advocates, evinces relatively little direct concern with population increases, since malnutrition is seen as a consequence of societal failings in the midst of planetary abundance. In this view, the challenge of properly nourishing everyone on the planet requires far-reaching social solutions rather than technical ones. Proponents of this position argue that if poor farmers were not so exploited by large multinational corporations, governments, and their local elites, they could provide enough food for themselves and their offspring. Their increased economic power would lead them to limit their own birth rates (as indeed has happened in earlier instances), completing the "demographic transition" away from overpopulation (Lappé and Collins 1978, 30–39).

From this perspective, the problem is neither overpopulation per se nor the supposed backwardness of the rural poor; it is the greedy policies and self-serving programs of the rich (see Magdoff, Foster, and Buttel 2000; Ross 1996; Lappé and Collins 1978). What is needed is not biotechnology to create another Green Revolution (which, these writers argue, mostly exacerbated the problems of the poor rather than improving their lot). Indeed, these thinkers are on the whole deeply suspicious of biotechnology and especially of the companies that largely control it.[6] They see instead a need for widespread land reform and fair trade policies to benefit small-scale cultivators.

If this vision of the future were to become a reality, agricultural laborers worldwide would own their own land, and they would curtail or cease their dependency on costly, industrially produced agricultural inputs (fertilizers, pesticides, herbicides, high-tech seeds, and machines) that bind agriculture to multinational corporations. Instead, the local wisdom of time-honored, largely preindustrial farming practices would prevail, and a much greater diversity of crops—for local consumption rather than for international export—would be planted (see Lappé and Lappé 2003, 126, 150). In practice, this low-tech, labor-intensive form of farming would make the growing of mass quantities of cheap animal feed difficult. The price of meat would presumably rise, and people would eat less of it. In consequence, Asians would increase the traditional soy products in their diets, and soy's genetic diversity would flourish on small farms throughout Asia. Meanwhile, cultivation of soy in the Western Hemisphere could be expected to fall sharply because demand for animal feed for meat would have dropped.

A fourth group of thinkers, the resource pessimists, often agrees with the social justice advocates on the need for organic farming or, at a minimum, for what Lang and Heasman (2004, 173–74) call "ecologically integrated" agriculture, which searches for "genuinely sustainable solutions within ecosystems" that might include some "soft" biotechnologies (see also Brown 2004, 78–79).

In contrast with the social justice advocates, however, the resource pessimists are quite alarmed about the growth in population and its effects on local natural and social environments (see R. Kaplan 2000; Homer-Dixon 1993).[7] These writers argue that population pressures are already creating serious social conflicts in areas with overtaxed natural resources, such as the Sahel region of Africa (Brown 2004, 26–29). Unless an urgent, concerted effort is made to address the food-and-population problem, they see wars over precious land, water, energy, and food itself as likely to become even more widespread. So too, they think, will other forms of suffering increase, for "if humans do not control their numbers, nature will do so through poverty, disease, and starvation" (Pimentel and Pimentel 1996, 297).

According to this view there are "limits to the earth's carrying capacity" (Pimentel and Pimentel 1996, 296). Environmental writer Lester Brown argues that even genetic engineering will not be able to raise crop yield potentials much due to intrinsic limits on plant production that we are already approaching (Brown 2004, 74–76). He therefore urges moving "quickly to a [universal] two-child family" to "try to stabilize world population at closer to 7 billion than the 9 billion currently projected" (39). Pimentel and his colleagues go further, recommending the reversal of population growth over the course of some one hundred years to reach an optimal two billion people on the planet. "Our suggested 2 billion population carrying capacity for the Earth is based on a European standard of living for everyone and sustainable use of natural resources" (Pimentel et al. 1999, 11).

Interestingly, although these writers predict far less consumption of meat in the future and far more plant-based protein in human diets (including from soy), they do not portray the production and consumption of meat in terms as negative as those of the social-justice advocates. Pimentel and Pimentel (1996, 290) see livestock as important converters of grasslands—that, given present technology, are unsuitable for crop production—into protein for human consumption. But soy does not figure much in this form of raising livestock.

By contrast, Lester Brown is impressed with the effectiveness of feeding soy to livestock. For metabolic reasons, particularly with pigs and chickens, "the incorporation of soybean meal into feed rations has revolutionized the world feed industry, greatly increasing the efficiency with which grain is converted into animal protein" (Brown 2004, 50). In this vision, soy has enabled a great worldwide rise in meat production and consumption and will likely continue to do so. Nevertheless, Brown also calls for the expansion of new models of animal protein distribution and production. These models, which have been successfully implemented in India and China, make better use of marketing possibilities and of fodder in the form of crop residues left over in fields after grain harvests (Brown 2004, 53–58).

For the resource pessimists, soy is thus potentially part of the answer to human nutritive needs—whether as animal feed or for direct human consumption—but a focus on population control is the real key to solving world food problems. Without that focus and without careful agricultural and resource planning, the positive aspects of soy could easily be overwhelmed by environmental problems associated with its production, particularly in Brazil (Brown 2004, 156–76; Kneen 2002, 125–30).

The fifth perspective, that of the neo-Malthusian biotechnologists, is a blend of steadfast optimism and resource pessimism. Malthus's eighteenth-century writings argued that population pressures could overwhelm resources and human productive capacity, at which point famine, disease, and wars would reduce the population. Neo-Malthusian biotechnologists argue that the primary solution to global population pressures is capitalist biotechnology, which, if left unencumbered, will succeed in feeding the world. Not surprisingly, this view is heavily promoted by companies invested in genetic engineering (see Stone 2002, 2005; Ross 1998). It should be noted, however, that not all who are concerned about population pressures and call for more biotechnology are as single-minded in their approach to world hunger (e.g., Borlaug and Carter 2005).

In none of these scenarios is soy an outright cure for malnutrition worldwide, nor, indeed, despite its healthful properties, is it a simple cure for hypernutrition in industrialized countries. But for most people soy is an excellent food when eaten in moderation,[8] and under any of the five scenarios above it would potentially be one part of the solution to world hunger, both in the present and the future. The future of soy is, of course, ultimately unknowable, since it depends on a vast multitude of decisions among humans and on events in nature, but it is extremely likely that in any scenario soy will continue to figure among the small handful of the most important crops on the planet. Indeed, its importance is likely to increase.

Shifting Soyfood Consumption

Even as the world as a whole may eat more soyfoods in the future, the amounts and recipes will vary with location. The chapters in this book show that such variability typified soy's lengthy history as a cultivated crop. Since the encouragement of soy agriculture and consumption in protein-deficient populations will often be a worthy goal and since soyfoods are generally a nutritious and environmentally responsible alternative to meat in well-fed populations, carefully contextualized understandings of the forces behind dietary change will be useful. By showing how soy has been adapted to many different cuisines, local rituals, social patterns, and economies, the essays in this volume point the way to intriguing possibilities for spurring soyfood consumption worldwide.

The historical and cultural details supplied by the contributors offer insights in three arenas. The first is the broad social, economic, and nutritional context of soyfood consumption; a detailed understanding of this context for each locale is essential. That knowledge must then be applied to the other two arenas. The second arena is soyfood product formulation in which genuine cultural sensitivity and creativity must be employed. The third arena—soyfood marketing—must also take sociocultural dynamics deeply into account (see Wansink 2005).

An example of nutritional context for soy is the matter of how soyfoods can fit into health-promoting cuisines. The pairing of legumes with cereals has been a very successful nutritious dietary strategy throughout human history. Although soy has the most complete protein of any cultivated legume and therefore can stand alone better than other legumes, human health will nevertheless be enhanced if soy can be promoted within a diet that is also rich in local whole-grain cereals.

The social context for eating is also very important and varies widely. One interesting observation from this volume is that soy served in institutional settings (schools, army bases, hospitals, and prisons) may be successful, at least for a time. Such settings provide occasions for trying new foods.

Similarly, the economic context for soy is a critical factor in its acceptance. Of concern is how soyfoods can be made more available economically for the poor in developing countries. In societies in which a large proportion of the population is engaged in subsistence farming, soy consumption stands a better chance of rising if soy is demonstrated to be an agronomically useful or valuable crop for small farmers. Working with farmers and entrepreneurs to find profitable ways to use the waste products of soy farming or processing can be particularly helpful in encouraging greater soy production. Greater production can be expected, in turn, to make soy more available or affordable for consumers.

The essays here have also afforded potentially useful insights for soyfood product development. The flavor and texture of soy protein pose challenges for product designers. Skillful basic processing, which makes soy easier and more healthful to digest, is therefore the first step in soyfood acceptance. Experimenting with local processing methods normally used for other foods is often a valuable approach. In addition, the people who will ultimately prepare the soyfoods, whether in industry or the home, must receive adequate training.

Soy products can be added to a diet in various ways. Modest amounts of soy protein can be unobtrusively included in recipes to enhance a food's nutritive value without changing its taste or texture. Soyfoods also have a good record of success when promoted as snacks or condiments. They are especially likely to be accepted when they can replace similar foods in the receiving culture. Adding either familiar flavors or fashionable foreign ones to soyfoods may also increase their consumption. Indeed, the entire hedonic experience of consuming soyfoods—including the perceptions of all five senses—matters greatly for consumption levels.

The hedonic experience needs to be predictable, however. Consistent quality and taste in soyfoods reassures consumers and can increase acceptance. By appealing to a wide range of hedonic preferences, the availability of a variety of soyfoods within a food system may also increase levels of consumption.

Convenience and price also matter. In nonindustrialized societies, soyfoods may be more readily adopted if they are cheaper or easier to store and prepare than parallel traditional foods. Similarly, in industrialized societies or among the elite in nonindustrial societies, soyfood consumption may rise if processing and packaging maximize convenience for the final consumer.

Long-range strategic thinking about soyfood product development can help as well. Development of new soybean varieties with nutritional or hedonic characteristics that appeal to consumers—whether through conventional breeding or genetic engineering—could make soyfoods more acceptable to certain populations. In some populations, however, soyfoods will be better accepted if they are made from organic (or at least not genetically engineered) soy—and if their packaging makes this fact clear. Similarly, some populations prefer soyfoods that explicitly lack the additive monosodium glutamate.

In the arena of soyfood marketing, we note first that many taste preferences are formed in childhood; this underlines the special importance of early encouragement of children to eat soy and other healthy foods in place of the sweet and fat-laden foods that are now fiercely marketed among youths worldwide. A reality-based marketing program stressing healthful aspects of soyfoods can encourage parents to buy them for themselves and for their families.

In addition to health, associating soyfoods with local history, heroes, myths, beliefs about good luck, or fine dining experiences can promote their consumption. Similarly, when soyfoods are connected to religion or mysticism, their prestige and consumption may increase.

Imbuing soyfoods with social cachet can also be very effective. Promoting soy among all socioeconomic and prestige strata within a society protects against soy becoming stigmatized as poor-man's food (and therefore not even preferred by the poor). Yet while it is helpful to impart to soyfoods an aura of prestige, if their preparation seems too complicated, expensive, or otherwise out of reach of the masses, popularization may be inhibited.

In the midst of these varied efforts, marketers should not neglect populations and subgroups that are most likely to be or become core soyfood consumers. For example, it should be borne in mind that those with an ethical commitment to vegetarianism may be especially receptive to new soyfoods. In addition, in societies where a tradition of soyfood consumption is being eroded by the presence of prestigious foreign foods, marketing soy as an aspect of cultural pride or nostalgia can help reduce or halt the decline. In societies with a soyfood tradition, marketers should also be alert during an economic downturn to the possibility that people will want to eat more soy instead of expensive meat.

Finally, the mode of marketing must be creative. For example, people may learn soy-preparation techniques best when they receive instruction directly from another person. Yet this mode of educating does not guarantee success. Success is perhaps most likely when the learning about soyfoods spreads through ethnic or religious communities, even though such communities can encompass a variety of natural environments and local cuisines.

These observations were culled from a careful reading of the contributions here to demonstrate the value of on-the-ground knowledge of soyfood processing and history for increasing broad awareness of these foods and for enlarging their use worldwide. The many inferences have been drawn with reference to soy, but they show basic principles of dietary change in general. What the case studies demonstrate concerning soyfood acceptance can prove useful as a burgeoning world population faces an uncertain future. Once again the soybean can prove beneficial to humanity, a resource with many potentials yet to be discovered.

Our aim in this book has been to increase and diffuse knowledge. We believe that the soybean and the potentialities it holds for world nutrition are far greater even than what many of its marketers have told us. But for a variety of reasons, some of which we have tried hard to spell out, soy's potentialities are also quite complex, particularly when an anthropological perspective on human welfare and environmental impacts is employed. We hope that we have made a contribution toward setting the record straight.

Notes

1. We offer our sincere thanks to Eric Ross, Ted Hymowitz, Glenn Stone, and George B. Du Bois Jr. for their careful comments on a draft of this conclusion.

2. We are aware of the intellectual and political hazards in terminology such as "the West," "Western," etc. But to make our points sometimes requires taking these risks.

3. American-style production of beef is substantially even less efficient due to cattle's high basal metabolism, large body mass, and long gestation and lactation periods (Glenn Stone, personal communication, 2005). However, there are alter-

native ways of feeding cattle that are less wasteful of resources. See Lappé (1991, xvi, 9–10, 67–70) and Brown (2004, 54–55). Cattle consume considerably less of the world's soy than pigs and chickens.

4. Similar effects of soybean farming have recently been reported for Paraguay. See GM Watch at http://www.gmwatch.org/archive2.asp?arcid=6959.

5. For example, scientists in the United States and China have been working for decades to develop hybrid soy. At present, hybrid soy only yields about 20 percent more than conventionally bred soy. Because of the higher cost of producing hybrid soy seed, this crop is therefore only just at the edge of commercial viability (see Palmer, Gai, Sun, and Burton 2001). But greater advances in the technology are certainly possible. In the early years of corn hybridization, many observers would not have guessed that the technology would advance to create the spectacular yield increases that it ultimately did (personal communication between Christine Du Bois and Hunt Wiley, research director, Dairyland Seed Company, 2006).

6. Distrust of biotechnology companies is, for example, quite evident in 2003 and 2005 reports by the ETC Group (Action Group on Erosion, Technology, and Concentration) on genetically engineered soy and maize and in the many writings of Indian activist Vandana Shiva (e.g., Shiva 2001).

7. See Peluso and Watts (2001)—especially the opening essay—for a political-economic critique of the assumptions of the resource pessimists.

8. Medical scientists are divided over whether soy is safe for postmenopausal women to eat in substantial quantities, as it may exacerbate preexisting hormone-dependent breast cancer. The evidence is unclear. At the same time, epidemiological evidence suggests that soy consumption among girls and premenopausal women could possibly help protect them from breast cancer.

References

Barkin, David, Rosemary L. Batt, and Billie R. DeWalt. 1990. *Food Crops vs. Feed Crops: Global Substitution of Grains in Production.* Boulder, CO: Lynne Rienner.

Berlan, Jean-Pierre, Jean-Pierre Bertrand, and Laurence Lebas. 1999 [1976]. "The Growth of the American 'Soybean Complex.'" *European Review of Agricultural Economics* 4(4): 395–416.

Borlaug, Norman, and Jimmy Carter. 2005. "Food for Thought." *Wall Street Journal,* October 14, p. A10.

Brown, Lester R. 2004. *Outgrowing the Earth.* New York: Norton.

Bruinsma, Jelle, ed. 2003. *World Agriculture: Towards 2015/2030. An FAO Perspective.* London: Earthscan.

d'Arcier, Constance Faivre. 2005. "Of Martian Dinners, Groggy Drivers, and Strawberries." *BusinessWeek,* July 4, p. 53.

ETC Group. 2003. "Patently Wrong!" May 7. http://www.etcgroup.org/en/materials/publications.html?pub_id=155.

———. 2005. "The Genetic Shell Game, or Now You See It! Now You Don't!" News release. August 11. Available at http://www.etcgroup.org/en/search.html?search=Shell+Game&search-button.x=7&search-button.y=14&search-button=Search.

FAO (Food and Agriculture Organization of the United Nations). 2005a. "The Top 10 World Food Produced Sources (Based on Energy)." October 11, 2005. http://www.fao.org/es/ess/chartroom/factoid04.asp.

———. 2005b. "Top Primary Food Commodities Imported (Ranked by Value)." October 11, 2005. http://www.fao.org/es/ess/chartroom/factoid18.asp.

Friedmann, Harriet. 1994a. "The International Relations of Food: The Unfolding Crisis of National Regulation." In Barbara Harriss-White and Sir Raymond Hoffenberg, eds., *Food: Multidisciplinary Perspectives*, 174–204. Oxford, UK: Blackwell.

———. 1994b. "Distance and Durability: Shaky Foundations of the World Food Economy." In Philip McMichael, ed., *The Global Restructuring of Agro-Food Systems*, 258–76. Ithaca, NY: Cornell University Press.

———. 2000. "What on Earth Is the Modern World-System? Foodgetting and Territory in the Modern Era and Beyond." *Journal of World-Systems Research* 6(2) (Summer/Fall): 480–515.

Geissler, Catherine. 1999. "China—the Soybean-Pork Dilemma." *Proceedings of the Nutrition Society* 58(2): 345–53.

GRAIN (Genetic Resources Action International). 1997. "Soybean: The Hidden Commodity." *Seedling* (June). http://www.grain.org/seedling/?id=28.

Homer-Dixon, Thomas. 1993. *Environmental Scarcity and Global Security.* Headline Series No. 300. New York: Foreign Policy Association.

Kaplan, Robert D. 2000[1994]. "The Coming Anarchy." In Robert D. Kaplan, *The Coming Anarchy: Shattering the Dreams of the Post Cold War*, 3–57. New York: Vintage Books/Random House.

Kneen, Brewster. 2002. *Invisible Giant: Cargill and Its Transnational Strategies*, 2nd ed. London: Pluto.

Lang, Tim, and Michael Heasman. 2004. *Food Wars: The Global Battle for Mouths, Minds, and Markets.* London: Earthscan.

Lappé, Frances Moore. 1991. *Diet for a Small Planet.* Twentieth Anniversary Edition. New York: Ballantine.

Lappé, Frances Moore, and Joseph Collins. 1978. *Food First: Beyond the Myth of Scarcity*, rev. ed. New York: Ballantine.

Lappé, Frances Moore, and Anna Lappé. 2003. *Hope's Edge: The Next Diet for a Small Planet.* New York: Jeremy P. Tarcher/Putnam.

Leathers, Howard D., and Phillips Foster. 2004. *The World Food Problem*, 3rd ed. Boulder, CO: Lynne Rienner.

Magdoff, Fred, John Bellamy Foster, and Frederick H. Buttel, eds. 2000. *Hungry for Profit: The Agribusiness Threat to Farmers, Food, and the Environment.* New York: Monthly Review Press.

McMichael, Philip, and Chul-Kyoo Kim. 1994. "Japanese and South Korean Agricultural Restructuring in Comparative and Global Perspective." In Philip Mc-

Michael, ed., *The Global Restructuring of Agro-Food Systems,* 21–52. Ithaca, NY: Cornell University Press.

Nelson, Randall. 2002. "Soybean Germplasm from Anhui to Zhejiang for BSR Resistance to Yield Improvement." http://agronomyday.cropsci.uiuc.edu/2002/bsr-resistance/.

Palmer, R. G., and J. Gai, H. Sun, and J. W. Burton. 2001. "Production and Evaluation of Hybrid Soybean." *Plant Breeding Reviews* 21: 263–307.

Peluso, Nancy Lee, and Michael Watts, eds. 2001. *Violent Environments.* Ithaca, NY: Cornell University Press.

Pimentel, David, O. Bailey, P. Kim, E. Mullaney, J. Calabrese, L. Walman, F. Nelson, and X. Yao. 1999. "Will Limits of the Earth's Resources Control Human Numbers?" http://dieoff.org/page174.htm.

Pimentel, David, and Marcia Pimentel. 1996. "Summing Up: Options and Solutions." In David Pimentel and Marcia Pimentel, eds., *Food, Energy, and Society,* rev. ed., 285–97. Niwot: University Press of Colorado.

Rosegrant, Mark W., Nancy Leach, and Roberta V. Gerpacio. 1999. "Alternative Futures for World Cereal and Meat Consumption." *Proceedings of the Nutrition Society* 58(2): 219–34.

Ross, Eric B. 1996. "Malthusianism and Agriculture Development: False Premises, False Promises." *Biotechnology and Development Monitor* 26 (March). http://www.biotech-monitor.nl/new/index.php?link=publications.

———. 1998. *The Malthus Factor.* London: Zed.

Shiva, Vandana. 2001. *Protect or Plunder? Understanding Intellectual Property Rights.* New York: Zed.

Shurtleff, William, and Akiko Aoyagi. 1979. *The Book of Tofu,* rev. ed. New York: Ballantine.

Simon, Julian. 1996. *The Ultimate Resource 2,* 2nd ed. Princeton, NJ: Princeton University Press.

Stone, Glenn D. (and commentators). 2002. "Both Sides Now: Fallacies in the Genetic-Modification Wars, Implications for Developing Countries, and Anthropological Perspectives." *Current Anthropology* 43(4): 611–30.

———. 2005. "A Science of the Gray: Malthus, Marx, and the Ethics of Studying Crop Biotechnology." In Lynn Meskell and Peter Pels, eds., *Embedding Ethics: Shifting Boundaries of the Anthropological Profession,* 197–217. New York; Berg.

United Nations. 2004. *World Population Prospects: The 2004 Revision.* Population Division of the Department of Economic and Social Affairs of the United Nations Secretariat. http://esa.un.org/unpp.

USDA (United States Department of Agriculture). 2006. "Briefing Room: Agricultural Baseline Projections: Global Agricultural Trade, 2006–2015." February. http://www.ers.usda.gov/Briefing/Baseline/trade.htm.

Wansink, Brian. 2005. *Marketing Nutrition: Soy, Functional Foods, Biotechnology, and Obesity.* Urbana: University of Illinois Press.

Appendix A
Scientific Names for Plants and Edible Fungi

adzuki bean—*Vigna angularis*
African locust bean tree—*Parkia biglobosa*
alfalfa—*Medicago sativa* subsp. *sativa*
allspice—*Pimenta dioica*
ang hua (red sorrel)—*Hibiscus sabdariffa*
apple—*Malus domestica*
apricot—*Prunus armeniaca*
arrowroot—*Maranta arundinacea*
asparagus bean—*Vigna unguiculata* subsp. *sesquipedalis*
bamboo—*Phyllostachys* spp., *Sinocalamus* spp., or *Bambusa* spp.
banana—*Musa* spp. and hybrids
barley—*Hordeum vulgare*
Bengal gram—*Cicer arietinum*
bitter gourd—*Momordica charantia*
bitter vetch—*Vicia ervilia*
black-eyed pea—*Vigna unguiculata* subsp. *unguiculata*
black gram—*Vigna mungo*
black moss (fat choy)—*Nostoc flagelliforme*
black mushroom (Chinese)—*Lentinus edodes*
black sesame (in China)—*Sesamum indicum*
broad bean—*Vicia faba*
broccoli—*Brassica oleracea* var. *italica*
buckwheat—*Fagopyrum esculentum*
cabbage—*Brassica rapa* subsp. *chinensis, Brassica oleracea* var. capitata
canola—*Brassica rapa* subsp. *oleifera*
carob—*Ceratonia siliqua*

carrot—*Daucus carota*
cashew—*Anacardium occidentale*
cassava—*Manihot esculenta*
caterpillar fungus—*Cordyceps sinensis*
catjang—*Vigna unguiculata* subsp. *cylindrica*
cauliflower—*Brassica oleracea* var. *botrytis*
celery—*Apium graveolens*
chickling pea—*Lathyrus sativus*
chickpea—*Cicer arietinum*
chili pepper—*Capsicum* spp.
chocolate (cacao)—*Theobroma cacao*
christophine (chayote)—*Sechium edule*
chrysanthemum—*Chrysanthemum* spp.
cilantro—*Coriandrum sativum*
cinnamon—*Cinnamomum* spp.
clove—*Syzygium aromaticum*
coconut palm—*Cocos nucifera*
coffee—*Coffea arabica*
common beans—*Phaseolus vulgaris*
coriander—*Coriandrum sativum*
corn (maize)—*Zea mays* subsp. *mays*
cotton—*Gossypium hirsutum*
cowpea—*Vigna unguiculata* subsp. *unguiculata*
cucumber—*Cucumis sativus* var. *sativus*
dracontomelum—*Dracontomelum* spp.
eggplant—*Solanum melongena*
einkorn wheat—*Triticum monococcum*
elm—*Ulmus* spp.
emmer wheat—*Triticum turgidum* subsp. *dicoccum*
fagara—*Zanthoxylum simulans*
fava bean—*Vicia faba*
flax—*Linum usitatissimum*
frijol—*Phaseolus vulgaris*
galingale—*Cyperus longus*
garbanzo—*Cicer arietinum*
garlic—*Allium sativum*
giant milkweed—*Calotropis procera*
ginger—*Zingiber officinale*
ginseng—*Panax ginseng*
gram—*Cicer arietinum*
grape (cultivated)—*Vitis vinifera*
grape (wild)—*Vitis* spp.

green gram—*Vigna radiata*
green onion (Asian)—*Allium fistulosum*
groundnut—*Arachis hypogaea*
guanábana—*Annona muricata*
hemp—*Cannabis sativa*
hot pepper—*Capsicum* spp.
indigo—*Indigofera tinctoria*
Jerusalem artichoke—*Helianthus tuberosus*
kelp (Japanese)—*Laminaria japonica*
koumo mushroom—*Tricholoma* spp. or *Calocybe gambosa*
lemon—*Citrus limon*
lemon grass—*Cymbopogon* spp.
lentil—*Lens culinaris*
lettuce—*Lactuca sativa*
lily bulb (tiger lily)—*Lilium tigrinum*
lily flower (daylily buds)—*Hemerocallis fulva*
lima bean—*Phaseolus lunatus*
lima bean (West Indian)—*Phaseolus lunatus*
lime—*Citrus aurantiifolia*
litchi—*Litchi chinensis*
locust bean—*Parkia biglobosa*
lot plant—*Piper lolot*
lotus—*Nelumbo nucifera*
maize (corn)—*Zea mays* subsp. *mays*
mallow—*Malva verticillata*
mango—*Mangifera indica*
manioc—*Manihot esculenta*
millet, panicum—*Panicum miliaceum*
millet, pearl—*Pennisetum* spp.
millet, setaria—*Setaria italica*
mold (white, like cat's hair)—generally *Mucor sufu* mixed with other *Mucor* species
mold ferment—a complex mixture of molds, yeasts, and bacteria. The most abundant mold is *Rhizopus oryza.*
mung bean—*Vigna radiata*
mustard (Chinese)—*Brassica rapa*
nang—*Manihot esculenta*
okra—*Abelmoschus esculentus*
olive—*Olea europaea* subsp. *europaea*
onion—*Allium* spp.
orange—*Citrus sinensis*
osmanthus—*Osmanthus fragrans*

palm (coconut palm)—*Cocos nucifera*
palm (for sugar)—*Arenga pinnata* or *Borassus flabellifer*
papaya—*Carica papaya*
pea—*Pisum sativum*
peach—*Prunus persica*
peanut—*Arachis hypogaea*
pear—*Pyrus* spp.
peony—*Paeonia* spp.
pepper (bell or chili)—*Capsicum* spp.
pepper (black)—*Piper nigrum*
pineapple—*Ananas comosus*
pinenut (Asian)—*Pinus koraiensis*
plum (wild)—*Prunus salicina*
polyanthus bean—*Phaseolus polyanthus*
potato—*Solanum tuberosum* subsp. *tuberosum*
pumpkin (in Chinese cooking)—*Cucurbita maxima*
qu—a complex mixture of molds, yeasts and bacteria. The most abundant mold is *Rhizopus oryzae.*
quinoa—*Chenopodium quinoa*
raspberry—*Rubus idaeus*
red bean (adzuki bean)—*Vigna angularis*
rice (Asian)—*Oryza sativa*
rice bean—*Vigna umbellata*
rosary pea—*Abrus precatorius*
rutabaga—*Brassica napus* var. *napobrassica*
saffron—*Crocus sativus*
scallion—*Allium fistulosum*
scarlet runner bean—*Phaseolus coccineus*
sesame—*Sesamum indicum*
shallot—*Allium cepa* var. *aggregatum*
sieva bean—*Phaseolus lunatus*
snow pea—*Pisum sativum* subsp. *sativum* var. *macrocarpon*
soursop—*Annona muricata*
soybean—*Glycine max*
spelt—*Triticum aestivum* subsp. *spelta*
squash—*Cucurbita* spp.
star anise—*Illicium verum*
star fruit—*Averrhoa carambola*
St. John's bread—*Ceratonia siliqua*
straw mushroom—*Volvariella diplasia* or *Volvariella volvacea*
strawberry—*Fragaria X ananassa*
string beans—*Phaseolus vulgaris*

sugar—*Saccharum officinarum*
sweet potato—*Ipomoea batatas*
tamarind—*Tamarindus indica*
tangerine—*Citrus reticulata*
tapioca—*Manihot esculenta*
taro—*Colocasia esculenta*
taro (Indian)—*Alocasia macrorrhiza*
tea—*Camellia sinensis*
tepary bean—*Phaseolus acutifolius*
tobacco—*Nicotiana tabacum*
tomato—*Lycopersicon esculentum* (= *Solanum lycopersicon*)
vang—*Aganonerion polymorphum*
vanilla—*Vanilla planifolia*
veo (red sorrel)—*Hibiscus sabdariffa*
walnut—*Juglans* spp.
water chestnut—*Eleocharis dulcis*
watercress—*Nasturtium officinale*
watermelon—*Citrullus lanatus*
wheat—*Triticum* sp.
yam—*Dioscorea* spp.
yam bean (jícama)—*Pachyrhizus tuberosus* (in South America) or *Pachyrhizus erosus* (in the tropics generally)
yeast (salt-tolerant)—primarily *Zygosaccharomyces rouxii, Candida versatili,* and/or *Candida etchellsii*

Christine Du Bois wishes to thank Lawrence Kaplan for his assistance with this appendix. Any errors are, however, hers.

Appendix B
More on Tofu in Chengdu

Nineteenth-Century Tofu Dishes

babao tofu (8-treasure tofu)
baihe tofu (lily bulb tofu)
baiye tofu (sliced tofu "leaf")
boli tofu (glassy tofu)
bosi tofu (Persian tofu) (This recipe has been lost, not handed down. It was probably a Muslim dish that used mutton rather than pork with tofu.)
Buddhist monk tofu
chunqiao tofu (spring and autumn tofu) (Tofu made both of green and of ripe yellowish soybeans, with green representing spring and yellow representing autumn.)
danfeng tofu (red phoenix tofu) (Tofu made in the shape of a phoenix.)
dong tofu (frozen tofu)
douchi tofu (tofu with fermented black soybeans)
dounao (jellied tofu)
duck web tofu
fasi tofu (black moss tofu)
fengzhu tofu (beehive tofu)
fried tofu
furong tofu (lotus tofu)
ganbo tofu (stirred dry-fried tofu) (The tofu is cut into small pieces. *Gan* means "dry," and *bo* means "stir constantly" to prevent the pieces from sticking together.)
gezi tofu (pigeon tofu)
guanxiang tofu (fragrant tofu)
guihua tofu (tofu with sweet-scented osmanthus flowers)

gusui tofu (marrow tofu)
haishi tofu (children's tofu) (The Sichuanese believe that ordinary tofu is difficult for children to digest; special, more digestible tofu is thus made for them.)
hebao tofu (poached tofu)
hudie tofu (butterfly tofu) (Another artistic dish. Here a big, thin slice of tofu is fried and then made into a butterfly shape. Beans and vegetable strips are added onto the "wings." After seasoning, the ensemble is steamed.)
huozhuo tofu (catching alive tofu) (A tofu block is cooked in boiling water and eaten directly with chopsticks. The name is given to make a simple way of eating seem special.)
jiaozi tofu (jiaozi dumpling tofu) (Dumpling that uses tofu "skin" to wrap minced meat.)
jiaxian tofu (stuffed tofu)
jilin tofu (fish scale tofu)
jinqian tofu (gold coin tofu)
jinyin tofu (gold and silver tofu)
jipi tofu (chicken skin tofu)
jisong tofu (shredded chicken tofu)
jixiang tofu (auspicious tofu) (Seasoned with peanut, fruit juices, mushrooms, pepper, and lily flower.)
juanjian tofu (curled tofu)
koumo tofu (koumo mushroom tofu)
lianzi tofu (lotus seed tofu)
lingjiao tofu (water chestnut tofu)
ma tofu (numbing tofu, i.e., fagara-flavored tofu)
Mapo tofu (numbing hot tofu)
mati tofu (horse-hoof tofu)
mixing tofu (tofu with minced rice)
mudan tofu (peony tofu)
nanjian tofu (southern fried tofu) (Tofu from southern China is considered firmer and better for frying.)
niurou tofu (beef with tofu)
oily tofu
pengliu tofu (quick-fried tofu)
qingsun tofu (tofu with lettuce)
qinxiang tofu (celery-flavored tofu)
ruyi tofu ("as you like" tofu) (This is an artistic dish in which tofu is made with one side that is round and big, while the other side is square and small.)
shijin tofu (tofu with assorted meats)
shouxing tofu (longevity tofu)
sliced tofu with rice wine

taiji tofu (*taiji* is the Ultimate Reality in Neo-Confucianism)
tao'er tofu (peach tofu)
tofu ball
wensi tofu (filamentary tofu)
wonton tofu
xiangyun tofu (auspicious cloud tofu) (Tofu made to look like clouds.)
xiangzi tofu (box tofu) (This is an artistic dish. Tofu is cut into square pieces and fried. A side edge is then taken out of each piece, and a hole is made and filled with minced meat. The edge is then put back to cover the hole. The dish is steamed and seasoned before serving.)
xiani tofu (tofu with shredded shrimp)
xiao tofu (small tofu)
xiapi tofu (tofu with dried small shrimp)
xiayou tofu (shrimp oil tofu)
xie'ao tofu (crab and pincers tofu)
xinglao tofu (apricot-cheese tofu)
xuehua tofu (snowflake tofu)
yinhe tofu (silver box tofu) (A late Qing dynasty recipe that was lost. Probably the dish included egg white.)
yinxiao tofu (silver knife tofu) (Tofu with minced chicken; *xiao* is the Sichuanese word for mincing with a knife.)
yinyu tofu (tofu with silver fish)
yulanpian lao tofu (hardened tofu with sliced dried bamboo shoots)
zaoyou tofu (tofu with distiller's grain in sesame oil)
zhengzhu tofu (pearl tofu) (Tofu prepared in small pieces described as "pearls.")
zicai tofu (seaweed tofu)

List provided by Jianhua Mao, with editorial assistance from Chee-Beng Tan and Christine Du Bois.

Contemporary Innovative Tofu Recipes

Provided by Jianhua Mao, with the editorial assistance of Christine Du Bois and Chee-Beng Tan.

Bear Paw Tofu (from the Chengdu Stone-Grinding Bean Curd Restaurant)

INGREDIENTS

tofu, fish, winter bamboo shoots, ham, fresh and tender vegetables, fine salt, black pepper powder, monosodium glutamate, and "refined oil" (a mixture of edible oils, such as peanut oil, canola oil, and corn oil)

PROCEDURE

(1) Finely mash tofu and fish, then fully mix them; add some salt, black pepper powder, and monosodium glutamate to the mixture; make the mashed ingredients into the shape of bear paws; put the "bear paws" into hot oil and fry until they are golden.
(2) Put some ginger juice, shallots, and water into a wok, then add sliced ham and winter bamboo shoots; heat the wok until the water boils, and put the "bear paws" into the soup; slowly heat the wok until the soup is almost evaporated, and add a little more salt and monosodium glutamate; place the dish in a plate and decorate with cooked fresh and tender vegetables surrounding the bear paws.

Cooking tips: The mashed tofu and fish should be mixed well.

Commentary: This dish is an innovation based on a more traditional preparation. Traditionally the dish was made by simply frying tofu with one or another sauce. Since fish has been added to the tofu, the tofu is now more delicious. The golden innovative bear-paw shape also looks very attractive.

Tender Tofu with Egg Yolk (from the Chengdu Restaurant)

INGREDIENTS

tofu, peeled shrimp, soaked sea cucumber, squid, fresh black mushroom, red chili, green chili, ham, salted yolk, fine salt, monosodium glutamate, potato starch, soup stock, and refined oil

PROCEDURE

(1) Cut tofu into small cubes; dice peeled shrimp, sea cucumber, squid, and black mushrooms into small granules, and quick-boil them; dice red chili and green chili as well as ham into small granules.
(2) Heat some oil in the wok, then fry and mash some egg yolk in the wok until fragrant; put some thick stock in the wok and add the prepared cubes and granules to the yolk; add some salt and monosodium glutamate; add water and then potato starch to thicken, and place the mixture in a soup bowl lined with tinfoil.

Cooking tips: The bottom of the bowl should be matted with about 500 grams of heated salt before the tinfoil is lined over it. This step will preserve the texture and tenderness of the dish.

Commentary: In this dish, vegetable protein and animal protein are cooked simultaneously. The dish is white and yellow, tastes delicious, and is tender and smooth, which is suitable for the elderly and the young.

Crispy Bean Curd with Pine Nuts (from the Chengdu New Waitan Restaurant)

INGREDIENTS

pine nuts, tofu, shredded ginger, garlic, shallot, shredded meat, vinegar, sugar, dark soy sauce, black soybean sauce produced in Pixian (a county in Sichuan), pickled red chili powder, potato starch, soup stock, red chili oil, and refined oil

PROCEDURE

(1) Cut tofu into rectangles and put some of the potato starch on them.
(2) Heat oil in the wok; fry tofu until crispy and then put on a plate.
(3) Fry the shredded ginger, garlic, shallot, shredded meat, vinegar, sugar, dark soy sauce, Pixian black bean sauce, and pickled red chili powder in the wok with a little oil. Add some soup stock, starch, and red hot oil and cook until the tofu is golden. Pour this sauce onto the fried tofu, and sprinkle with pine nuts.

Cooking tips: Control the temperature of the oil when frying the tofu to avoid splitting it.

Commentary: The dish is crispy outside and tender inside, with a fragrance of pine nuts.

Contributors

DR. KATARZYNA J. CWIERTKA is a lecturer at the Centre for Japanese and Korean Studies, Leiden University. She is the editor of *Asian Food: The Global and the Local* (2002), and her most recent publications include *Modern Japanese Cuisine: Food, Power and National Identity* (2006); "Western Food and the Making of the Japanese Nation State" in *The Politics of Food* (2004); and "Cuisine and Culinary Culture" in *A Companion to the Anthropology of Japan* (2005).

DR. IVAN SERGIO FREIRE DE SOUSA is a sociologist and senior researcher at Embrapa (the Brazilian State Corporation for Agricultural Research) and a member of the Institute for Food and Agricultural Standards of Michigan State University. He is finishing a book on food history (production and consumption) in Brazil. He has published on soybeans with Lawrence Busch in *Rural Sociology.*

DR. CHRISTINE M. DU BOIS is an anthropologist and a manager of the Johns Hopkins Project on Soybeans. In 2004 she published *Images of West Indian Immigrants in Mass Media: The Struggle for a Positive Ethnic Reputation.* She has also coauthored articles on food with Dr. Sidney Mintz in the *Annual Review of Anthropology* and in Scribner's *Encyclopedia of Food.*

DR. H. T. HUANG is retired from the Needham Research Institute at Cambridge University, where he was the deputy director. He was also a program director at the National Science Foundation. Dr. Huang's recent book on the history of food science in ancient China was part of the Cambridge University Press's Science and Civilisation in China series.

DR. LAWRENCE KAPLAN is an emeritus professor of biology at the University of Massachusetts and a former editor of the journal *Economic Botany.* He has published articles and extended chapters on the prehistory of bean agriculture in *Chiles to Chocolate* (edited by Nelson Foster and Linda S. Cordell), in *The Cambridge World History of Food,* in *Conquista y Comida: Consequencias del Encuentro de dos Mundos* (edited by Janet Long), and in various journals.

DR. YING LIU is a lecturer at the School of Literature and Journalism at Sichuan University in Sichuan Province, Chengdu, China.

PROFESSOR JIANHUA MAO is deputy dean of the Faculty of Literature and Mass Communication at Sichuan University in Sichuan Province, Chengdu, China. He is a specialist on Sichuan food.

DR. SIDNEY W. MINTZ is an emeritus professor of anthropology at Johns Hopkins University. He has published numerous books on Caribbean ethnology and on food consumption patterns, including *Sweetness and Power* (1985) and *Tasting Food, Tasting Freedom* (1996). He is the principal investigator of the Johns Hopkins Project on Soybeans.

MS. AKIKO MORIYA is a PhD student at the Graduate University for Advanced Studies (Japan) and is currently conducting fieldwork in Korea in affiliation with the Center for Social Sciences of Seoul National University. Her project examines postwar transformation of food-related practices in South Korea.

DR. CAN VAN NGUYEN is a researcher at the Chinese Studies Institute, National Academy of Social Sciences and Humanities, Hanoi, Vietnam.

MR. DUONG THANH NGUYEN is a master of science student in Environmental Science and Technology at Vrije Universiteit in Brussels.

DR. DON Z. OSBORN is the former associate director for agriculture with the Peace Corps in Niger. He currently coordinates an international project and a major Internet resource, Bisharat.net, on the use of African languages in information technology. He has done research on farming systems and soy processing in West Africa.

DR. ERINO OZEKI is an associate professor of anthropology at Osaka International University. Her most recent publications include "Philippine Dento Orimono Sangyo no Fukko ni Kansuru Jirei Kenkyu: Piña no Saisei ni Kiyoshita Hitobito ["Revival of a Traditional Textile Industry: A Case Study of Philippine Piña"] in the *Osaka International University Journal of International Studies* (2003) and "Philippine-san Orimono 'Nipis' no Bunkateki Imihen'yo wo Megutte" ["On the Cultural Meanings of 'Nipis,' a Philippine-Made Fabric: Its Change and Continuity] in *Hen'yosuru Tohnan'ajia Shakai: Minzoku, Shukyo, Bunka no Dohtai* [*Southeast Asian Societies in Transformation: Ethnicity, Religion, and Culture in Their Dynamics*] (2004).

DR. MYRA SIDHARTA is a retired lecturer from the Faculty of Letters at the University of Indonesia. She has published "The Silent Invasion of Tofu" and "The Chinese Touch on Indonesian Cooking," both in the journal *Latitude.*

DR. CHEE-BENG TAN is chair of the Department of Anthropology at the Chinese University of Hong Kong. His publications on food include *Changing Chinese Foodways in Asia,* coedited with David Y. H. Wu (2001); "Bean-Curd Consumption in Hong Kong," with Sidney W. Mintz, in *Ethnology* (2001); and "Family Meals in Rural Fujian: Aspects of Yongchun Village Life," in the *Taiwan Journal of Anthropology* (2003).

DR. RITA DE CÁSSIA MILAGRES TEIXEIRA VIEIRA is an agricultural economist and senior researcher at Embrapa (the Brazilian State Corporation for Agricultural Research). She is also the agribusiness general coordinator for the Brazilian Ministry of Development, Industry, and Foreign Trade.

DR. XIAOLU WANG is a professor at the School of Literature and Journalism, Sichuan University, Chengdu, China.

Index

Accelerator Mass Spectrometry (AMS), 31–33
ADM. *See* Archer, Daniels, Midland Company
adzuki bean, 40
Afghanistan, 38
Africa, 18, 29, 41–42, 92n15, 305; East, 279; West, 19–20, 38, 276–97, 294n20. *See also individual countries*
African locust bean, 19, 280–82, 289–91, 293n7
Algeria, 277
allergies. *See* health, human: allergies
Amaggi, Ltd., 244–46
Amazon region, 244–45
American Heart Association, 221
American Revolution, 209
American Soybean Association, 213, 262, 271n12
amino acids, 8, 27, 90, 138, 147, 168; in Bangladesh, 263; in soy sauce, 171. *See also* lysine
analogs. *See* soy, as substitute for other foods
Anderson, Eugene N., 35, 59, 69n11, 69n15, 109
Andoh, Elizabeth, 60, 70n16
Angola, 42
animal feed. *See* feed, animal
Aoyagi, Akiko, 5, 69n15, 70n16, 101, 108; on Bangladesh, 259; on meat, 301; on tamari, 158n15; on tofu, 220; on United States, 211, 214
Archer, Daniels, Midland Company (ADM), 213, 226, 245
Argentina, 6, 18, 234–243, 251–52; trade with Bangladesh, 264. *See also* genetic engineering
Asia, 70n22. *See also individual countries*
Aspergillus species, 167, 170
Australia, 79–80, 115
Aventis, 78
awara. *See* bean curd

Bacillus natto, 60
Bacillus species, 167, 281
Bangladesh, 18–20, 257–75
bean curd, 19–20, 282–92, 294n13. *See also* tofu
Benin, 42, 277, 293n11
Biafra War, 279
Bill and Melinda Gates Foundation, 90
biodiesel, 223, 228n6, 303
biotechnology. *See* genetic engineering
black-eyed pea. *See* cowpea
Bolivia, 240
Borlaug, Norman, 90, 307
Botswana, 42
Bovine Spongiform Encephalopathy (BSE), 85, 239, 248
Bradyrhizobia. *See Rhizobiacae*
Brazil, 5–6, 18, 234–56, 306; North American farmers in, 240; trade with Bangladesh, 264. *See also cerrado*; genetic engineering; poverty: in Brazil

Brazilian Agricultural Research Corporation (EMBRAPA), 250–51
Brazil nuts, 78
Britain, 33, 83, 140–41, 195, 209, 267
broad bean, 35, 37
Brown, Lester, 305–6, 311n3
Bruinsma, Jelle, 301, 304
BSE. *See* Bovine Spongiform Encephalopathy
Buddhism, 9, 15, 64, 138, 148, 150–51; in Vietnam, 183–87. *See also* vegetarianism: and Buddhism
Bunge, Ltd., 223, 226, 245
Burkina Faso, 39, 277, 280
B vitamins, 68n6, 200, 265, 281

Cameroon, 277, 285, 289
Canada, 88, 107–8, 197, 259
capitalist agriculture, 2–6, 239, 243, 304
Cargill, 226, 244–45
Central America, 32–33
cereals, paired with legumes 27, 30, 40–41, 70n21, 248, 307–8; in Africa, 280, 293n5. *See also* core-fringe-legume hypothesis
cerrado, 18, 236, 238–39, 251–52, 301, 304
chang, 16, 161–81
chemistry, 4–5, 56–58, 63, 190; and agricultural inputs, 239, 270, 301; and processed foods, 155, 171–73, 178n22. *See also* soy, industrial uses
Chicago Board of Trade, 213
chicken, 18, 123, 134, 185; consumption levels, 217, 247, 268; expanding production, 235, 248, 267; fed soy meal, 196, 218, 258, 270. *See also* feed, animal
chickling pea, 28, 37–38
chickpea, 38, 265
Chile, 31, 33
chili paste, 146, 166–69, 173–75
China, 20, 45–55, 99–143, 148, 306; ancient history, 59, 64; fermentation in, 59, 62–64, 68n8, 69n9, 69n15, 116n5; genetic engineering in, 86–87, 89, 92n13; landraces in, 82; prehistory, 29, 35, 37, 39–40, 58; relations with Vietnam, 183–187, 193; and soy imports, 208. *See also* dietary change: in China; dietary cultural norms: in China; Hong Kong; Li Shizhen; Macau; poverty: in China; Sichuan; Sino-Japanese War; soy: domestication; soy: early history; tofu
Chinese-Japanese War (1894–95), 210
Chinese migration. *See* migration: Chinese
coagulants. *See* curdling agents
Colombia, 41
colonialism, 19, 161; in Africa, 277–78, 280; in Bangladesh, 267; in Indonesia, 195–97, 205; Japanese, 170–72, 178n18
Columbian Exchange, 1–4
competitive advantage, 83, 243–44, 246
consolidation, economic, 173, 224–27
convenience, consumer, 16, 112, 154, 309
core-fringe-legume hypothesis, 8, 66
core tofu culture area, 14, 17, 115
Côte d'Ivoire, 277–78
cowpea, 38–39
crop rotations, 108, 187
crop testing, 79–80
cultural norms. *See* dietary cultural norms
cultural packaging, 15, 121, 124–138
Cultural Revolution (China), 130–31
curdling agents, 20, 102–5, 107, 188–89, 192; in Africa, 283–84, 293n12
Cwiertka, Katarzyna, 16, 161–81

daddawa, 19–20, 279–82, 289–92, 293n6, 293n8
dashi, 14, 147–49, 152, 154–55
debt, farmer, 87, 89, 271n3
Democratic Republic of the Congo, 279, 294n20
diet: and choice, 10, 137, 156, 175, 220–21; and gatekeepers, 10; and inequality, 10–11, 89, 267–70. *See also* dietary change; dietary cultural norms
diet, and food prices, 8, 19, 137, 153, 172, 182; in Africa, 294n13, 294n19; in Bangladesh, 259, 263, 266; in Brazil, 236, 247, 249; in Indonesia, 204, 205; in the United States, 219–20
diet, and income, 41, 136–37, 150–51, 169, 175, 310; in Africa, 283; in Bangladesh, 266; in Brazil, 239–40, 247, 302
dietary change, 2, 7–11, 18–21, 71n27, 307–10; in Africa, 276–97; in Bangladesh, 259–61, 269; in Brazil, 234–35, 245–47, 252; in China, 270, 300; in Europe, 70n24, 115, 217; and genetic engineering, 80; in Indonesia, 195, 204; in Japan, 148,

152–53, 155, 157n5, 170, 217; in Korea, 146, 157n6, 162–66, 169, 172, 175; in legume consumption, 41, 300; in Mexico, 21n2, 209; in United States, 64–66, 69n11, 70n20, 209, 221; in Vietnam, 185, 187
dietary cultural norms, 9, 16, 56–57, 64, 116, 209; in Bangladesh, 261, 266; in Brazil, 242; in China, 100, 109–13, 121–24; in Indonesia, 200, 204; in Korea, 163; in Southeast Asia, 111. *See also* standard taste
differentiation, culinary, 60, 62, 70nn17–18, 110, 147, 243; in Bangladesh, 266; in Britain, 140–41; in China, 299; in Indonesia, 202; in Japan, 151–52; in Korea, 166, 169, 178n16; in Sichuan, 125, 137; in Vietnam, 190, 192
differentiation, social, 16, 114, 309; in Bangladesh, 266–67; in Brazil, 238, 249, 252; in Britain, 140–41; in Korea, 169, 176; in Sichuan, 125, 137; in Vietnam, 192. *See also* diet: and inequality; poverty
domestication, plant, 30, 34. *See also* soy: domestication
Dreyfus, Louis (company). *See* Louis Dreyfus (company)
Du Bois, Christine M., 1–23, 74–96, 108, 208–33, 257–75, 299–313
Dunlop, Fuchsia, 140–41
Dupont, 75–76, 91n4, 223, 226

ecology, 8, 21, 21n5, 75, 248, 305; and Amazon, 244–45; in Bangladesh, 260, 270; and *cerrado*, 238, 252; and genetic engineering, 81–83
Egypt, 34
El Tejar (company), 246
EMBRAPA. *See* Brazilian Agricultural Research Corporation
energy bars. *See* soyfoods: energy bars
environment, natural. *See* ecology
Ethiopia, 38
Europe, 37, 60, 65, 67, 85–86; and soy imports, 208, 210; and World War II, 216. *See also* Bovine Spongiform Encephalopathy; dietary change: Europe; European Union; precautionary principle; *and individual countries*
European Union, 85
evolution, biological, 8
export crops, 2–4, 21n4, 108, 196, 208, 302; in Africa, 280, 289–90, 292; in Brazil, 239, 242, 246; after World War II, 216. *See also* rice, long-grain; trade

famine, 38, 85–86, 186, 305; in Bangladesh, 263, 267, 269–70. *See also* soy: famine relief
FAO. *See* United Nations: Food and Agriculture Organization
favism, 34
FDA. *See* United States Food and Drug Administration
feed, animal, 6, 20, 21n4, 77, 118n20, 301–3; nutritional value, 78, 306; in South America, 234, 247. *See also* chicken: fed soy meal; fish: fed soy meal; forage crops; soy: processing wastes; soy meal
fermentation, 15–17, 48–50, 56–73, 116n2, 147–60, 165–81; in Africa, 280–82; in Indonesia, 199–200, 203; in Vietnam, 191. *See also* China: fermentation in; *daddawa;* Huang, H. T.; miso; soyfoods: *natto*; soyfoods: *oncom*; soyfoods: relish; soyfoods: tamari; soy paste; *tempe*; *and names of Asian countries*
fish, 17, 58, 110–11, 134–35, 148, 152; for *dashi*, 14, 149, 152; fed soy meal, 218, 272n16; fermented, 146, 157n5; raw, 145–46, 156n3, 157n4; sauce, 67n2, 147–48, 192
food aid, 85, 216–17, 267. *See also* soy: as famine relief
Food for Peace. *See* Public Law 480
food labeling, 84–86, 92nn10–12, 224; in Brazil, 242
food prices. *See* diet, and food prices
food production, household, 16, 20, 102–6, 151; in Indonesia, 201–2; in Korea, 162, 166–69, 172–73, 177n6, 178n14; in Vietnam, 187, 189–90, 192
food production, industrial, 16, 78, 85, 102, 105–6, 140; in Korea, 162, 169–74, 178n19
forage crops, 5, 27, 57, 210, 212, 215
Ford, Henry, 4, 214
France, 33, 60, 157n7
Freedom to Farm bill, 224
Friedmann, Harriet, 3, 301–2
Fulani, 293n11
functional foods. *See* health food movement; soy: nutraceuticals

Gambia, 277
gender, 10, 20, 167–68, 261–66; in Africa, 280, 283–85, 291–92, 294n18
gene jumping, 81–82
genetic engineering, 14, 18, 74–96, 115, 118n20, 228n8; in Argentina, 240; and crop yields, 75, 305; and international trade, 225; and population pressures, 306–7; and social-justice advocates, 304, 311n6. *See also* Dupont; Monsanto; Roundup
Gepts, Paul, 32
Ghana, 277, 293n11
globalization, 8, 21n4, 86, 107, 110, 112; ambivalence toward, 163; and commerce, 139–142, 162, 240; and local adaptations, 115; resistance to, 153, 156
global warming, 270
glyphosate. *See* Roundup
GMO. *See* genetic engineering
Golden Rice, 89
Goody, Jack, 110
government: officials, 114, 150, 183–86, 193, 197–98; regulation, 77–79, 82–85, 172, 227, 240–42; support for traditions, 175–76. *See also* trade: government policies
government support for agriculture, 75, 90; in Bangladesh, 257, 260–61; in Brazil, 235–36, 243–44; in United States, 209, 216, 224–45, 235, 239
gram. *See* chickpea
Great Depression, 213–14
Greece, 34–35, 38
green manure, 5, 213
Green Peace, 84–85
Green Revolution, 89–90, 92n15, 263, 268, 270, 272n14; and social-justice advocates, 304
green soybeans, 279. *See also* soyfoods: *edamame*
Guinea, 277, 293n11
Guinea-Bissau, 277

Hausa, 19, 280, 284, 291
health, human, 115, 183; allergies, 76–80, 82, 91n4, 92n7; Alzheimer's disease, 117n19; cancer, 117n19, 221, 311n8; cardiac, 77, 80, 91n4, 117n19, 141, 221–23; diabetes, 141, 197; osteoporosis, 221. *See also* nutrition, human
health food movement, 17, 100, 115, 153–55, 262
Heasman, Michael, 305
hishio. *See* soy paste
Hong Kong, 106–10, 112, 116n1, 117n19
Huang, H. T., 12–15, 45–55, 58–60, 268; on fermentation, 62–63, 69n9, 69n13, 116n2, 165–66; on tofu, 102
hybrid soy, 311n5
Hymowitz, Theodore, 4, 13, 92n7, 214
hypernutrition, 21, 141, 307

identities, 16, 163, 173–76, 242, 248
identity-preserved crops, 91n6, 92n10
imports. *See* trade
India, 29, 36, 38–41, 59, 61–62, 306; exports to Bangladesh, 258, 262, 264; and genetic engineering, 87–89
Indonesia, 17, 59, 61–62, 110–11, 116n3, 195–207
inequality. *See* diet: and inequality; differentiation, social
infant formula. *See* soyfoods: infant formula
inoculant, 260–61. *See also Rhizobiacae*
intellectual property, 88, 90, 92n7
intercropping, 108–9
International Institute of Tropical Agriculture (IITA), 19, 278–79, 282–83, 290–91
International Soybean Program (INTSOY), 259, 278, 280
Iran, 38, 58
iru. *See* daddawa
Ishige, Naomichi, 147–48, 158n15, 170–71, 177n5, 248
isoflavones, 117n19, 221. *See also* health, human
Italy, 41, 153

James, Clive, 86–87, 89
Japan, 40–42, 69n15, 70n17, 106, 108; exports, 107; fermented foods in, 14, 59–60, 62, 147–60; and genetic engineering, 85; and soy imports, 208, 236; tofu in, 102, 117n12, 140. *See also* Chinese-Japanese War; colonialism: Japanese; dietary change: in Japan; Russo-Japanese War; Sino-Japanese War
Japanese International Cooperation Agency (JICA), 19, 283, 290–91

Japanese migration. *See* migration: Japanese
Java War, 196
jiang. *See* soy paste

kanjang. *See* soy sauce
Kaplan, Lawrence, 8, 12, 27–44, 57
katsuo-bushi. *See* fish: for *dashi*
kelp, 14, 147–48, 152, 157n10
Kikkoman, 71n25, 217
koch'ujang. *See* chili paste
kombu. *See* kelp
Korea, 20, 22n8, 40, 42, 146, 161–81; fermented foods in, 16, 59, 61; tofu in, 14, 102. *See also* dietary change: in Korea; meat: in Korea; migration: Korean
Korean War, 161, 171, 216
Kublai Khan, 22n9, 197–98
k̄wai-da-k̄wai. *See* bean curd

lactose intolerance, 227
Ladizinsky, G., 35–36
land, distribution of, 238, 272n17
landraces, 81–82
Lang, Tim, 305
Laos, 193
Lappé, Frances Moore, 220, 268, 272n14, 301, 304–5, 311n3
lecithin. *See* soy: lecithin
legumes, 8, 12, 27–44, 57–73, 293n3, 300; in Bangladesh, 263, 265–66; in Indonesia, 204; in United States, 35, 39, 41–42. *See also* soy; soyfoods
Le Huu Trac, 183, 186, 188
lentil, 34–36, 265
Le Quy Don, 183–84
Liberia, 277
Li Shizhen, 13, 101, 104
Liu An, 52, 101–2
Liu KeShun, 90, 212
locust bean. *See* African locust bean
Louis Dreyfus (company), 245
lysine, 27, 248, 281

Macau, 112
mad cow disease. *See* Bovine Spongiform Encephalopathy
Malaysia, 100, 106–7, 110–13, 115, 116n3, 117n13
Mali, 39, 277, 293n8, 293nn10–11
malnutrition, 10–11, 21, 74, 80–81, 88–91; and activists, 220, 304; in Africa, 280; in Bangladesh, 263, 271n12; in Brazil, 248–49
Malthus, Thomas, 306–7
Mao Jianhua, 14–15, 121–43, 320–24
Mao Zedong, 127, 129–30
margarine, 5, 17, 215–16, 219, 247, 249
mass media, 153, 158n16, 173, 179n29, 204
mass production. *See* food production, industrial
Mauritania, 39
McDonald's Corporation, 84, 115, 163
McMichael, Philip, 3, 302
meal, soy. *See* soy meal
meat, 17–18, 65, 110, 148, 301–2; capitalist production of, 3, 218; consumption levels, 42, 204, 205n5, 217, 222, 263; demand for, 270, 300, 306; and income elasticity, 240; in Korea, 302; prices, 270. *See also* soy, as substitute for other foods
mechanization of farming, 212, 226, 235
Mennonite Central Committee (MCC), 18, 260–62, 269, 271n9
menopause, 221
Mexico, 31–33, 38, 40, 42; and soy imports, 208. *See also* dietary change: in Mexico
migration, Chinese 13, 15, 17–18, 115, 197; to Brazil, 251; to Britain, 141; to Indonesia, 195, 198, 202; to Southeast Asia generally, 106–7, 110–13, 116n3, 117n13; to Vietnam, 182–83
migration: Eurasian, 197; Indian, 115; Japanese, 18, 151, 169–71, 251; Javanese, 201; Korean, 150; Old World, 3; to the United States, 213, 221; Vietnamese, 183–85
Mintz, Sidney, 1–23, 56–73, 106, 108–9, 111–12, 299–313
miso, 14, 59–60, 62, 65–67, 70n16; and Japanese standard taste, 147, 151–52, 155; in Korea, 170
modernity, 1, 6, 13–14, 105, 115, 300; in Bangladesh, 262; in Brazil, 240, 245, 251
monarch butterfly, 82
monoculture, 260, 263, 300–1
monosodium glutamate (MSG), 140, 192, 309, 322–23
Monsanto, 75, 87–88, 91n4, 223

Moriya, Akiko, 16, 161–81
Mozambique, 85–86
MSG. *See* monosodium glutamate
mung bean, 39–40

nata de soya, 203
nationalism, 175–76, 205, 216
Native Americans, 1–4, 30–33
Near East, 29–30, 34–38, 40, 68n8
nematodes, 76, 82
Nestle, Marion, 82, 84–85, 91, 227
Netherlands, the, 196–97
New World. *See* Western Hemisphere
New Zealand, 115
NGOs. *See* non-governmental organizations
Nguyen, Can Van, 15, 182–94
Niger, 19–20, 277, 283–92, 293n6, 293n9; and promotion of soy, 294n14
Nigeria, 19, 68n4, 277–85, 289–92, 293n6
nitrogen fixation, 4–5, 19, 108, 210, 264
Nixon, Richard, 18, 236
nodulation. *See Rhizobiacae*
non-governmental organizations (NGOs), 257, 259–60, 271n12
North America, 115. *See also individual countries*
nostalgia, culinary, 153–56, 163–64, 175, 310
no-till farming, 83, 239
nutraceuticals. *See* soyfoods: nutraceuticals
nutrition, animal. *See* feed, animal
nutrition, human 7–8, 27–44, 57, 68n6, 138–39, 308; activists, 76; in Bangladesh, 264–65; in Brazil, 245, 249; in historic texts, 183, 186, 196–97; in *tempe*, 200. *See also* hypernutrition; malnutrition

oil, 222–23. *See also* soy oil
oncom. *See* soyfoods: *oncom*
organic foods, 84, 92n11, 305. *See also* soyfoods: organic
Osborn, Donald Z., 18–20, 276–97
Ozeki, Erino, 11–15, 144–60

Pakistan, 267
Paraguay, 240, 311n4
Pauling, Linus, 21n7
pea, 37–38; genetically engineered, 79–80
Peace Corps (U.S.), 291, 294n18
Peru, 33, 40
Philippines, 61, 158n17, 204
photoperiodism, 211, 236, 239, 264, 278
phytoestrogens. *See* isoflavones
Pimentel, David, 305–6
Pinstrup-Anderson, Per, 78, 82, 87–89, 91
Pollan, Michael, 228n5
population pressures, 11, 21, 205, 222, 303–7, 310; in Bangladesh, 263, 268, 270
poverty, 17, 88–91, 301, 304; in Bangladesh, 257–58, 262, 266–70; in Brazil, 247, 302; in China, 100, 105, 107, 113–14; in Indonesia, 196; in Korea, 161. *See also* diet: and inequality; differentiation, social; malnutrition
precautionary principle, 85
prehistory, 27–44
prices, food. *See* diet, and food prices
processed foods, 6–7, 16, 71n26; in Bangladesh, 266; in Brazil, 235, 241, 251–52; canned tofu, 140; in Japan, 151, 154–55; in Korea, 162, 169, 177n6; and trans fats, 76, 223; in United States, 224
processors, food (corporate), 226, 245–46
protein, 19, 41–42, 64, 67n3, 68nn6–7, 90; in Bangladesh, 258, 260. *See also* amino acids; legumes; malnutrition; meat; soyfoods; soy meal
psychology, 9
Public Law, 480, 216–17, 257, 259, 262
pulses. *See* legumes
Pythagoras, 34

radiocarbon dating, 31, 42n1
recipes, 190–92, 322–24
religion, 9, 279; Seventh Day Adventist, 213, 220, 259. *See also* Buddhism; soy: and religion
restaurants, 18, 69n11, 71n29, 110, 115; luxury, 114, 121–43, 322–24; and trans fats, 76, 223; in United States, 217
Rhizobiacae, 4–5, 53n1, 278, 293n3
Rhizopus mold, 199–200
rice, long-grain, 79
Romance of the Three Kingdoms, 128, 132
Ross, Eric, 21n5, 304, 307
Roundup, 74–75, 77, 81, 83, 91nn3–5, 92n8
Rozin, Elizabeth, 11, 14
Rozin, Paul, 7, 9
Russia, 37, 210
Russo-Japanese War, 210

savannah, Brazil. *See cerrado.*
Schiøler, Ebbe, 78, 82, 87–89, 91
Schmeiser, Percy, 88
school feeding programs, 85, 219, 249–50, 262, 308
Senegal, 277
shi. See soyfoods: relish
Shiva, Vandana, 87, 311n6
shoyu. See soy sauce
Shurtleff, William, 4–5, 69n15, 70n16, 101, 108; on Bangladesh, 259; on meat, 301; on tamari, 158n15; on tofu, 220; on United States, 211, 214
Sichuan Province (China), 12, 14–15, 107–10, 112–13, 116n1, 121–43; recipes from, 320–24
Sidharta, Myra, 22n9, 112, 195–207
Sierra Leone, 277
silkworms, 106
Simoons, F. J., 34–35, 40, 105, 108
Singapore, 110–12, 116n3
Sino-Japanese War (1937–45), 172
slow food movement, 153, 155–56
soil erosion, 83
Solae, 226, 272n13
Sousa, Ivan Sergio Freire de, 14, 18, 74–96, 234–56
South Africa, 89
South America, 29, 38, 68n4, 197, 258–59. *See also individual countries*
Southeast Asia, 111, 115, 116n1, 116n3, 148. *See also individual countries*
soy, agronomic characteristics, 19, 75, 81, 106, 187, 210–12; in Africa, 278; in Bangladesh, 260, 264; in Brazil, 236
soy: and controversy, 74, 84, 224–27; cultivation of, 75, 83, 196, 239, 260–64, 292; domestication, 1, 13; early history, 12, 45–55, 100–1, 299; extruded, 6, 222; as famine relief, 10–11, 48, 59, 187, 216; and flatulence, 48, 52, 57, 90, 266; genome, 76; lecithin, 5–6, 92n11, 208, 213; marketing, 121–43, 307, 309–10; military consumption, 215, 217, 220, 308; processing wastes, 103, 105–6, 199–200, 203, 285, 308; and religion, 113, 185–86, 193, 309; symbolic associations, 113–14, 117n18, 205, 309; texture, 141, 219–20, 222, 250. *See also* export crops; food production, household; food production, industrial; genetic engineering; Roundup
soy, flavor of, 48, 52, 65, 90, 136, 262; in Bangladesh, 266; in Brazil, 248, 250–51; in United States, 209, 214–15, 219. *See also chang;* standard taste
soy, herbicide-tolerant. *See* Roundup
soy, industrial uses, 5, 80, 203, 234; in United States, 208, 210–11, 214–15, 224
soy, introduction of, 4, 18, 195, 209–10; in Africa, 276–79, 291–92, 293n3
soy, promotion of, 115, 196, 201, 210–11, 214; in Africa, 279, 290, 294n14; in Bangladesh, 261, 266, 271n8
soy, roasted, 16, 19, 64, 165, 197; in Africa, 279, 294n20; in Bangladesh, 258, 266
soy, as substitute for other foods, 6, 64–65, 101, 114, 116, 141; in Africa, 282–83, 285, 289–90, 293n5; in Bangladesh, 267; in Indonesia. 199–200, 204–5; in United States, 210, 214, 219–22, 227, 300; in Vietnam, 190, 193
soy consumption levels, 42; in Bangladesh, 257–58, 271n3; in Brazil, 246; in China, 300; in Indonesia, 201, 204; in Japan, 218; in Korea, 173; in United States 71n25, 217–19, 221
soy custard, 99–100, 102, 104, 106–7, 112–13, 115; in Indonesia, 203; in Sichuan, 121; in Vietnam, 192
soy digestibility, 12, 47–48, 52, 57, 59, 63; in Bangladesh, 266; in Indonesia, 197
soyfoods, 77: chips, 64, 198; *edamame,* 59, 64, 69n11, 107, 203, 226; energy bars, 17; flour, 16, 20, 165, 197, 203–4, 285–86; fortified biscuits, 19, 258, 262; infant formula, 6, 17, 92n6, 213; *natto,* 59–60; noodles, 209, 266; nutraceuticals, 6–7, 17, 221; *okara,* 67, 69n15, 199; *oncom,* 17, 59, 61, 196, 199; organic, 77, 84, 226, 309; relish, 48–49, 59, 61, 70n19, 100; sprouts, 50–51, 110–11, 164, 187; tamari, 64, 151, 158n15; *yuba,* 153–54. *See also* miso; soy custard; soymilk; soy pulp; soy sauce; *tempe*; tofu
soygurt, 203-4
soy meal, 6, 196, 210-12, 217-18, 222, 253n3; demand for, 300; exports of, 236; standardization of, 241
soymilk, 13, 16-17, 51-52, 99, 107, 112; in Africa, 293n4; in Bangladesh, 266; in

soymilk (*continued*)
Brazil, 249-50; early history, 102; globalization of, 115; household production, 102-6; in Indonesia, 203; in Korea, 165; in schools, 85, 219, 249; sweets made from, 154; in United States, 221, 227; in Vietnam, 192-93
soy oil, 4-6, 17-19, 61, 75-77; in Africa, 280; in Argentina, 236; in Bangladesh, 257-58, 262, 264, 269; in Brazil, 235, 247, 252; exports, 236; in Indonesia, 204; in United States, 208-10, 213, 215-19
soy paste, 6, 50, 59, 61, 66-67, 70n19, 101; in Indonesia, 203; in Japan, 150-52; in Korea, 166-71, 173, 175
soy production levels, 74-75, 86, 108, 151, 246; in Africa, 292, 294n21; in Bangladesh, 258, 271n4, 271n11; in Brazil, 236-39; in United States, 208, 211-16, 225; in Western Hemisphere, 235, 305
soy pulp. *See* soyfoods: *okara*
soy sauce, 59-60, 62; in Indonesia, 17, 195, 202; in Japan, 14, 117n12, 147, 150, 152, 154-55; in Korea, 16, 166-75, 178n12, 178n16, 178n19; in Malaysia, 114; manufacturing, 171-72; in United States, 209, 217; in Vietnam, 185, 190, 192-93; in Western cuisines, 64-65, 70n24. *See also* Kikkoman
Stahl, A. B., 28
standardization, 18, 139-41, 151, 172, 212, 308; in Brazil, 240-43. *See also* standard taste
standard taste, 144-60, 299
Starlink corn, 78
Stone, Glenn, 87, 89-90, 303, 307, 310n3
sumbala. See daddawa
Syria, 38

Taiwan, 100, 105, 108, 111-12, 116n1, 117n13; and soy imports, 208
Tan, Chee-Beng, 1-23, 99-120, 70n19
taoco. See soy paste
taste (sensation), 64, 66-67, 68n6, 70n24, 71n28, 156n2; in Bangladesh, 259; in Brazil, 242; and commercial agriculture, 243; and genetic engineering, 76, 80; in Indonesia, 17; in Japan, 14, 60, 69n15; in Korea, 166-68, 172, 176; in Sichuan, 122-24; in United States, 217. *See also* soy, flavor of; standard taste
tempe, 17, 59, 61-62, 197, 199-202; with bean sprouts, 110; early history, 201-2; production of, 112, 117n15, 196
Thailand, 166, 204
toenjang. See soy paste
tofu, 13-18, 99-143, 320-24, 197; in Africa, 293n10; in Brazil, 251-52; early history, 101-2, 182-86, 197-98; foods derived from, 64-65, 69n15, 71n29, 99, 188; in Indonesia, 195, 199; invention of, 52; in Korea, 165; in Vietnam, 182-94. *See also* core tofu culture area
Togo, 277, 293n4, 293n11
tourism, 137, 140, 153-54, 198
trade: disputes, 74, 86, 225, 227; government policies, 18, 109, 240; local, 100, 104-8, 111-12, 187, 198-203; multinational corporations, 18, 238, 240, 302, 304-5; networks, 19, 234, 241, 252, 291; tariffs, 213, 240. *See also* export crops
trade, international, 86-87, 140, 195-96, 202-3, 300; and Bangladesh, 258-59, 262, 264, 269-70; and Brazil, 243; and China, 216, 300; and United States, 208-10, 214, 216, 225, 236, 302
traditions. *See* dietary cultural norms; government: support for traditions
trans fats, 75-76, 223, 228nn7-8
transgenic crops. *See* genetic engineering
trypsin inhibitors, 28, 48, 52
Turkey (country), 38

umami cultural area, 147-48
Union of Concerned Scientists (UCS), 80, 82, 92n9
United Nations, 303; Food and Agriculture Organization (FAO), 10-11, 41, 205n5; World Food Programme (WFP), 262, 271n12; World Health Organization (WHO), 76
United States, 4-7, 17-19, 31-33, 108, 208-39; and Bangladesh, 257, 259, 262, 266-67, 269, 271n7; and Indonesia, 195, 197. *See also* dietary change: United States; genetic engineering; legumes: in United States; soy, industrial uses: United States; soy consumption levels: United

States; soy production levels: in United States; trade, international: and United States; United States Department of Agriculture; United States Food and Drug Administration
United States Department of Agriculture (USDA), 80, 84, 219, 227, 262; early soy research, 210, 268
United States Food and Drug Administration (FDA), 221, 227
urbanization, 107, 112, 161-62, 172-73, 177n3, 178n14
USDA. *See* United States Department of Agriculture

vegetarianism, 15, 41, 64, 110, 115-16, 139; and Buddhism, 148, 186-87, 300; and New Age movement, 220; in Sichuan, 124; and *tempe*, 200; in United States, 220, 222; in Vietnam, 183, 190-93; and world hunger, 302
Venezuela, 41
Vieira, Rita de Càssia Milagres Teixeira, 18, 85, 234-56
Vietnam, 14-15, 20; tofu in, 102, 106, 182-94
Vietnamese migration. *See* migration: Vietnamese

wagashi, 19, 283, 289, 291
Wansink, Brian, 10, 307
war, 11, 182-83, 193n3, 198, 305. *See also* soy: military consumption; *and names of particular wars*
wara. See wagashi
Warnken, Philip, 236
weaning foods, 68n5
weeds, 75, 82-83. *See also* gene jumping; Roundup
Western cuisines, 59-67, 69n11, 69n14, 115, 141, 153; in Korea, 177n6. *See also* Europe; *and individual countries*
Western Hemisphere, 30-33, 300-301. *See also individual countries*
WHO. *See* United Nations: World Health Organization
World Trade Organization, 86, 225, 241
World War I, 210
World War II, 5, 214-17, 267

yeasts, 168

Zambia, 85-86
Zimbabwe, 85-86, 279-80
Zohary, D., 35-39

THE FOOD SERIES

A History of Cooking *Michael Symons*
Peanuts: The Illustrious History of the Goober Pea *Andrew F. Smith*
Marketing Nutrition: Soy, Functional Foods, Biotechnology, and Obesity
Brian Wansink
The Banquet: Dining in the Great Courts of Late Renaissance Europe *Ken Albala*
The Turkey: An American Story *Andrew F. Smith*
The Herbalist in the Kitchen *Gary Allen*
African American Foodways: History and Culture
Edited by Anne Lieberman Bower
The Complete Vegetarian: The Essential Guide to Good Health
Edited by Peggy Carlson
The World of Soy *Edited by Christine M. DuBois, Sidney Mintz, and Chee-Beng Tan*

The University of Illinois Press
is a founding member of the
Association of American University Presses.

Composed in 10.5/13 Adobe Minion Pro
with FF Meta display
by BookComp, Inc.
for the University of Illinois Press
Designed by Kelly Gray
Manufactured by Thomson-Shore, Inc.

University of Illinois Press
1325 South Oak Street
Champaign, IL 61820-6903
www.press.uillinois.edu